Mealtime Manual for People with Disabilities and the Aging

Mealtime Manual for People with Disabilities and the Aging

Judith Lannefeld Klinger, OTR, MA

With the Howard A. Rusk Institute of Rehabilitation Medicine
New York University Medical Center

Foreword by Mathew H. M. Lee, MD, FACP

Publisher: John H. Bond
Editorial Director: Amy E. Drummond
Creative Director: Linda Baker
Editorial Assistant: Viktoria Kristiansson

Printed in the United States of America

Klinger, Judith Lannefeld.
    Mealtime manual for people with disabilities and the aging/by Judith Lannefeld Klinger; with the Howard A. Rusk Institute of Rehabilitation Medicine; New York University Medical Center; foreword by Mathew H.M. Lee.--3rd ed.
        p. cm.
    Includes bibliographical references and index.
    ISBN 1-55642-341-1
    1. Cookery for the physically handicapped.
I. Howard A. Rusk Institute of Rehabilitation Medicine. II. Title.
    [DNLM: 1. Cookery. 2. Disabled. 3. Aged. 4. Cooking and Eating Utensils. TX 652 K65m 1997]
TX652.K4697 1997
641.5'087--dc21
DNLM/DLC
for Library of Congress   97-16056

This book is a companion to *Meal Preparation and Training: The Health Care Professional's Guide*. Anyone who wishes to obtain a copy can contact the publisher listed below.

Published by: SLACK Incorporated
                6900 Grove Road
                Thorofare, NJ 08086-9447 USA
                Telephone: 609-848-1000
                Fax: 609-853-5991
                World Wide Web: http://www.slackinc.com

Contact SLACK Incorporated for more information about other books in this field or about the availability of our books from distributors outside the United States.

An earlier edition of this book was published by Campbell Soups as *Mealtime Manual for the Aged and the Handicapped*.

Last digit is print number: 10 9 8 7 6 5 4 3 2 1

DEDICATION AND ACKNOWLEDGMENTS

This third edition is again dedicated to those courageous homemakers who, although limited by physical problems, are unbounded in their ability to love and care for their families; to readers of the first and second editions who offered their comments and insights; to clients of the Visiting Nurse Association, Incorporated, of Ridgefield, CT, who helped by testing procedures and providing new answers; and last but not least to both my mom and my husband, Herb, one who started me off right so that I love working with people and foods, and the other who supports my efforts and adds his own special flair.

I wish to thank all those who helped with the preparation of this third edition, including Sophie Chiotelis, OTR, MA, Occupational Therapy Director, for her warm professionalism and confidence, and Lucy Beck, MA, CHE, home economist who reviewed the manuscript, both of whom are at the Howard A. Rusk Institute of Rehabilitation Medicine, New York University Medical Center; the Campbell Soup Company for their initial support; plus Greg Kaplowitz, who printed many of the photos; Greg Klinger, who provided illustrations; and Laurie Klinger who assisted in the research.

Judith Lannefeld Klinger, OTR, MA

CONTENTS

SECTION ONE
LIVING WITH A DISABILITY

SECTION TWO
IN AND AROUND THE KITCHEN AND THE HOME

SECTION THREE
KITCHEN UTILITIES, TOOLS, AND APPLIANCES

SECTION FOUR
MEAL PLANNING

SECTION FIVE
PREPARING AND SERVING, AND APPENDICES

FOREWORD

It is with sadness that I must write in the foreword that Dr. Rusk passed away in November 1989. The author of the previous forewords for this book, he was truly the "Father of Rehabilitation Medicine." With the founding of the Institute of Rehabilitation Medicine, now renamed the Howard A. Rusk Institute of Rehabilitation Medicine of New York University Medical Center, he pioneered the idea that people with disabilities could be rehabilitated rather than hidden. With the third edition of *Mealtime Manual*, we have seen much change in the world since 1968, the date of the first edition, but we have also witnessed Dr. Rusk's beliefs about rehabilitation not only confirmed, but becoming a part of the fabric of our society. With the passage of the Americans with Disabilities Act in 1990, we, as a country, for the first time, wholeheartedly affirmed the right of people with disabilities to participate fully and equally in our society.

This was the promise for the first *Mealtime Manual*: enabling homemakers to return to full participation in their families. Now, with this edition, it is the family that has changed—the person we hope to empower with enabling techniques is no longer necessarily the wife and mother of the family. It is just as likely to be a husband and father, or a single person of either sex. Let there be no mistake, although fewer people may identify themselves as "homemakers" these days, someone is still performing those tasks!

Begun as a research project 29 years ago, this book can be considered an unequaled source of information on the most effective and useful techniques for meal management for anyone who must cope in spite of some physical challenge. It is the distillation of Mrs. Klinger's experience in the field, of the extensive feedback from readers of earlier editions, and of our own experience in our Home Management Unit of the Occupational Therapy Department at the Rusk Institute. The techniques, equipment, and suggestions in this book are, more than usual, the result of working with real people to solve real problems. This is the true goal of rehabilitation therapy, and as we approach the 21st century, we believe this book will continue to be a gold mine of solutions that are useful for the lay reader and health-care workers.

Mathew H. M. Lee, MD, FACP
Professor and Acting Chairman
Howard A. Rusk Institute of Rehabilitation Medicine
New York University Medical Center

INTRODUCTION

The *Mealtime Manual for People with Disabilities and the Aging* is designed for you, the consumer, so that information you need is easily available. We all want to streamline tasks. If, however, you have a physical disability, efficient methods, tools, and safe short-cuts become essential. This third edition of the *Mealtime Manual*, like the previous editions, is for people who are just learning to live with a disability and for those with long-standing conditions caused by disability or aging. There is always a new trick we can learn.

If you are reading this book for the first time, you might be interested in its background. In May 1968, the Howard A. Rusk Institute of Rehabilitation Medicine, New York University Medical Center, received a grant from the Campbell Soup Fund to study the meal preparation problems of the handicapped and elderly. Our research concentrated on the packaging of convenience foods as well as the design and use of portable appliances. Testing focused on opening the most popular types of packages and finding techniques that would make handling these containers easier. Appliance testing focused on design features that offered the most versatility and help in meal preparation. No affiliation with or endorsement of any company was, or is, intended by the selection of specific appliances.

In the 26 years since the first edition, appliances have improved in safety and multiplied in variety. Much of the food packaging, however, continues to lock flavors in and those with hand limitations out. Simple aids and techniques can help solve packaging problems.

Much of the equipment described in this book may be found in local stores. Suggested retail prices are stated with the understanding that they may change. The same items are often available at a discount or on sale. Shipping costs are not included in the pricing information.

Your own physician, visiting nurse service, occupational and physical therapists, extension service, school, or other local organizations are your first lines of information. Groups that can offer additional help are found in Appendix B, Helpful Organizations and Agencies.

If you face serious problems, ask your doctor to refer you to a rehabilitation team or center, or talk to your local health department or a hospital outpatient service.

This manual contains a wide range of tools and techniques. Choose the ones you wish to use according to your own needs.

If you have any questions about an appliance, consult your health team before you buy. Refer to Chapter 25 for tips on shopping by mail.

A companion *Meal Preparation and Training: The Health Care Professional's Guide* is available for health care professionals working with people with disabilities and the aging. It provides techniques for teaching clients and other health professionals, for kitchen planning, and resources for further study. For information, write to the publisher: SLACK Incorporated, 6900 Grove Road, Thorofare, NJ 08086. Slides of illustrations in the manual are also available. For information, write to Living Media, Inc. **Source**: 243.

We wish you creative cooking, joyful meals, and good health. And we look forward to receiving your ideas and comments on the Suggestion Page at the end of the manual.

HOW TO FIND WHAT YOU NEED

Each of the products described in the *Mealtime Manual* is followed by a list of numbers indicating the manufacturers and sources of the product. These numbers are keyed to the addresses listed under Appendix A, Sources for Equipment and Tools. Companies and addresses were current as of the date of publication.

We hope you do not find the numbering system confusing, as it saves many pages of repetition. Most of the toll-free numbers given here are for out-of-state calls; if the company or organization is within your state, call information for the local number.

Whenever possible, you should purchase the item from a local retailer or mail-order firm. If you cannot locate one, then contact the manufacturer for your nearest retail source. If you have no luck locating an item, write to us on the Tear-Out Suggestion Card, and we will try to help.

PREFACE
IF YOU ARE THE CAREGIVER

You, as the caregiver, may want to use *Mealtime Manual* for your family member or other person who has a disability or is handling problems related to aging. If your spouse is recovering from a stroke, for example, he or she may not be able to read the Manual. You can learn and demonstrate the techniques in this book. Training may take many repetitions. Remember that the individual you care for needs motivation before he or she can fully function.

If the person you are caring for lives alone and is not eating properly, you can help by shopping, planning meals to eat together, and making up meals ahead of time. Many factors can affect one's appetite—from lack of interest due to diminished sense of taste to poorly fitting dentures, medications that depress appetite, and the sadness of eating alone. Some suggestions for enlivening meals are presented in Chapter 11. When you are unable to help due to distance or other circumstances, contact the local Visiting Nurse Association or Office of Aging.

The kinds of help mentioned in many of the chapters is available through your town hall, local hospital, and self-help groups. We urge you to talk with your physician, a nurse, therapist, or social worker about long-term needs. If you have a parent who is unable to function safely, ask your physician about a home evaluation which will provide you with suggestions for home modifications to increase independence.

At times you must feel a great deal of stress in trying to provide help for a loved one. There are self-help support groups for you, too, where you can talk out your feelings, discover new ways to cope, and find new friends who care and understand what you are going through. The effects are felt by everyone. Do not carry the burden alone. Share your feelings, and explain your needs.

This Manual has a companion volume, *Meal Preparation and Training: The Health Care Professional's Guide*. It provides methods of training as well as additional resources.

GOING FURTHER

Addresses are listed in the Appendices.

About Homemakers and Home Health Aides. (1988). South Deerfield, MA: Channing L. Bete Co. Booklet available free from your Visiting Nurse Association, physician's office. $1.25 per copy. **Source:** 62.

Carter, F., with Golant, S. K. (1994). *Helping Yourself Help Others: A Book for Caregivers.* New York: Times Books, Random House.

Coughlan, P. B. (1993). *Facing Alzheimer's: Family Caregivers Speak.* New York: Ballantine.

Gruetzener, H. (1992). *Alzheimer's: A Caregiver's Guide and Sourcebook.* New York: John Wiley.

Lustbader, W., & Hooyman, N. (1994). *Taking Care of Aging Family Members: A Practical Guide.* New York: Free Press.

Mace, N. L., & Rabins, P. V. (1991). *The 36-hour Day: A Family Guide to Caring for Persons with Alzheimer's Disease, Related Dementing Illness, and Memory Loss in Later Life* (rev. ed.). Baltimore: Johns Hopkins University Press.

Rob, C., with Reynolds, J. (1991). *The Caregiver's Guide: Helping Elderly Relatives Cope with Health and Safety Problems.* Boston: Houghton-Mifflin.

Strong, M. (1988). *Mainstay: For the Well Spouse of the Chronically Ill.* New York: Penguin Books.

Susik, D. H. (1995). *Hiring Home Caregivers: The Family Guide to In-home Elder Care.* San Luis Obispo, CA: American Source Books.

Section One

LIVING WITH A DISABILITY

Working with One Hand, After a Stroke, or with Incoordination

Whether you have the use of one hand, are living with the effects of a stroke, or have incoordination, keeping active will help you function better and enjoy life more.

If you are unsure of your ability to handle kitchen tasks, ask your physician, therapist, nurse, or local Visiting Nurse Association for advice. An occupational or physical therapist or rehabilitation home economist can show you ways to ensure your safety, increase efficiency, and can help you adapt or select kitchen equipment.

WORKING WITH ONE HAND AFTER A STROKE

Thousands of people who use one hand are able to care for themselves and their families by using a few simple techniques and aids.

A stroke, or cerebral vascular accident (CVA), may cause hemiplegia, the complete or partial paralysis of one-half of the body. If you are recovering from a stroke, have limited use of one hand, are using a wheelchair or walking with a cane, relearning tasks may seem difficult. You are not alone. Stroke is the leading cause of adult disability in the United States. Today, more than two million people in the United States are coping with the effects of a stroke.

The limitations imposed by your stroke may affect more than your arms and legs. Perception and awareness, as well as vision, are sometimes altered. It may seem confusing or difficult to remember how you used to do things or even to know exactly what you want to do now. It helps to write notes or to have someone write them for you. You may find it easier if you divide each activity into smaller steps.

If a traumatic injury or stroke has caused you to become left-handed, there are companies that specialize in products for the left-hander. Some of these include scissors, pot holder mitts, knives, and vegetable peelers. **Source:** 233.

Additional information on living with a stroke, including referral to a local stroke survivors support group, is available from the American Heart Association, the National Aphasia Association, the National Institutes of Neurological Disorders and Strokes, and the National Stroke Association. Addresses are given in Appendix B.

WORKING WITH INCOORDINATION

Incoordination may be caused by fatigue after a long illness, or it may be a symptom of diseases such as Parkinson's disease, multiple sclerosis (MS), or cerebral palsy. Your coordination may vary, depending on tiredness, amount of light in the room, your position (whether you are sitting or standing), your emotional state, and other factors.

You may find that when you tire, incoordination seems to increase. Allow yourself enough time for each activity.

Conserving energy is essential. Do your housework in short shifts with rests in between. Apply energy-saving techniques: slide items instead of lifting them, use convenience foods and labor-saving appliances. Avoid carrying hot water or pots.

Prepare familiar dishes that do not require a cookbook; work up gradually to more complicated recipes and menus. Prepare meals in advance so that you can rest before adding the final touches. This will leave you more zest for eating.

Multiple Sclerosis (MS) is the most prevalent central nervous system disease among young adults in the United States. Symptoms differ from person to person. These may include weakness, tingling in the arms and legs, numbness in hands and feet, impaired sensation for hot and cold, poor coordination, unsteady balance, difficulty in remembering or speaking, spasticity, or stiffness. Visual problems may include blurring, double vision, or rapid involuntary eye movements. Despite all these symptoms, about two-thirds of individuals diagnosed with MS are still able to walk, with or without a walking aid. The Multiple Sclerosis Society has chapters in many cities that offer assistance in finding treatment programs, support groups, and

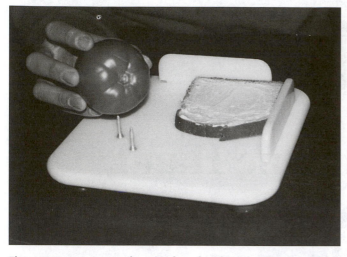

Figure 1-1. A waterproof cutting board with two stainless-steel or aluminum nails holds foods in place. (Photo by J.K.)

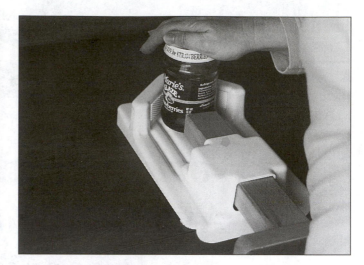

Figure 1-3. The Belliclamp secures packages, cans, and jars. (Unit by North Coast Medical, Inc., San Jose, CA. Photo by J.K.)

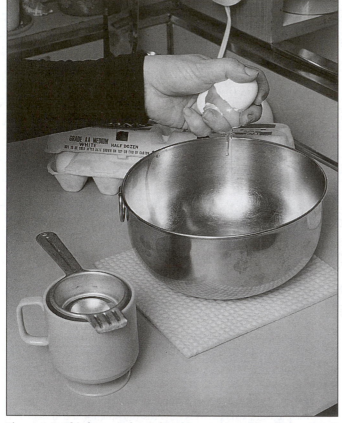

Figure 1-2. This homemaker is breaking an egg with one hand and using an egg separator. (Photo courtesy of the O.T. Dept., Howard A. Rusk Institute of Rehabilitation Medicine.)

adapted equipment. See Appendix B. Suggestions in some of the other chapters, including Chapter 2, Chapter 4, and Chapter 9, may also be beneficial.

If you have cerebral palsy, the joint protection techniques in Chapter 2 may be helpful. Studies have found that older individuals with cerebral palsy tend to develop arthritis. Using methods to protect your joints now may benefit you later.

STABILIZING

While you work, make it your first task to keep foods and containers stationary. Stabilizing one or both arms on a solid surface may give you greater control. For pouring, try supporting your arm on the edge of the counter or on your wheelchair arm. Rest on your elbow, and use it as a pivot. Experiment with straight-arm pouring—practice at the sink until you find the best solution. Use your knees to anchor boxes or bags to be opened.

A waterproof cutting board with two stainless-steel or aluminum nails holds foods in place while you peel or cut them (Figure 1-1). A raised ledge at one corner of the board keeps bread from moving while you spread and cut it. Rubber suction cups, rubber pads, or a damp sponge cloth under the board keep it from sliding. Polyethylene boards are lighter and easier to clean than wooden ones. Some boards have handles for easy lifting. **Manufacturer:** 103. Cost is $12 and up from self-help firms. **Sources:** 5, 13, 16, 108, 120, 155, 238, 247, 252, 261, 264, 290, 368, 383, 408. For additional adapted boards, see Chapter 21.

A damp sponge cloth placed under a bowl or plate becomes your second hand, keeping the bowl stationary while you combine ingredients (Figure 1-2). The absorbent cloth is easily cleaned. **Manufacturer:** 102. Cost is about $1 a pair from grocery and variety stores.

Dycem® Non-Slip can be used to hold a bowl, plate, or cutting board in place. This product is non-toxic, lasts for years, and is easily washed—just wipe it clean with a damp cloth. Dycem® Non-Slip products include mats, trays, cup holders, self-adhesive strips, and tray liners. It is also available in a continuous roll or netting that can be cut to a desired size. **Manufacturer** of Dycem®: 104; distributor: 103. Available from self-help firms. **Sources:** 1, 5, 13, 104, 120, 155, 238, 252, 261, 264, 290, 368, 408.

One-handed egg beaters cost about $4 and up from housewares stores and mail-order firms. See Chapter 28.

The Belliclamp secures packages, cans, and jars up to 4 1/2" in diameter for one-handed opening (Figure 1-3). You lean against the wooden ram, which is set in a plastic, non-slip frame. Cost is about $30 from self-help firms. **Sources**: 5, 120, 252, 290, 408.

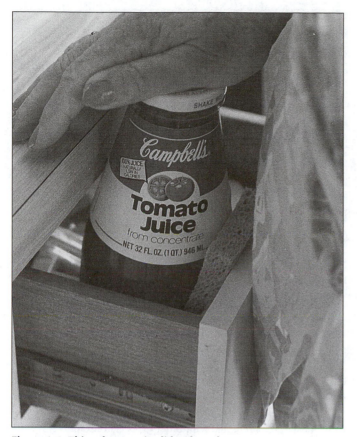

Figure 1-4. This releases a jar lid. (Photo by J.K.)

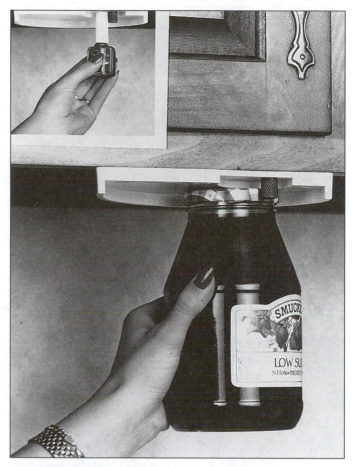

Figure 1-5. A wedge-type opener simplifies opening a jar with one hand. (Photo courtesy of Multi Marketing & Manufacturing, Inc., Littleton, CO.)

To release a jar lid, place it inside a drawer with a damp sponge cloth between the glass and the side of the drawer (Figure 1-4). Press against the drawer with your hip as you turn the top.

Opening a jar with one hand is easy with a wedge-type opener (Figure 1-5). Steel teeth grasp the cover as you turn the jar. The Un-Skru® jar opener mounts under a cabinet. A hardened, steel knob in the wedge-type opener holds the lid as you turn the jar with one hand. It opens both narrow- and wide-mouthed jars, toothpaste tubes, and pill bottles with child-proof caps. **Manufacturer:** 281. Cost is about $10 and up from mail-order and self-help firms. **Sources:** 16, 71, 120, 238, 240, 252, 264, 281, 368, 370, 408, 415.

A workbench vise can be handy in the kitchen. Because it is heavy, you may not need to secure it to the counter. You will find clamps and vises in assorted styles and sizes to suit your needs in hardware stores and hobby catalogs. **Sources:** 234, 430.

Lightweight and rechargeable, a cordless one-handed electric can opener is easily operated (Figure 1-6). It requires no pressure to continue operation once you push the "power pierce cutter" button. The opener cuts around the lid, then shuts off automatically. It stores in its wall-mounted recharger, saving counter space. **Manufacturers:** 41 (pictured), 94. Cost is $27 and up from housewares stores and self-help firms. **Sources:** 5, 13, 120, 261, 290, 359.

See other can, jar, and container openers in Chapter 20 and Chapter 21.

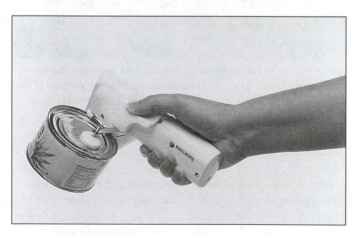

Figure 1-6. This cordless one-handed electric can opener is easily operated. (Can opener by Black and Decker, Inc. Photo courtesy of North Coast Medical, Inc., San Jose, CA.)

CUTTING

A board with two nails to stabilize food is the preferred cutting base. Always use a serrated knife for cutting and chopping. The sawtooth edge permits greater control and is less likely to slip than a straight-edged blade. To control excess motion while cutting, try

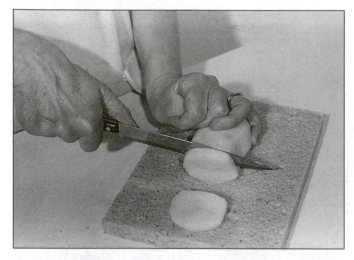

Figure 1-7. This homemaker with cerebral palsy positions the knife on the potato before bringing her hand down to hold it. (Photo courtesy of the O.T. Dept., Howard A. Rusk Institute of Rehabilitation Medicine.)

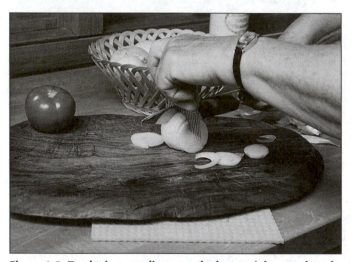

Figure 1-8. To obtain even slices, use the long stainless-steel teeth of an onion holder to guide the knife blade. (Photo courtesy of the O.T. Dept., Howard A. Rusk Institute of Rehabilitation Medicine.)

to keep the blade point-down on the board. Cutting aids designed for the blind are also helpful if you have incoordination. See Chapter 9.

People with cerebral palsy can rest fruits and vegetables on a damp sponge to anchor them so that they do not slide when cut (Figure 1-7). Position the knife on the fruit or vegetable before bringing your hand down to hold it. Another way to keep fingers clear of a knife is to hold the food down with a fork.

To obtain even slices, use the long, stainless-steel teeth of an onion holder to guide the knife blade (Figure 1-8). **Manufacturers:** 142, 289. Cost is $1.25 and up from housewares stores and mail-order firms. **Sources:** 5, 231, 270.

A knife with a curved blade cuts with a rocking motion, using one hand, without moving the food (Figure 1-9). Also known as a skinning knife, it costs $10 and up from sporting goods stores and self-help firms. A textured board also helps prevent slipping of foods while cutting. **Sources** for knife: 5, 120, 252, 264, 290.

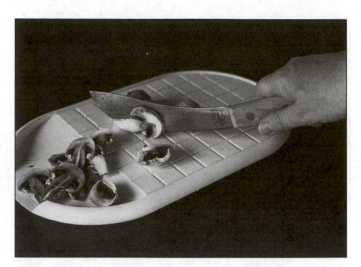

Figure 1-9. A knife with a curved blade cuts with a rocking motion, using one hand, without moving the food. (Photo by J.K.)

A one-blade chopper is safer to use than a knife if your hands are incoordinated (Figure 1-10). The handle keeps fingers completely away from the blade.

Choppers with more than one blade are not as safe as single-blade models, because food often gets caught between the blades. It is dangerous to remove the food if you have tremors or involuntary movements. Single-blade choppers come with or without bowls from housewares stores and mail-order firms. **Manufacturers:** 142, 181. Cost is $3 and up. **Sources:** 65, 71, 231, 261.

Other cutting utensils and tools are described in Chapter 21.

SELECTING UTENSILS

Heavier utensils can reduce tremors or add control. However, if you have weakness and poor coordination, choose implements that are heavy enough to counteract tremors, yet light enough to handle easily.

When purchasing kitchen utensils, check the attachments to make sure they can sustain the sudden or added force you put on them. Some kitchen tools designed for forceful use are guaranteed against breakage. Wood, Teflon-coated, or non-metal tools are preferred, as they will not scratch the coatings on non-stick pans. Utensil **manufacturers** include 142, 273, 289.

Unbreakable dishes come in a variety of attractive designs and styles from housewares stores. **Manufacturers:** 79, 343.

To protect dishes, line your sink and the top of a wheeled cart with a rubber mat—Dycem® non-slip or rubber mesh matting (Figure 1-11). Mats cost $1.50 and up from housewares and hardware stores (see Figure 1-2). **Sources** for sink mats: 185, 231, 242.

Non-slip materials also cushion shelves and drawers to help prevent breakage and to hold an object in place until you have a secure grasp. **Manufacturers** of rubber mesh matting and non-slip materials: 314, 333, 343. A roll is about $7 and up from housewares stores and mail-order firms. **Sources:** 185, 410.

A sink rack safely holds wet dishes but allows water to flow through. Made of steel with an epoxy coating, it comes in two sizes: 12" x 16", and 10" x 12". Cost is about $5 from mail-order firms. **Sources:** 231, 378.

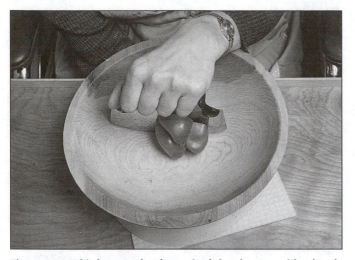

Figure 1-10. This homemaker has paired the chopper with a bowl to hold diced food. She seeds and cores the pepper after she has started to cut it. The single blade chopper also works on a board when dicing meat. (Photo courtesy of the O.T. Dept., Howard A. Rusk Institute of Rehabilitation Medicine.)

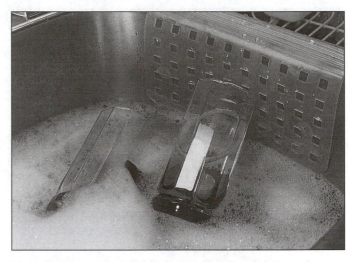

Figure 1-11. To protect dishes, line your sink and the top of a wheeled cart with a rubber mat. (Photo by J.K.)

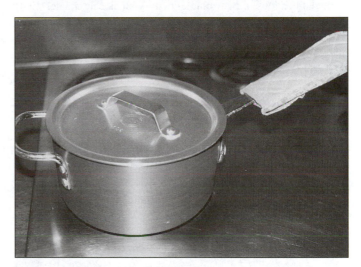

Figure 1-12. If you use both hands, look for pots with two handles, such as this saucepan. (Photo by J.K.)

If your major problem is incoordination not combined with weakness in your upper extremities, heavier pans may make it easier for you to work safely (Figure 1-12). If you use both hands, look for pots with two handles. **Manufacturers:** 72, 84, 257. Cost is $25 and up from department stores and gourmet specialty firms. **Source:** 65.

A pot handle cover replaces a hot pad and stays in place so you do not have to grasp so tightly. Handle covers are available in rubber, leather, or fabric. Silicone rubber "Cool Handles" are heat-resistant rubber grips, available in three sizes to slip over the handles of most industry fry, sauce, and sauté pans. **Manufacturer:** 339. Cost is about $3 each from housewares stores and mail-order firms. **Sources:** 65, 231. Fabric pot handle covers are about $2.50 a pair from housewares stores and mail-order firms. **Sources:** 185, 261, 270. One can be made of fabric by folding a standard square pot holder in half and whip-stitching the edges.

For cooking and serving with one hand, you can pick up and release food more easily with tongs than with a fork (Figure 1-13). Tongs with spatula blades slip under food easily. **Manufacturer:** 112. Cost is $4 and up from housewares stores, self-help and mail-order firms. **Sources:** 16, 65, 196, 247, 261, 270.

SAFE CARRYING, AVOIDING SPILLS

- Slide, do not lift; wheel, do not carry. Suggestions on organizing your kitchen and choosing a wheeled cart to minimize carrying are given in Chapter 16.
- To minimize the chances for spills, measure liquids beside where you are cooking. Stabilize your pouring arm by holding it close to your body (Figure 1-14).
- Let pans cool on the range, before moving them to the sink.
- After returning from the grocery store, ask your family or a neighbor to transfer items packaged in glass bottles into unbreakable containers.
- If you are using a hand-held can opener, place the can to be opened inside a large pan or bowl to catch potential spills.
- Never install a jar opener on a wall with only the floor or sink beneath it, because the jar may accidentally fall and break. Instead install it over a counter or shelf.
- A pan equipped with a strainer basket reduces the chances of spilling hot water when draining the contents of a pot. Alternatively, ladle the contents into a serving container.

GOING FURTHER

Addresses are listed in the Appendices.

STROKE AND WORKING WITH ONE HAND INFORMATION

Publications

American Heart Association. Free publications from the American Heart Association include materials on nutrition, quitting smoking, high blood pressure, exercise, and weight control. Audiovisual materials are also available for use by groups. Your

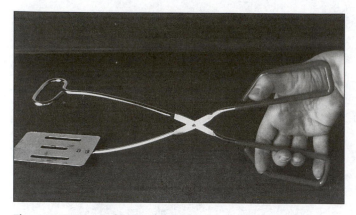

Figure 1-13. For cooking and serving with one hand, you can pick up and release food more easily with tongs. (Photo by J.K.)

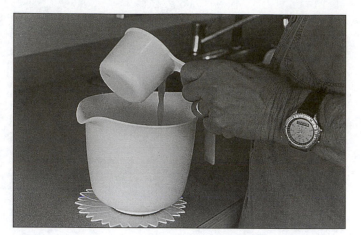

Figure 1-14. This cook stabilizes the pouring arm by holding it close to the body. (Photo by J.K.)

local chapter may have information on nearby stroke clubs where you can share ideas and solve problems with others. The following free publications are available (call your local chapter first): *Aphasia and the Family*, #50-002A (1988); *How Stroke Affects Behavior*, #50-1019 (1989); *Recovering from a Stroke*, provides daily routines to make life easier; *Strokes: A Guide for the Family*, #50-1017, suggestions for patient care.

About Living After A Stroke. (1984). South Deerfield, MA: Channing L. Bete Co. Easy-to-understand, illustrated booklet available from your physician or directly from company for $1.25 per copy. **Source:** 62.

Be Stroke Smart. National Stroke Organization. Series of 20 one-page articles for stroke survivors, their families, and the public. $7.50.

Burnett, P. (1990). *Independent Living: Functioning with the Use of One Hand in a Two-Handed World*. Thorofare, NJ: Slack, Inc. (Out-of-print, check with library.)

Caplan, L. R., Dyken, M. L., & Easton, J. D. (1994). *American Heart Association: Family Guide to Stroke Treatment, Recovery, and Prevention*. New York: Times Books, Random House. Spotting the signs of a stroke, changing your lifestyle to prevent a stroke, how to receive the best treatment, getting the most out of rehabilitation in the hospital and at home, involving the family, and finding a support network. **Source:** 326B.

Josephs, A. (1992). *The Invaluable Guide to Life After Stroke: An Owner's Manual*. Portland, OR: Amadeus Press. **Source:** 19A.

The Road Ahead: A Stroke Recovery Guide. (1986). The National Stroke Association. Descriptions of stroke impairments with practical suggestions and solutions for coping. $12.50 plus $2 postage and handling.

Sarton, M. (1988). *After the Stroke: A Journal*. New York: Norton. **Source:** 290B.

Shimberg, E. F. (1990). *Strokes: What Families Should Know*. New York: Random House. **Source:** 326.

Single-Handed?: A Book for Persons with the Use of Only One Hand, #1480. Bloomington, IL: Accent. Devices and aids, special techniques, how-to tips, other helpful publications. $3.50 plus handling. **Source:** 3.

Stroke Connection. Free bimonthly newsletter by and for stroke survivors and their families, from Stroke Connection.

Ask your therapist about the availability of videos and films that show other homemakers with use of one hand or incoordination managing their daily self-care and homemaking activities. These are best viewed with your therapist or nurse so that questions you have may be raised and answered properly.

INCOORDINATION INFORMATION

Publications

American Parkinson Disease Association, Inc. Free publications distributed through their east and west coast offices include Clapcich, J., Goldberg, N., & Walsh, E. (1993). *Be Independent!: A Guide for People with Parkinson's Disease*; Wichmann, R. (1990). *Be Active: A Suggested Exercise Program for People with Parkinson's Disease*; Levin, S. (Ed.). *Coping With Parkinson's Disease*; Carter, J. *Good Nutrition in Parkinson's Disease*; Johnson, M., (1994). *Let's Communicate: A Speech and Swallowing Program for Persons with Parkinson's Disease*; Leiberman, A. N., Gopinathan, A. N., & Goldstein, M. *Parkinson's Disease Handbook—A Guide for Patients and Their Families*; *Speech Problems and Swallowing Problems in Parkinson's Disease*; *34 Helpful Hints to Ease the Daily Life of Parkinson's Disease Victims*.

Atwood, G. W., & Hunnewell, L. G. (1991). *Living Well with Parkinson's*. New York: Wiley. Upbeat guide to living a full life with Parkinson's disease. **Source:** 426.

Carroll, D. L., & Dorman, J. (1993). *Living Well with Multiple Sclerosis: A Guide for Patient, Caregiver, and Family*. New York: Harper-Perennial, HarperCollins. **Source:** 172.

Carroll, D. (1992). *Living with Parkinson's: A Guide for the Patient and Caregiver*. New York: HarperCollins.

Cristall, B. (1992). Coping When a Parent Has Multiple Sclerosis. New York: The Rosen Group. **Source:** 338.

Duvoisin, R. C., & Sage, J. (1991). *Parkinson's Disease: A Guide for Patient and Family* (4th ed.). Philadelphia: Lippincott/Raven Press. **Source:** 242B.

Graham, J. (1992). *Multiple Sclerosis: The Self-Help Guide* (3rd ed.). New York: HarperCollins. Mother and career woman who was diagnosed with MS 15 years ago provides overview of treatments and methods for coping with daily life.

Lieberman, A. N., & Williams, F. L. (1993). *Parkinson's*

Disease: The Complete Guide for Patients and Caregivers. New York: Simon & Schuster. **Source:** 364B.

National Multiple Sclerosis Society provides services through local chapters including referrals, clinics, equipment loans, support groups, and free publications. Publications include *Coping With Stress*; *Food for Thought: MS and Nutrition*; *Living with MS*; *Multiple Sclerosis and Your Emotions*; *Positive Nutrition*; *Plaintalk: a Booklet About MS For Families*; *Solving Cognitive Problems*; *Someone You Know Has Multiple Sclerosis: a Book for Families*; *Taking Care: a Guide for Well Partners*; *Things I Wish Someone Had Told Me*; *What Everyone Should Know About Multiple Sclerosis*.

National Parkinson Foundation, Inc., provides services and information on diagnosis, research, treatment, and care for individuals with Parkinson's and related neurological diseases. Free publications include: Pengilly, K. *Introduction to Speech and Swallowing Problems Associated With Parkinson's Disease*; Carlton, L. *Practical Pointers for Parkinsonians*; *The Parkinson Handbook: A Guide for Parkinson Patients and their Families*; *The Parkinson's Patient: What You and Your Family Should Know*.

Pierce, J. R. (1989). *A Patient's Perspective: Living with Parkinson's Disease or Don't Rush Me! I'm Coping as Fast as I Can*. Knoxville, TN: Spectrum Publications.

Scheinberg, L. C., & Holland, N. J. (1987). *Multiple Sclerosis: A Guide for Patients and Their Families* (2nd ed.). New York: Raven Press. See Lippincott/Raven. **Source:** 242B.

Shuman, R., & Schwartz, J. (1994). *Living with Multiple Sclerosis: A Handbook for Families*. New York: MacMillan. **Source:** 251B.

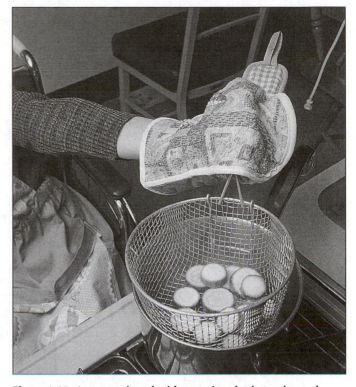

Figure 1-15. A pan equipped with a strainer basket reduces the chances of spilling hot water when draining the contents of a pot. (Photo courtesy of the O.T. Dept., Howard A. Rusk Institute of Rehabilitation Medicine.)

If You Have Arthritis or Upper Extremity Weakness

Homemaking tasks provide light exercises that help keep your joints limber and your muscles active.

ARTHRITIS

If you have arthritis, it is very important that you protect your joints from stress. Simple aids can help reduce strain on your joints, reduce bending, and extend your reach. To work efficiently without overusing your joints, follow these principles:

- Avoid fatigue. Set up a balanced schedule of work and relaxation. Your physician, nurse, or therapist will tell you which activities you can do, which you can do with new methods or aids, and which you should totally avoid. An occupational or physical therapist can teach you how to conserve energy, protect your joints by adapting tools or techniques, and will provide a daily home exercise program for you to follow.
- Organize your kitchen. Place your most frequently used items within reach. If you have difficulty bending or reaching, use tongs for stretching and a long-handled dustpan and brush for cleaning. A long fireplace match or butane match lighter simplifies lighting an older style gas oven.
- Keep your weight down. Excess pounds place unneeded stress on arthritic joints. To maintain a healthy weight, eat a balanced diet, exercise daily within your capabilities, and maintain a balanced schedule of activity and rest.
- Always hold tools correctly. Grasp tools with your fingers completely encircling the handle, and extend your thumb to meet your fingers (Figure 2-1). Do not slip the handle between two fingers, because this forces your fingers to the little finger (or ulnar) side, eventually causing more problems.
- Keep fingers extended while working. Scrub dishes, clean counters, and dust furniture with your fingers extended.
- Wear comfortable shoes. How your feet feel affects your posture and your ability to walk. Always, even at home, wear well-fitting shoes. A well-made sneaker or an oxford-style shoe with no more than a 1" heel will provide good support.

Avoid slippers and shoes with wedge-type heels.
- Sit while you are working. Prolonged standing puts unneeded stress on your hips, legs, and feet. Select a strong, comfortable chair that supports your back; be sure the seat is wide enough. Add a back support to improve posture and comfort, if necessary. Always alternate sitting with standing or some other movements. If you have arthritis in your arms and hands, use a chair with arm supports. See Chapter 5.
- Use a higher chair with foot supports or a foot stool at the kitchen counter to keep your ankles at right angles, especially if you have arthritis in your hips, legs, and feet. Adjustable-height chairs are available from artist and office supply firms. For more information on chairs, see Chapter 4.

A multipurpose chair with large casters rolls easily for gathering food and equipment or for sitting comfortably while working (Figure 2-2). The glider chair should have brakes to prevent it from moving as you stand up or sit down. **Manufacturer:** 12. Manufacturers of similar units: 125, 249, 428. Cost is $200 and up from hospital supply firms.

When getting up and down from a seated position, a higher chair reduces stress on the hips and knees. Adding a foam cushion or chair leg extenders are two answers. See Chapter 5.

The artherapedic chair is designed for the person with limited hip motion (Figure 2-3). A lever manually retracts the footrest so you can rise from the higher seat when you are ready to stand. When sitting, the lever is moved in the opposite direction. **Manufacturer:** 411.

UPPER EXTREMITY WEAKNESS

If you have weakness in your upper extremities, some of the principles for the person with arthritis may apply to you. If you have post-polio syndrome, you must especially avoid overtiring yourself and stress on muscles and joints. If the weakness is progressive, as with multiple sclerosis, joint and muscle protection is paramount. See Chapter 10.

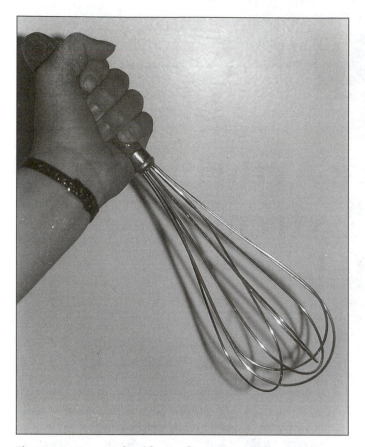

Figure 2-1. Grasp tools with your fingers completely encircling the handle, and extend your thumb to meet your fingers. (Photo by J.K.)

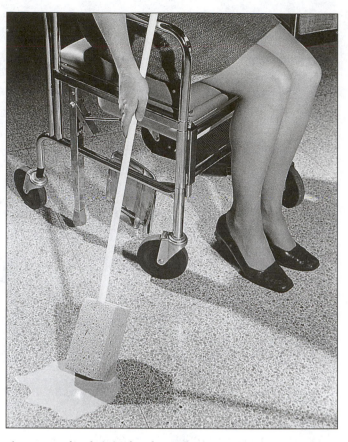

Figure 2-2. The chair in the photo also converts to a commode chair. (Photo courtesy of the O.T. Dept., Howard A. Rusk Institute of Rehabilitation Medicine.)

There are more than 641,000 U.S. survivors of paralytic polio. As an increasing number of these individuals have developed post-polio syndrome, organizations have become available to assist with information and research. Some of these include the International Polio Network, the Post-Polio Program at the National Rehabilitation Hospital, the Polio Society in Washington, and the Post-Polio Study, National Institutes of Health. Addresses are listed in Appendix B.

- Use substitute motions. Releasing the plastic top on a can, such as for coffee or peanuts, is easier when you hold the can against your body with one arm. Push the lid up with the heel of your other hand. To open a hot cooking bag, place it in a bowl, cut it open, and let it stand until cool enough to handle. Press one hand against your other hand on the bottom of the bag, and lift the bag to empty its contents into the bowl.
- Use your strongest motions (Figure 2-4). The quadriplegic in the photo finds operating an electric can opener with his elbow provides the power he needs.
- Do not strain yourself. Instead of brute strength, use tools and appliances, such as a jar opener, electric can opener, food processor, and electric mixer. See Chapter 20 and Chapter 21.
- Select lightweight utensils. Look for attractively designed, plastic and aluminum tools for cooking and serving. Rather than lift a glass or cup, use a long straw. Carry your eating aids in a bag to use when eating out.

If you have very weak grasp or no grasp, turn your hand over,

palm up, to pour or shake grated cheese, salt, or spices (Figure 2-5). Your thumb will provide enough weight to keep the shaker from slipping.

Interweaving a utensil between your fingers and supporting it with your thumb may let you turn and handle foods with no additional adaptations (Figure 2-6).

WORKING WITH ARTHRITIS OR UPPER EXTREMITY WEAKNESS

These suggestions will help compensate for weakness in your hands and arms while protecting them from strain:

- Use large, strong joints instead of small ones. Close cupboards with the palms of your hands, rather than with your fingers.
- If you have arthritis, keep your fingers extended whenever possible, such as when scrubbing dishes or dusting.
- Avoid holding anything for prolonged periods. Prop your book on a stand while reading. Take breaks from holding vegetables while peeling. Even better—do not peel if you do not have to. Stretch your fingers frequently to give them a chance to relax.
- Use both arms and hands when possible. Lift and slide items with two hands; dust with both arms.
- Slide, don't lift, whenever possible (Figure 2-7). If you must lift, slide both hands under a pan to transfer the weight from your fingers and palms to your wrists and elbows.

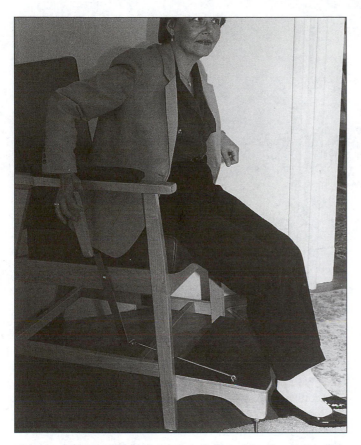

Figure 2-3. This artherapedic chair is designed for the person with limited hip motion. (Chair from Viva Medical Sciences Corp., Ogdensburg, NY. Photo by J.K.)

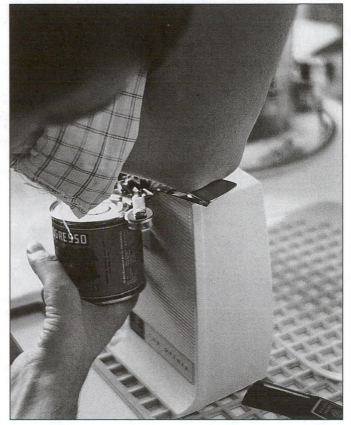

Figure 2-4. This quadriplegic finds operating an electric can opener with his elbow provides the power he needs. (Photo by J.K.)

- Put a loop of cloth around the handle of the refrigerator or oven door, and slip your arm through the loop to open the door with your forearm and upper body muscles. See Chapter 14.
- Begin an activity only if you can call a halt to it. If you feel too much pressure on your hands, wrists, or elsewhere, immediately stop what you are doing.
- Find new ways to transport items. Push, rather than lift. Wheel groceries to your car and into your house. If you must carry, use a lightweight basket that you can hold over your arm or a shoulder bag supported by the trunk of body. Create smaller loads, rather than one big one. See Chapter 16.
- Let others lift and carry heavy items for you. Do not be afraid to ask. Save your energy for important events like family and social activities.

HANDLING EQUIPMENT

Increasing the friction on the handles of kitchen utensils decreases the need for a strong grip. Utensils can be dipped into a liquid rubber coating. The coating also helps insulate the handle. Handles of wood or plastic utensils may be dipped. Cost is about $10 per pint from hardware stores and mail-order firms. **Source:** 49.

A large handle is more comfortable to grasp than a small one (Figure 2-8). Utensils with built-up handles are manufactured by

181, 273, 301. Cost is about $4 to $13 each from housewares and self-help firms. **Sources:** 5, 65, 238, 261, 290.

Adhesive-backed foam tape or a wide elastic band spiral-wrapped around the utensil handle increases both the friction and diameter of the handle. **Manufacturer** of foam tape: 390. Cost is about $2 and up per roll from hardware stores.

Handles of utensils may also be built up with foam padding or foam curlers (Figure 2-9). Foam padding is available from self-help firms. Cost of foam padding is $5 and up. **Sources:** 5, 13, 16, 120, 130, 264, 290, 368, 369, 408.

If grasp is totally lacking, loops of 1" wide elastic can be added to a universal cuff to hold kitchen utensils (Figure 2-10). **Manufacturers** of universal cuff include 103. **Sources:** 5, 13, 16, 120, 130, 264, 290, 368, 369, 408.

A multipurpose, continuous strap may be cut to fit cutlery, grooming aids, and appliance knobs (Figure 2-11). Slip the first hole over the handles, draw the strap over the back of your hand, slip the most convenient hole over the end of the handle, and cut the strap. Cost is about $3 per yard from self-help firms. **Sources:** 13, 368.

Opening jars can be stressful and potentially harmful. Always use a jar opener that grasps the lid firmly as you twist the jar. Use both hands to reduce stress. Jar openers are illustrated in Chapter 1 and Chapter 27.

To open a milk or juice carton, use the heels of your hands to push back the sides, then use a fork to pry open the spout (Figure

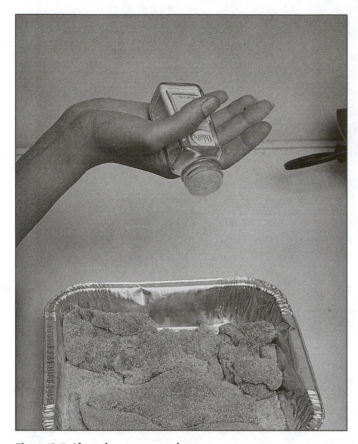

Figure 2-5. If you have very weak grasp or no grasp, turn your hand over, palm up, to pour or shake grated cheese, salt, or spices. (Photo courtesy of the O.T. Dept., Howard A. Rusk Institute of Rehabilitation Medicine.)

2-12). Do not use your thumbs; they will be forced backward, which may stretch the ligaments, causing pain and joint instability.

To pour the contents of one bowl into another, place both elbows on the counter for better leverage (Figure 2-13). Bring the bowl close to your body while pouring, to reduce the weight of lifting.

Always pour hot liquids away from yourself. A bowl or pitcher with a wide handle makes lifting easier. See Chapter 28 and Chapter 30.

CUTTING

Using an angled knife reduces stress on your wrist when you have arthritis and decreases the force required to cut by up to 80% (Figure 2-14). You use your shoulder and upper arm motion, rather than the wrist, to cut. **Manufacturer:** 122. Cost is $15 and up from self-help firms. **Sources:** 5, 13, 120, 122, 290, 408. A folding model is also available, so you can take it with you.

When your grasp is weak, a knife with a hole in the handle allows you to use both hands while cutting for better control (Figure 2-15). **Manufacturer:** 122. Cost is about $20 from self-help and specialty gourmet firms. **Sources:** 5, 13, 122, 261, 264, 290, 368, 408.

The quad meat cutter knife in Figure 2-16 slips over the palm of your hand. The plastic-coated steel cuff bends to fit your hand.

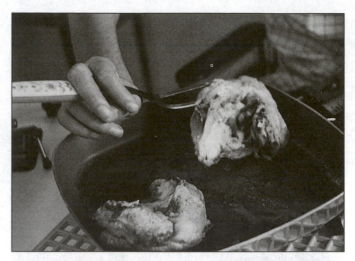

Figure 2-6. Interweaving a utensil between your fingers and supporting it with your thumb may let you turn and handle foods with no additional adaptations. (Photo by J.K.)

The sharp, stainless-steel blade cuts by rocker action and is useful if your wrist is stable. Cost is about $7 from self-help firms. **Sources:** 5, 120, 252, 264, 290, 408. A similar deluxe quad meat cutter has a serrated blade.

Additional knives and cutting aids are described and illustrated in Chapter 21 and Chapter 28.

Adapt your kitchen as fully as possible to your physical needs (Figure 2-17). A wall oven may be set at the proper height for you to handle pans with minimal lifting. An oven shovel can extend your reach. See Chapters 13, 28, and 29.

REACHING

Reaching devices are helpful if you have difficulty bending and/or extending your arms or are confined to a wheelchair. They should, however, only be used to lift lightweight, nonbreakable items.

A child's hoe is a handy tool for pulling items from the back of the counter (Figure 2-18). The hoe is usually found in a set of three tools sold in department stores, especially in the spring season, for $4 each and up. Sturdier, heavier hoes are carried by garden supply mail-order firms. **Source:** 367.

If your grip is weak, a locking reacher is recommended (Figure 2-19). The EZ-Reacher® II clamps onto the object being lifted. Rubber suction cups help secure the object in place; then the tongs of the reacher lock around an item, so you do not have to maintain pressure. Slight pressure on a lever by the pistol grip handle releases the item when it is within reach or placed where you desire. An optional wrist support reduces pressure on your wrist while you lift. Reacher comes in three standard non-folding models (20", 30", or 40" long), a lighter weight Light Touch E-Z Reacher® with a built-in wrist support and easier pull trigger (20" or 30" long), and two folding models (30" folding, or 30" folding and locking) for easier portability when shopping or traveling. **Manufacturer:** 32. Cost is about $30 and up from mail-order and self-help firms. **Sources:** 3, 5, 13, 32, 120, 130, 151, 155, 252, 264, 290, 368, 370, 374, 408, 410.

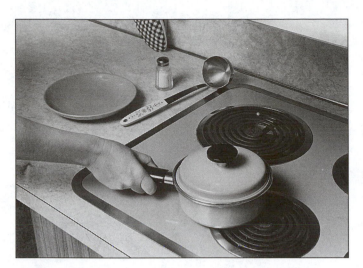

Figure 2-7. Slide, don't lift, whenever possible. (Photo courtesy of the O.T. Dept., Howard A. Rusk Institute of Rehabilitation Medicine.)

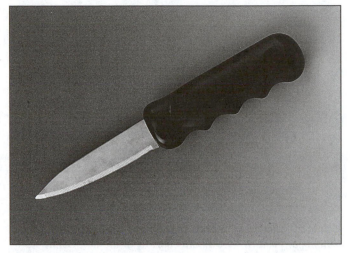

Figure 2-8. A large handle is more comfortable to grasp than a small one. (Photo courtesy of Hoan® Products Ltd., Dayton, NJ.)

ORTHOSES

An orthosis or brace may be very simple, such as one designed to keep your hand from deviating to the ulnar side (which is a common problem where there is arthritis) your thumb web space open for grasping, or your wrist supported to compensate for loss of muscle power. A splint may also be complex, requiring power from batteries. Some are so sophisticated that they have electrical implants to activate paralyzed muscles.

Any orthosis should be prescribed by your doctor or therapist; it is not a device to select on your own.

Custom-made cuffs are designed to reduce ulnar deviation and wrist strain if you have arthritis, especially during vacuuming, sweeping, or mopping (Figure 2-20). Elastic wrist supports have a removable aluminum bar that adjusts for added wrist flexion (Figure 2-21). It is helpful if you have slight weakness in your wrist. Velcro® closures make it easy to put on or remove. This type of support is helpful if you have slight weakness, arthritis, or carpal tunnel syndrome in your wrist(s). **Manufacturers:** 38, 218. Cost is about $15 and up from hospital supply firms. **Sources:** 1, 13, 16, 290, 368, 389.

Wrist supports with a palmar clip let you slide a utensil handle into the pocket so you may use shoulder or upper arm motion for stirring and handling foods (Figure 2-22). The degree of wrist extension is adjusted by bending an inner metal bar. **Manufacturer:** 202. Cost is about $16 and up from self-help firms. **Sources:** 5, 16, 120, 202, 264, 290, 368, 408.

The tenodesis orthosis transfers the extension of the wrist to flexion of the fingers, enabling you to grasp and hold objects (Figure 2-23). To obtain a custom-made splint and training in its use, talk with your occupational therapist or physician.

An arm support makes working easier if your shoulders and upper arms are weak (Figure 2-24). This plastic trough pivots for holding, mixing, and cutting foods, and for feeding yourself, within a limited range. Cost is about $50 from self-help firms. **Sources:** 5, 120, 252, 264, 290, 408.

Balanced forearm orthoses can help those with severe weak-ness due to paralysis or muscular dystrophy (Figure 2-25). The adjustable brackets for the metal arms attach to the back uprights of a wheelchair. The arms are adjusted to reduce gravity and provide movement away from or toward the body. **Manufacturer:** 202. **Sources:** 8, 120, 202, 290, 408.

OTHER HELPFUL TECHNIQUES AND AIDS

These items may also help if you have limited motion or limited strength in your arms, hands, and wrists:
- Single control faucets and tap turners: See Chapter 17.
- Eating aids including scoop plate and swivel spoon; and drinking aids: See Chapter 22.
- Pump tops for condiments: See Chapter 27.
- Bowl stabilizers, double handled pans, kitchen roll-about to reduce lifting, Kettle tilter: See Chapter 28 and Chapter 29.
- Wraparound pot holder: See Chapter 12.
- Hot water heater: See Chapter 20.

GOING FURTHER

Addresses are listed in the Appendices.

ARTHRITIS

Publications

Publications about arthritis are available from your local chapter of the Arthritis Foundation. The following publications are free, except where indicated: *Arthritis: The Basic-Facts*; *Arthritis: Diet Guidelines & Research*; *Arthritis Today*, a bimonthly magazine available with a donation of $20 or more; *Guide to Independent Living for People with Arthritis,* Self-help techniques and aids, with sources, 1988, (out-of-print, request loan from local AF chapter); *Home Care Programs in Arthritis: Manual for Patients,* includes exercises; *Osteoarthritis—Handbook for Patients*; *Rheumatoid Arthritis—Handbook for Patients.*

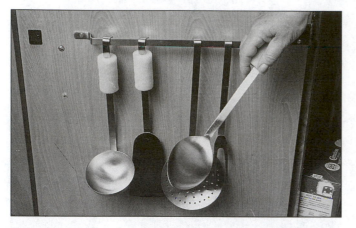

Figure 2-9. Handles of utensils may also be built up with foam padding or foam curlers. (Photo courtesy of the O.T. Dept., Howard A. Rusk Institute of Rehabilitation Medicine.)

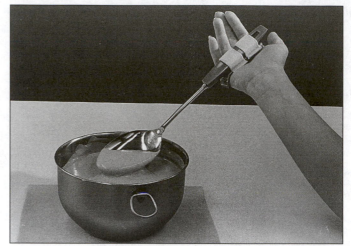

Figure 2-10. If grasp is totally lacking, loops of 1″ wide elastic can be added to a universal cuff to hold kitchen utensils. (Photo courtesy of the O.T. Dept., Howard A. Rusk Institute of Rehabilitation Medicine.)

Brewer, E. J., & Angel, K. C. (1994). *The Arthritis Sourcebook*. Chicago: Contemporary Books. **Source:** 76B.

Fries, J. F. (1995). *Arthritis: A Take Care of Yourself Health Guide* (4th ed.). Reading, MA: Addison-Wesley. **Source:** 13B.

Learning to Live with Osteoarthritis. (1983). Available from your physician or for $3 from Medicine in the Public Interest, Inc. **Source:** 266.

Lorig, K., & Fries, J. F. (1986). *The Arthritis Helpbook: A Tested Self-Management Program for Coping with Your Arthritis* (rev. edition). Reading, MA: Addison-Wesley. $13. Recommended by the Arthritis Foundation for use in its classes. **Source:** 13B.

The Remedy Arthritis Newsletter. Westport, CT: Rx Remedy, Inc. Bimonthly newsletter, $18 per year.

Shen, H., & Solimini, C. (1993). *Living with Arthritis*. New York: Penguin Books. **Source:** 308B.

Swezey, R. G. (Ed.). (1985). *Straight Talk on Ankylosing Spondylitis*. Spondylitis Association of America.

What Everyone Should Know About Arthritis, and Living With Arthritis. (1972). South Deerfield, MA: Channing L. Bete Co. Easy-to-understand illustrated booklets. $1.25 per copy, or available from your physician. **Source:** 62.

WEAK UPPER EXTREMITIES

Publications

Accent on Living. Quarterly periodical. $12 per year. Information on equipment daily living with disabilities, sources for additional information. **Source:** 3.

Corbet, B. (1980). *Options: Spinal Cord Injury and the Future*. Denver, CO: A.B. Hirschfeld Press. Available through the National Spinal Cord Injury Foundation, and **Source:** 96.

Halstead, L. S., & Grimby, G. (1995). *Post-Polio Syndrome*. Philadelphia: Hanley & Belfus. **Source:** 169B.

How to Live with a Spinal Cord Injury: An Accent Guide. Bloomington, IL: Accent on Living. Written by a paraplegic, book gives realistic information about how this disability affects one's life and what you can do about it. $6.95 plus handling. **Source:** 3.

Post Polio: An Accent Guide (#3204). Bloomington, IL: Accent on Living. Post-polio syndrome, what it is, its effects, what can be done. $3.95 plus handling. **Source:** 3.

Spinal Network. Extra. Periodical. Miramar Communications. See Appendix C. Maddox, S. *Spinal Network*. Both with extensive overview from medical aspects of spinal cord injury to rights, recreation, and resources. **Source:** 5.

Ask your therapist about available videos and films on living with arthritis and spinal cord injury that will give you information on ways to increase your own independence.

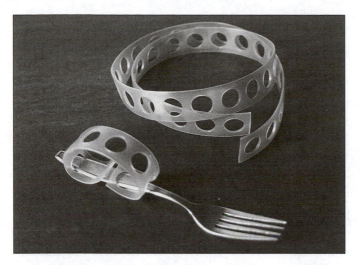

Figure 2-11. This multi-purpose, continuous strap may be cut to fit cutlery, grooming aids, and appliance knobs. (Photo by J.K.)

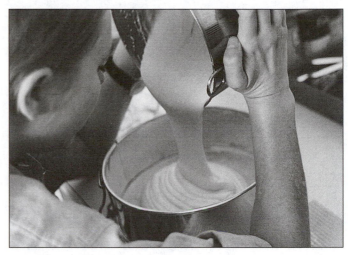

Figure 2-13. This quadriplegic homemaker has no grasp in her fingers, so she presses her palms against the sides of the bowl to hold it. (Photo by J.K.)

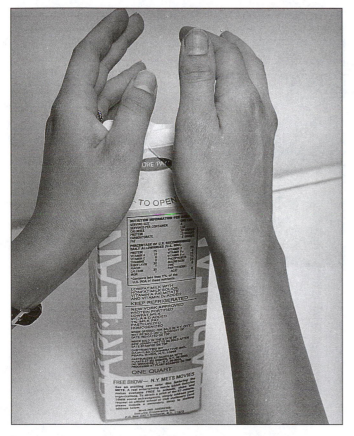

Figure 2-12. To open a milk or juice carton, use the heels of your hands to push back the sides, then use a fork to pry open the spout. Do not use your thumbs. (Photo courtesy of the O.T. Dept., Howard A. Rusk Institute of Rehabilitation Medicine.)

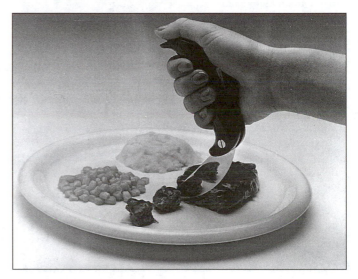

Figure 2-14. Using an angled knife reduces stress on your wrist when you have arthritis and decreases the force required to cut by up to 80%. (Photo courtesy of AliMed®, Inc., Dedham, MA.)

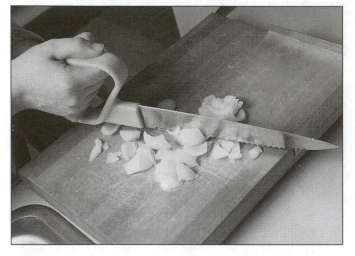

Figure 2-15. The design of this knife with a hole in the handle allows you to use both hands while cutting for better control. (Photo courtesy of the O.T. Dept., Howard A. Rusk Institute of Rehabilitation Medicine.)

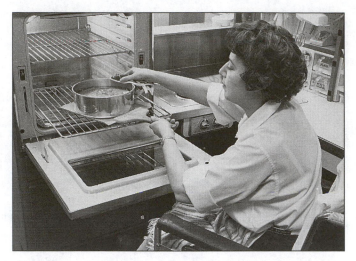

Figure 2-17. Adapt your kitchen as fully as possible to your physical needs. (Photo courtesy of the O.T. Dept., Howard A. Rusk Institute of Rehabilitation Medicine.)

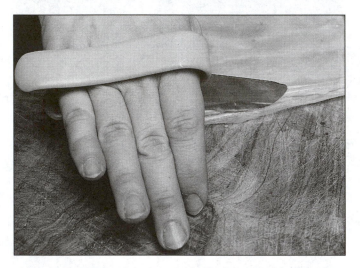

Figure 2-16. This quad meat cutter knife slips over the palm of your hand. (Photo courtesy of the O.T. Dept., Howard A. Rusk Institute of Rehabilitation Medicine.)

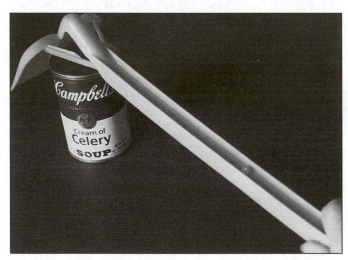

Figure 2-18. A child's hoe is a handy tool for pulling items from the back of the counter. (Photo by J.K.)

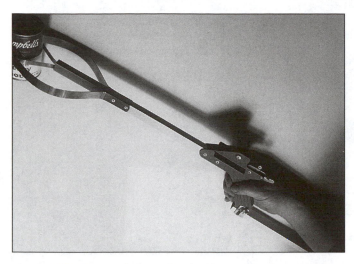

Figure 2-19. If your grip is weak, a locking reacher is recommended. This EZ-Reacher® II clamps onto the object being lifted. (Arcmate Industries, Escondido, CA. Photo by J.K.)

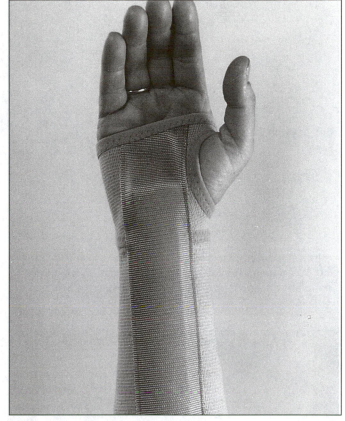

Figure 2-21. This elastic wrist support has a removable aluminum bar that adjusts for added wrist flexion. (Photo courtesy of AliMed®, Inc., Dedham, MA.)

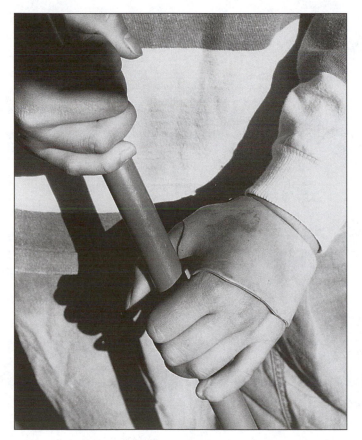

Figure 2-20. This custom-made cuff is designed to reduce ulnar deviation and wrist strain if you have arthritis. (Photo by J.K.)

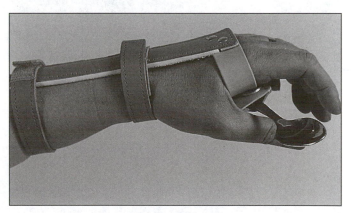

Figure 2-22. This wrist support with a palmar clip lets you slide a utensil handle into the pocket so you may use shoulder or upper arm motion for stirring and handling foods. (Photo courtesy of AliMed®, Inc., Dedham, MA.)

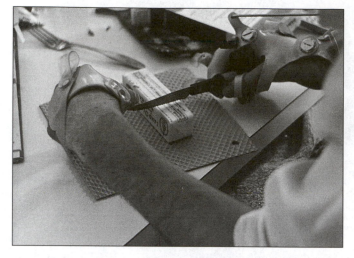

Figure 2-23. A spinal cord injury left this young man with a complete loss of grasp. He does, however, have enough wrist extension to bring his wrist up with a tenodesis splint and hold it in position, thus flexing his fingers. (Photo by J.K.)

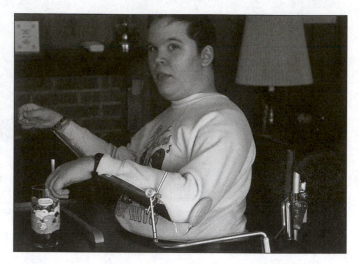

Figure 2-25. This teenager with muscular dystrophy uses balanced forearm orthoses. (Photo by J.K.)

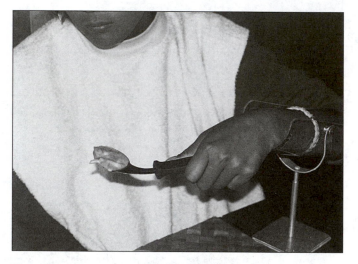

Figure 2-24. An arm support makes working easier if your shoulders and upper arms are weak. (Photo by J.K.)

If You Are an Upper Extremity Amputee

Learning to use an upper extremity prosthesis takes time and practice. Once you have received training, mastered the basic controls, and know how to position utensils securely, you'll be able to efficiently manage most meal preparation and home-making tasks. In the kitchen, a hook is preferable to a cosmetic hand because it is less prone to damage by heat, water, oil, and food colors.

For tips on stabilizing food and equipment, see Chapter 1. In selecting kitchen utensils that require the use of two hands, be certain that you can grip the handles safely and comfortably. Rubber-coated, large handles are easier to grasp. **Manufacturers:** 273, 301. See Chapter 21.

When choosing electrical appliances, such as mixers, can openers, knives, and skillets, check that the controls extend out far enough for you to manipulate them easily. A double-handled electric skillet is easier to lift and carry, but make sure that you can position the hook on your prosthesis to grasp the skillet handle securely.

If you have two prostheses, positioning is even more important. For lifting, which is difficult, you might adapt some of the ideas in Chapter 2.

To cut food, hold the knife in your non-prosthetic hand, or if you have two prostheses, in your more dominant device.

Position the fork so that the handle rests on the outer surface of the hook's thumb. Rotate your wrist until the top of the fork rests evenly on the cutting surface.

If kitchen utensils tend to slip, add another elastic band to your terminal device or wrap the utensil handles with electrician's or foam tape. **Manufacturer:** 390. Flat-handled utensils fit more securely in hooks.

Hold a large object by positioning the hook so that the tips are straight up or down. Secure the item with the rounded part of the hook. A damp sponge cloth or a piece of Dycem® Non-Slip under the object helps stabilize it. **Manufacturer** of Dycem®: 104. **Sources:** 5, 13, 16, 103, 108, 120, 130, 155, 238, 252, 290, 368, 408.

If it is impossible to exert enough force to open a jar, use a jar opener. See Chapter 1 and Chapter 27.

To carry a tray or cookie sheet, position the hook fingers so that they are parallel with the tray at waist level. Grasp the edges with hook fingers and hand. For maximum security, slide the edge all the way into the opening of the terminal device. If you have an above-elbow amputation, make sure the prosthetic elbow is locked.

For transporting many items at once, use a wheeled table or cart to save time and energy. See Chapter 16.

To wash dishes, hold the dish in your non-prosthetic hand and the scrubbing mop or sponge in your prosthetic device. Avoid detergents, which can dissolve lubricating oils in the hook and wrist mechanism. If you wash dishes often, make sure you frequently clean and oil the threads and bearing of the hook.

GOING FURTHER

Addresses are listed in the Appendices.

PUBLICATIONS

Ability, AMP, and *In Motion* are three periodicals written by and for amputees.

Winchell, E. *Living with Limb Loss.* New York: Avery. **Source:** 34B. Also available from **source** 13.

Ask your therapist about videos and films done by and for people who have had an amputation. They give suggestions on how to increase your independence.

If You Use a Cane, Crutches, or Other Walking Aid

The use of any walking aid should be evaluated by your physician, therapist, or nurse. Correct fitting and proper instruction are vital to your safety. If you use a cane, crutches, walker, or other ambulation aid, you should organize activities to conserve energy in your lower extremities. You should find a way to keep your walking aid within reach at all times and devise a way to carry things.

To avoid extra steps, before starting, gather together everything you need for meal preparation, cleanup, or other tasks. You may cook meals with electric appliances right at the table, so there is no need to transfer hot pans. Organize your kitchen so that the most frequently used items are at the correct work areas. Keep all measuring and baking items within reach in one area, and store all cutting and peeling items near the sink.

CANES

Just like crutches and wheelchairs, a cane should be measured for you by your physician or therapist. If it is too short, you will have to bend over to walk, and you will feel pain in your back. If it is too long, you will not have the optimum support, and your shoulder, arm, and wrist will tire more quickly.

Canes come with a variety of handle shapes to accommodate different grips. If you have arthritis or weakness in your hands, look for a cane with an ergonomically designed handle that provides padded comfort to your palm and a built-up grip for your fingers. **Manufacturers:** 122, 163. Cost is about $25 and up from self-help and hospital supply firms. **Sources:** 13, 50, 120, 264, 265, 370, 408.

A quad cane has four legs, so it can remain upright beside you while you work (Figure 4-1). **Manufacturers** include 163. Cost is $35 and up from hospital supply and self-help firms. **Sources:** 120, 240, 247, 264, 290, 261, 370, 408.

Ask your therapist if any of the new ergonomic canes would be helpful for you. Some are designed with curves for better balance; others have a bend that allows you to use it for assistance when rising from a seated position.

Keeping your walking aid close at hand is a primary safety consideration. A cane clip or holder stays on your cane, allowing you to hang the cane securely within your reach on any open-edged flat surface, such as a countertop or table. If you have weakness or arthritis in your hands, ask a friend to put the clip on your cane. Cost is about $5.50 and up from self-help firms. A cane loop lets you keep the cane on your arm as you reach for an object. Cost is about $7 from self-help firms. **Sources** for both items: 5, 50, 100, 120, 261, 264, 370, 408.

WALKERS

A walker may be prescribed as an ambulatory aid if you need more support than a cane or crutch offers, need assistance to maintain balance within the home and while traveling, or just need an aid for stability when waking during the night to go to the bathroom. A folding walker is preferred, because it is easier to handle when going shopping or doing other activities. Make sure that the walker has good rubber tips to prevent sliding. Your therapist will help determine the correct height of the walker for you and will teach you to walk without excess lifting the walker off the floor. Walkers are also available with wheels or casters on the two front legs, but the decision to add them should always be discussed with your physician and therapist. They will know how much weight-bearing you should be doing and whether the casters will decrease your safety. Make sure that you can handle the unlocking mechanism if you must fold and stash the walker yourself. **Manufacturers:** 163, 342, 428. Walkers are carried by the same sources as canes, see above.

Walker or crutch pads cushion your grasp, help prevent blisters, and absorb perspiration while providing a non-slip grip. They are made of machine-washable terry cloth or synthetic sheepskin with Velcro® closures to fit a round rail. **Manufacturer:** 58. Cost is about $7 to $15 per pair from self-help firms. **Sources:** 5, 58, 120, 252, 264, 270, 290, 370, 408.

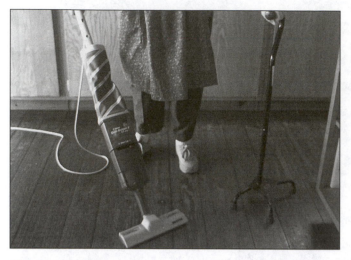

Figure 4-1. A quad cane has four legs, so it can remain upright beside you while you work. An attached bag will carry light items like glasses, pens, notepad, and tissues. (Photo by J.K.)

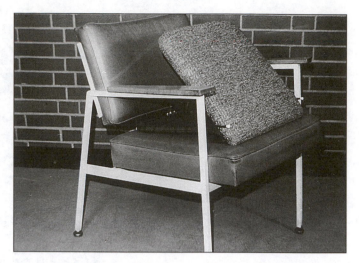

Figure 4-3. Specialized chairs, such as this manually operated spring-action lifter chair, gently elevate you from a sitting to standing position. (Photo courtesy of Maddak, Inc., Pequannock, NJ.)

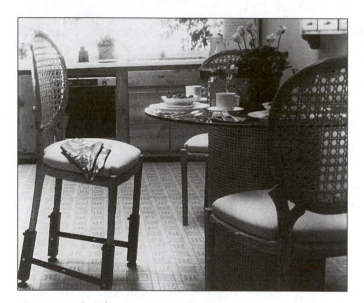

Figure 4-2. Chair leg extenders reduce stress on your hips and knees when you get up or down. (Photo courtesy of RoLoke Co., Culver City, CA.)

SEATING

Whenever possible, work while seated. Save your energy for getting from place to place. Your chair should be stable and should allow your feet to rest flat on floor or on a stool. A backrest provides trunk support and comfort. See Chapter 5.

It is easier to lower your body into and rise from a taller chair. A higher seat also allows you to sit comfortably at the counter while preparing or cleaning up meals.

Chair leg extenders reduce stress on your hips and knees when you get up or down (Figure 4-2). Extenders that raise your chair to a comfortable height are $40 and up per set from self-help firms. **Manufacturer:** 337. **Sources** of similar leg extenders: 120, 408.

A foam seat cushion makes it easier to rise and sit, and may be moved from place to place. Some have shoulder straps for carry-

ing. **Manufacturers:** 16, 103. Cost is $8 and up from mail-order and self-help firms. **Sources:** 13, 16, 59, 100, 120, 252, 270, 290.

Chairs that promote good posture, chairs with higher seats, and those with seats that lift you to a standing position are available in a variety of styles. Also see Artherapedic Chair in Chapter 2.

Electrically operated lift seats reduce stress on knees and hips; but for people with lower extremity weakness, they are only recommended after evaluation and training with a therapist. **Manufacturers:** 43, 51B, 297.

Specialized chairs, such as a manually operated spring-action lifter chair, gently elevate you from a sitting to standing position (Figure 4-3). A side lever activates a spring action that expands the seat to a 45° angle. It comes in a two-spring model for individuals up to 150 pounds and a three-spring model for people up to 220 pounds, but should be used only after training with a therapist and then with a chair that has arms. Cost is about $280 from self-help firms. A seat insert is also available. **Sources** for both: 120, 252, 261 290.

A lightweight mobile stool permits you to stand with reduced pressure on your hips, legs, feet, and back (Figure 4-4). It supports up to 90% of your weight. The height of the padded seat adjusts from 27" to 34", so that you can work at a standard counter. Casters allow you to propel the stool with your feet. Before you buy a stool, discuss it with your therapist or physician, and try it out at a local self-help or hospital supply firm. Cost is $70 and up from business supply and self-help firms. **Sources:** 13, 120, 158, 264, 370, 408.

CARRYING

A cart can be pushed with your hands or your body. It helps you organize and gather everything you need for meal preparation, laundry, or cleaning. You can even carry an infant secured in a small bed or infant seat firmly attached to the cart top. See Chapter 16.

Swivel casters on a cart allow you to push it with your body while walking with crutches. If you need to replace the casters, take one from your cart to a hardware store to find the correct size. **Manufacturer:** 363.

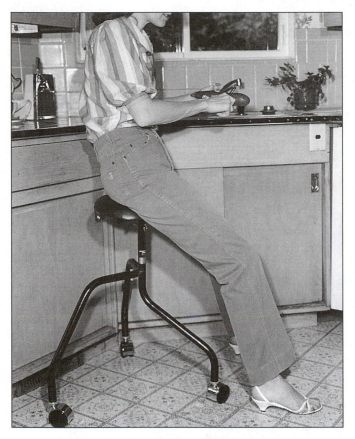

Figure 4-4. This lightweight mobile stool permits you to stand with reduced pressure on your hips, legs, feet, and back (Photo courtesy of Bissell® Healthcare Corp., Inc., Jackson, MI.)

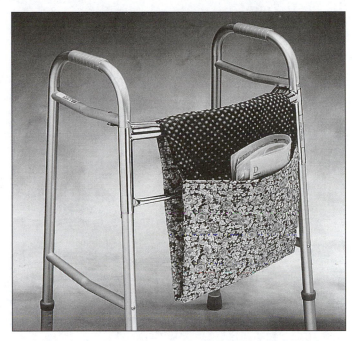

Figure 4-5. A walker bag carries eyeglasses, tissues, and other small items. (Photo courtesy of North Coast Medical, Inc., San Jose, CA.)

A walker basket is the best choice for transporting utensils and food. See Chapter 25.

Caution: Transporting items on a walker tray is more difficult than in a basket, because objects tend to slide. Carried liquids should always be covered to avoid spills.

A walker bag carries eyeglasses, tissues, and other small items (Figure 4-5). In single and multiple pocket styles, and in a variety of colors and washable fabrics, most bags attach to walkers with Velcro® straps. **Manufacturers:** 14, 36, 125, 163. **Sources:** 5, 14, 16, 36, 50, 120, 125, 252, 261, 264, 290, 370, 408.

If you tire while walking, try a walker with a seat. The seat flips down when needed, and the walker folds flat for travel. Cost is $95 and up from hospital supply and self-help firms. Seats are also available as optional accessories for some walkers. Talk to your therapist before purchasing one of these items.

A wheeled walker or walking aid reduces the stress of lifting if your arms are weak or affected by arthritis (Figure 4-6). You and your therapist together must evaluate the safety of a wheeled unit. **Manufacturer:** 414 (pictured), 25, 122, 163. Cost is about $275 and up. **Sources:** 13, 25, 100, 120, 122, 247, 290, 414.

The Swedish-designed Avant Walker has a fold-down seat so that you roll it up close and sit to work, then walk with support (Figure 4-7). **Manufacturer:** 122. See another Etac walker in Chapter 25.

When shopping, a shoulder bag pocketbook leaves your hands free to manage your walking aid and to open doors.

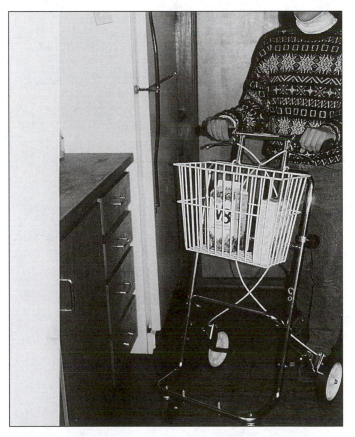

Figure 4-6. This wheeled walker has adjustable height handles, folds for transporting and storage, and has hand-controlled rear wheel brakes and a basket. The large front casters swivel easily. (Walk Away Walker, LLC. Photo by J.K.)

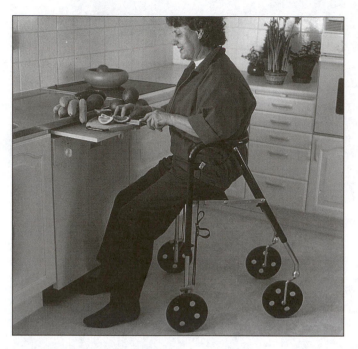

Figure 4-7. This Swedish-designed Avant Walker has a fold-down seat so that you roll it up close and sit to work, then walk with support. (Photo courtesy of Etac USA, Waukesha, WI.)

A small pocketbook may be adapted with leather loops to fit over a contoured or T-handle cane. Ask your local shoe repairer to make the alterations.

When shopping or traveling, attach a small bag to your crutch to leave your hands free. Bags snap under the hand grips and should be purchased by the pair to equalize the load. Do not overload the bags—the added weight will affect your balance. **Manufacturer:** 14. Cost is about $10 each from self-help equipment firms. For additional carrying aids, see Chapter 25.

If You
Have Back Pain
or Chronic Pain

More than 80% of Americans suffer from back or chronic pain at some time in their lives. The severity can range from an occasional, mild ache to constant, chronic distress. Back pain may be caused by excess weight, poor posture, weak abdominal muscles, ruptured disks, physical or emotional stress, illness, or injury resulting from incorrect bending and lifting. See your physician if your back pain is accompanied by pain, weakness, or numbness in one or both of your legs; if it is the result of a fall or injury; if it is accompanied by a fever; or if it has lasted longer than six weeks.

Chronic pain may be a symptom of many diseases, such as arthritis, fibromyalgia, other rheumatic illnesses, chronic fatigue and post-polio syndromes, multiple sclerosis, and aging. Often, the pain may be reduced through relaxation techniques. Talk with your physician and therapist about a "Pain Busters" support group, a pain clinic, or write to the American Chronic Pain Association or the National Chronic Pain Outreach Association. Addresses are in Appendix B.

Chronic headaches may be the result of poor posture, eye strain, stress, or physical factors, including diet. You may reduce the severity of your headache by applying relaxation techniques, such as deep breathing, physical exercise, massage, acupressure, meditation, and biofeedback. If headaches are limiting your ability to handle daily life, talk to your physician. Headache clinics are available through many hospital centers.

If your back is to serve you well, you must learn the correct ways to stand, sit, lie, lift, reach, and even walk. Back care education programs are offered through hospitals and rehabilitation centers, sports medicine clinics, and the YMCA or YWCA. Videos demonstrating back exercises are also available; check with your physician or therapist.

The following suggestions will assist you in meal preparation and homemaking tasks; however, they do not replace a thorough evaluation by your doctor or the daily exercises prescribed by a therapist:

- To protect your back, avoid carrying heavy loads. Use a wheeled cart, or divide loads into smaller bundles. See carts in Chapter 16. Ask others to help carry heavy items.
- When lifting, bend your knees instead of your back. Avoid twisting your body. Stop if the item is too heavy.
- Always wear comfortable shoes that correctly support your feet.
- Adjust your eyeglasses so that they do not slip. Wrap tape around the ear pieces to keep them in place or have the frames adjusted. As strange as it sounds, poorly fitting eyeglasses can lead to poor posture and resulting pain in your back, shoulders, and even your jaw. If your glasses slip down your nose, you may be slouching forward to see and to keep them in place. Slouching causes neck strain and improper breathing. Be sure to breathe through your nose rather than your mouth.
- Take breaks from sitting to stand, stretch, and walk a little. Sitting is harder on your back than standing.

The largest single contributing factor to comfort while you work is your chair. For your chair to properly support you, the chair seat must be wide enough to accommodate your full buttocks and deep enough that it extends to within 1" of the crease behind your knees.

Your thighs should be parallel to the floor when sitting in a standard-height chair; a foot stool may be used to achieve this on a higher chair (Figure 5-1). A portable foot rest permits you to maintain proper sitting posture at home, work, or when traveling. Cost is about $22 from office supply and self-help firms. **Source:** 13.

The back of the seat should be just a bit higher than the front, so you lean backward slightly, achieving good posture. If you have poor trunk balance, however, the seat may need to be higher in front to maintain your balance.

The chair back should be approximately 2" above the lower tip of your shoulder blades and should tilt about 10° back. The ideal chair is one that tilts and swivels so that you can move in it. Ergonomic chairs feature back supports and adjustable height and foot support. Visit a business furniture or art supply firm, and try several models to find the one most comfortable for you. Check pricing through office furniture catalogs. **Sources:** 52, 144, 153, 158, 179, 293, 377.

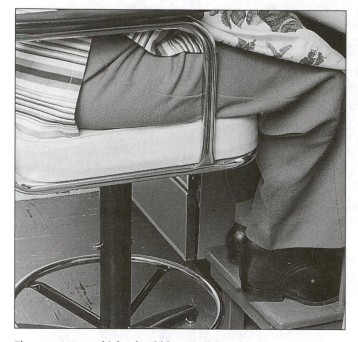

Figure 5-1. Your thighs should be parallel to the floor when sitting in a standard-height chair. (Photo courtesy of the O.T. Dept., Howard A. Rusk Institute of Rehabilitation Medicine.)

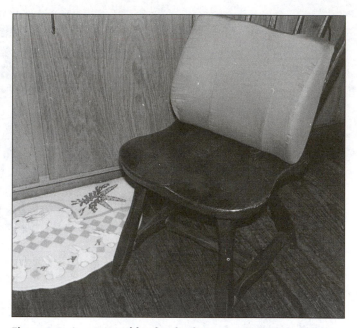

Figure 5-2. A contoured lumbar back support eases fatigue by maintaining alignment to keep the lower back muscles relaxed. (Photo by J.K.)

A contoured lumbar back eases fatigue by maintaining alignment to keep the lower back muscles relaxed (Figure 5-2). Use it in the office, at home, and in the car. **Manufacturers** include 103, 246. Cost is about $15 and up from self-help and mail-order firms. **Sources:** 21, 120, 138, 169, 261, 270, 290.

A padded rug at your sink or where you stand to work helps reduce pressure on your feet, legs, and back. Make sure the underside is rubberized to prevent slipping when wet. **Manufacturers** include 35. Cost is about $5 and up from department stores and mail-order firms. **Sources:** 242, 245, 270, 378.

The Obus Forme® is molded to provide lumbar as well as lateral support to your back (Figure 5-3). Use with or without the lumbar pad, which adjusts with a Velcro® strip to the position that feels best for you. An elastic strap holds the Obus Forme® in place on your chair, wheelchair, or car seat. Cover is removable for washing. **Manufacturers:** 56, 292. Cost is $99 and up through self-help and mail-order firms. A molded seat by Obus is $70 and up. **Sources:** 56, 120, 138, 292.

The Back Machine® contains a roller bar that adjusts the bend of the lumbar spring-steel ribs to nine positions (Figure 5-4). Foam padding covers the ribs, and a soft cover removes for washing. It may be used in any chair and weighs two pounds. Take it with you in the car or even on a plane. **Manufacturer:** 221. Cost is about $40 from self-help and mail-order firms. **Sources:** 49, 263 (similar unit), 410.

A seat wedge may add comfort and support. A center groove helps ease pressure on your tail bone. See Chapter 7.

The Back Joy® or Relaxo-Bak® is a molded seat that cups your buttocks so you don't lean on your spine (Figure 5-5). This reduces strain and pressure on the muscles and ligaments of your back. **Manufacturer:** 271. Cost is about $50 from self-help firms. **Source:** 21.

Sitting on a gel cushion disperses pressure to reduce stress on your back. The gel absorbs vibrations so is especially helpful for use in a wheelchair or when traveling. The 16" square cushion comes with a breathable, non-stick Lycra® cover with a slip-resistant nylon bottom. **Manufacturer:** 372. Cost is about $100 from durable medical distributors and self-help firms.

GOING FURTHER

Addresses are listed in the Appendices.

PUBLICATIONS

American Chronic Pain Association. Write for a list of publications and information on support groups.

Arthritis Medical Information Series: *Back Pain* and *Managing Your Pain*. Booklets free from your local chapter of The Arthritis Foundation.

Caplan, D. (1987). *Back Trouble: A New Approach to Prevention and Recovery*. Gainesville, FL: Triad Communications, Inc. **Source:** 402.

Caplan, D., et al. (1988). *The Fit Back: Prevention and Recovery*. Alexandria, VA: Time-Life Books. Back structure, correct posture, exercises (which should be checked with your therapist), day-to-day back care and aids. **Source:** 397A.

Caudill, M. A. (1994). *Managing Pain Before It Manages You*. New York: Guilford Press. Guide/workbook to living with chronic pain, based on clinically tested program. **Source:** 164.

Coping With Pain: Arthritis Medical Information Series. Free from your local chapter of the Arthritis Foundation.

Duckro, P., Richardson, W. D., & Marshall, J. E., et al. (1995). *Taking Control of Your Headaches*. New York: Guilford Press. **Source:** 164.

Hendler, N. (1993). *How to Cope with Chronic Pain* (rev. ed.).

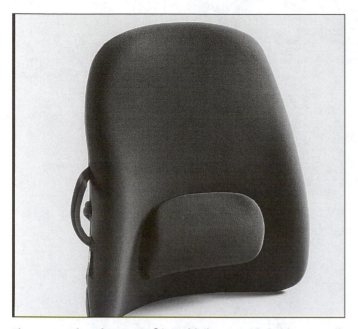

Figure 5-3. The Obus Forme® is molded to provide lumbar as well as lateral support to your back. (Photo courtesy of Obus Forme®, Toronto, ON.)

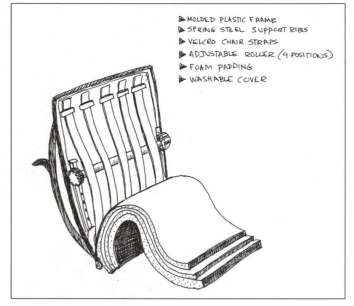

- MOLDED PLASTIC FRAME
- SPRING STEEL SUPPORT RIBS
- VELCRO CHAIR STRAPS
- ADJUSTABLE ROLLER (9 POSITIONS)
- FOAM PADDING
- WASHABLE COVER

Figure 5-4. The Back Machine® contains a roller bar that adjusts the bend of the lumbar spring-steel ribs to nine positions. (Illustration by G.K.)

Boca Raton, FL: Cool Hands Communications. Practical suggestions and steps to follow for relief. Designed for clients, their families, and physicians. **Source:** 77B.

McIlwain, H. H., et al. (1994). *Winning with Back Pain: A Complete Program for Health and Well-Being.* New York: Promotheus. **Source:** 322.

Melnik, M. *Fibromyalgia—Getting Healthy*, Jeanne Melvin; *Occupational Therapy in the Relief of Foot Pain*; and *Understanding Your Back Injury.* Consumer guides from the American Occupational Therapy Association, Inc. Available through your occupational therapist.

National Chronic Pain Outreach Association. Send for list of publications and support groups.

Sarno, J. E. (1991). *Healing Back Pain.* New York: Time-Warner Books, Random House. Author believes that most back pain is the result of stress and teaches how to overcome it. $9.95. **Source:** 326B.

Spondylitis Association of America. Materials available on request.

You and Your Back: How to Prevent Injury and Maintain Health. (1996). and *The ABCs of Moving and Lifting Things Safely.* (1996). Both booklets from South Deerfield, MA: Channing L. Bete. Available through your physician or therapist or $1.25 each. **Source:** 62.

Ask your therapist about videos, films, and relaxation tapes that teach how to cope with back and chronic pain.

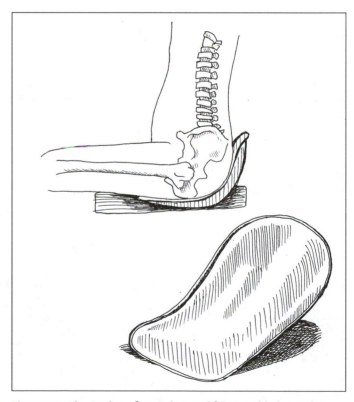

Figure 5-5. The Back Joy® or Relaxo-Bak® is a molded seat that cups your buttocks so you don't lean on your spine. (Illustration by G.K.)

If You Have
Loss of Sensation

Loss of sensation may affect any part of your body. It may be limited to the inability to discern hot and cold, or may include loss of the sense of touch. The cause may be a spinal cord injury, neurological involvement after a stroke, a severed nerve, or a disease, such as multiple sclerosis.

If you have loss of sensation, you must take safety precautions when working in the kitchen. Here are a few helpful tips:

- Be careful. Always watch what you are doing.
- Use padded pot holders when handling hot pans from the range, oven, and microwave. You may also want to use them to remove items from the freezer. See Chapters 12 and 29.
- Slide rather than lift pans, whenever possible, to prevent spilling.
- Use kitchen utensils with large, easy-to-grip, non-slip handles.
- Select pans and utensils with insulated handles for working at the range. The handle of a non-insulated cooking utensil could quickly burn you without your feeling it.
- Ladle hot liquids instead of pouring them to avoid spills. Remove hot foods with a strainer basket or slotted spoon instead of lifting the pot to drain or pour.
- Use cooking thermometers to help determine when a desired temperature is reached.
- If you use a wheelchair, a lapboard with a raised rim will help you to more safely carry hot pots and casseroles. Do not put hot dishes directly onto your lap.
- When you are cutting, stabilize the food on a breadboard that has two nails. This will help keep your fingers out of the way. See Chapter 1.
- Ask for help to move heavy, hot pans from the oven or range. If there is no one around, transfer the contents into smaller containers, and leave the pans to cool before moving them.
- Ask someone to check the temperature of your hot tap water. If your tap water is hot enough to cause burns, have the thermostat turned down. If this is not possible, wear protective gloves and use a faucet turning aid. Faucets are also available with thermostatic controls.

- Use a dishwasher, if possible. It is not only a great convenience, but also a safety aid. Otherwise, wear insulated rubber gloves when you do dishes. See Chapter 17.
- If you are remodeling your kitchen so you can sit at the sink to work, make sure that your legs are protected from contact with the water and drain pipes under the sink. The pipes may be enclosed or wrapped with foam pipe insulation, which is available from the plumbing section of your local hardware store.

A hand protector insulates and helps you maintain a secure grip on slippery, cold, or hot glasses, pans, and cups (Figure 6-1). Thumb and fingers fit in the end pockets. The surface is made of many small suction cups. The rubber hand protector keeps its flexibility from 170° to 500° F. Cost is about $10 from self-help firms. **Sources:** 252, 261, 264.

Use a thermo-probe thermometer to check the interior temperature of meat or poultry (Figure 6-2). The temperature is displayed on a dial located on the thermometer's insulated handle. It is dishwasher safe and contains no glass that could break.

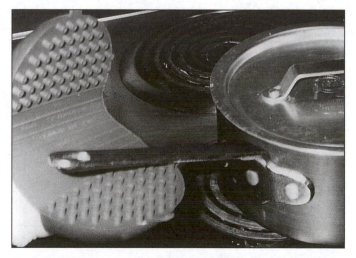

Figure 6-1. Hot Hands, a hand protector, insulates and helps you maintain a secure grip on slippery, cold, or hot glasses, pans, and cups. (Photo by J.K.)

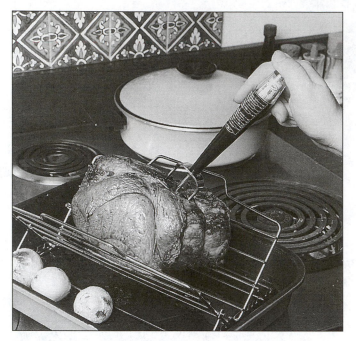

Figure 6-2. Use a thermo-probe thermometer to check the interior temperature of meat or poultry. (Photo courtesy of the O.T. Dept., Howard A. Rusk Institute of Rehabilitation Medicine.)

Manufacturer: 396. Cost is about $12 each from gourmet specialty firms.

The Scaldsafe® Faucet Aerator is a hot water sensor that turns off automatically when water reaches 114° F. It resets at the touch of a button. Cost is about $8 from plumbing suppliers and self-help firms. **Source:** 3. Models of Scaldsafe® are also available for tub and shower areas and are required in these places in homes built by the Veterans Administration. UltraFlo®, a one-line push button plumbing system with pre-set temperatures, also eliminates the need to turn faucet knobs. **Source:** 406. See Chapter 13.

When drinking, use thermal mugs or insulated glasses to protect your hands. Both are available through housewares stores (look in the leisure and seasonal sections) and through mail-order firms. **Sources** of insulated tumblers: 152, 270, 343. See also Chapter 22.

CHAPTER

7

If You Use
a Wheelchair

The designs of your wheelchair and of your home, including your kitchen, have a major effect on your ability to work comfortably and efficiently. Preparing foods on the counter, reaching the sink and refrigerator, operating the range, and retrieving items from storage may be accomplished more easily with careful planning.

Appliances should be arranged to permit safe use from your wheelchair. A lowered, drop-in surface cooking unit allows sliding instead of lifting. Legs and footrests can roll under, giving more usable floor space. Controls may be placed on the side or front, with light and fan controls also located within easy reach. Wall ovens can be installed at the most convenient height for you, providing access to controls while seated or standing. In addition, some side-opening microwave and convection ovens have pull-out boards beneath them. Dishwashers should have easy loading, slide-out upper and lower racks, as well as a removable flatware basket.

A side-by-side refrigerator allows the fullest access to both refrigerator and freezer from a wheelchair. Check door bin design, because this is the easiest area to reach and the easiest position from which to lift items back and forth. Shelves that adjust in height and pull out increase wheelchair-accessible areas of the refrigerator. In-door dispensers for ice and water are a bonus. **Manufacturers** of major appliances include 20, 34, 147, 150, 156, 205, 222, 303, 356, 380, 385, 395, 424, 425.

Jockeying around cabinet and regular doors in a wheelchair is frustrating; remove the doors! Rearrange contents of cabinets so that you can reach one item without having to shuffle through others. Remember to insulate hot pipes under your sink to prevent burning your legs.

Your work surface should be high enough to allow the arms of your wheelchair to roll under the counter. This means the countertop should be about 31" high with a 29½" clearance from the floor; check the measurements of your own chair because dimensions vary. Always keep the area under the counter open to facilitate turning your chair. One long counter stretching from the refrigerator to the range, including the sink, lets you slide items instead of carrying them.

You will find descriptions of specific appliances, storage aids, and helpful techniques in Chapters 12 through 20.

In a wheelchair kitchen at Ballard Green Housing, Ridgefield, CT., the undersurface of the counter just clears the wheelchair arms (Figure 7-1). A pullout board to the left of the sink provides an extra work area. It is slightly lower than the counter, which makes cutting and mixing easier.

The stainless-steel sink is only 6" deep, so it clears the legs of someone sitting at it. The bottom of the sink is insulated to prevent burns. A 5½" deep sink with an offset drain to the right or left is also available. **Manufacturers** of sinks suitable for use from a wheelchair include 115.

If you must cook from a wheelchair but cannot adapt your kitchen work surfaces, add a lower work area. For example, a standard kitchen table of the proper height is available from department stores and wood-working firms.

A wheelchair-height counter can be completely open underneath (Figure 7-2). The microwave oven is placed above a pull-out board to reduce lifting and prevent spilling while carrying.

The pull-out board is used as a resting place, which makes transferring food to and from the microwave oven simpler and safer. An over-the-drawer board holds appliances while in use. A portable socket strip allows easier access to electrical plugs.

WHEELCHAIR CONSIDERATIONS

Your physician or therapist will help you select a wheelchair. It should have removable or swing-away arms, removable swinging foot rests, and brakes that you can operate. Non-removable arms interfere with safety, transfers, ease, and independence. Specialized seating units and other modifications selected for your individual needs will make your chair more functional, safer, and more comfortable.

Manufacturers of wheelchairs include 12, 119, 122, 125, 146, 163, 200, 249, 295B, 328. You may send for catalogs or brochures from any of these companies, but you should actually try the

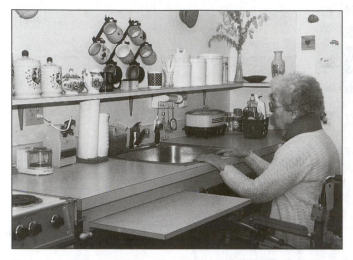

Figure 7-1. The wheelchair rolls under the counter in this kitchen at Ballard Green Housing, Ridgefield, CT. (Photo by J.K.)

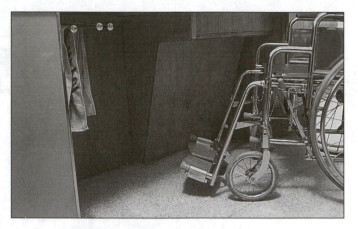

Figure 7-3. Desk arms, arms that are lower in front, permit you to roll your chair up under a table or counter. (Photo courtesy of the O.T. Dept., Howard A. Rusk Institute of Rehabilitation Medicine.)

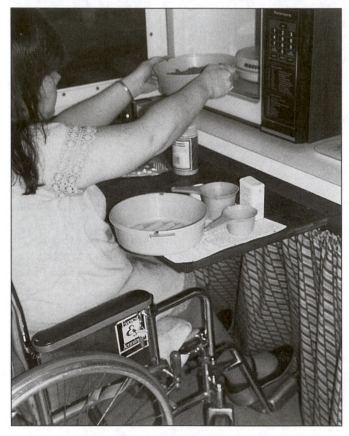

Figure 7-2. This wheelchair-height counter, also at Ballard Green Housing, Ridgefield, CT., is completely open underneath. (Photo by J.K.)

Many new wheelchairs are made of materials about half the weight of older models. If you are choosing a new wheelchair, consider these questions:

- Can you use your legs to help propel the chair? If so, removing the foot rests while you work in the kitchen reduces the chair's weight and allows you to use your legs. It also permits a closer approach to furniture or equipment and more mobility in narrow spaces.
- Do your elbows rest on the armrests without hunching your shoulders? Do you need to support your arms while working because of poor trunk balance or arm weakness? If so, adjustable height wheelchair arms come in a variety of styles.
- Do your hips and back get tired while you are in the chair? If so, check your posture with your physician, nurse, or therapist. A molded seat or backrest helps stabilize your trunk and keeps your body aligned. A wheelchair cushion increases comfort and protects your skin. If you are of average height or taller, a cushion might even raise you high enough to use standard-height kitchen equipment.
- Do you propel with one arm? A one-arm drive wheelchair with a double-hand rim will let you move in a straight line by moving just one wheel.
- Are your hands weak or affected by arthritis? If so, use knobs or spacers on the wheels to transfer work of the fingers to the palms of your hands.

Desk arms, arms that are lower in front, permit you to roll your chair up under a table or counter (Figure 7-3). Moving closer to your work is especially crucial if you have poor trunk balance or must support your arms while working. Adjustable-height arms help improve your posture and accommodate a variety of activities.

A custom-contoured wheelchair cushion increases comfort and reduces the chances of skin breakdown (Figure 7-4). Gel-filled cushions also shift with your weight to equalize pressure and minimize your risk of developing sores. Any cushion should have a solid base underneath it. The base may be cut out to reduce pressure on the end of your spine. If sitting is not comfortable, talk with your physician, nurse, or therapist. **Manufacturers** of cushions include 11, 103, 116, 125, 203, 217,

wheelchairs. Your therapist can arrange for wheelchair venders to come to your home or place of therapy, or you may visit the showrooms of local durable medical equipment suppliers.

If you have some use of your lower extremities or work in an area small enough to allow you to pull yourself around with your hands, a glider chair may be appropriate for maneuvering in your kitchen. See Chapter 2.

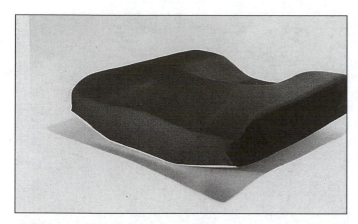

Figure 7-4. A custom-contoured wheelchair cushion increases comfort and reduces the chances of skin breakdown. (Photo courtesy of AliMed® Inc., Dedham, MA.)

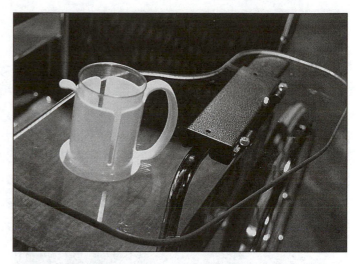

Figure 7-5. This clear acrylic tray locks securely onto desk or standard wheelchair armrests for carrying small items or for eating. (Photo courtesy of Consumer Care Products, Inc., Sheboygan, WI.)

310, 372. Price ranges from $6 for a simple foam cushion to more than $200 for a molded unit. **Sources:** 13, 16, 50, 116, 120, 130, 155, 203, 217, 252, 264, 290, 310, 368, 370, 408.

Custom-made cushions are often covered by Medicare and other insurance if cushions are ordered when purchasing a wheelchair. Your therapist can arrange for vendors of custom-made cushions to come to your place of therapy for fitting.

A wedge-shaped cushion keeps you from sliding forward in the seat and gives you better posture and weight distribution. Of contoured foam, it comes with a fabric cover and an optional solid insert. **Manufacturer:** 139. Cost is $35 and up from self-help firms. **Sources:** 5, 13, 120, 264, 290, 368, 408.

LAPBOARDS

A lapboard may be used as a work surface, for organizing what you need at the preparation area or table, and for safely carrying items, such as hot dishes. If you use a wall oven, the main shelf may be set at the same level as your lapboard, so that you can slide pans to and from the oven without lifting them. If sliding pans onto a lapboard, the surface must be heat-resistant or protected with a pad.

A clear acrylic tray that locks securely onto desk or standard wheelchair armrests can be used for carrying small items or for eating (Figure 7-5). This type of tray is not designed for carrying heavy or hot items. **Manufacturer:** 75. Cost is $34 and up from self-help firms. **Sources:** 5, 13, 120, 264, 290, 368, 370, 408.

You may have a lapboard made to fit your wheelchair (Figure 7-6). The board should have a slight rim to prevent objects from sliding off or spills from landing in your lap. Custom-made trays may be attached to your desk-arm wheelchair with metal supports.

Ask your therapist or a carpenter to help design the best lapboard for your needs. Some self-help firms will make you a custom tray. **Source:** 393. If buying a ready-made tray, be sure that it correctly fits the dimensions of your chair.

A laptop cutting board can be designed to be used on your lap or placed in a drawer (Figure 7-7). Each surface has a cutout to hold a bowl: one an 8" stainless-steel bowl, the other a 5" con-

tainer. Cut food can be slid directly into the receptacle, rather than picked up and transferred. The dowelled food-holding cage allows one to slice and dice with two weak hands or one hand. A local craftsman could build a similar unit for you.

While a lowered tray is better for mixing, cutting, and other meal preparation activities, you may want a higher armrest tray for writing, reading, and related tasks. **Manufacturers:** 75, 103, 125. Cost depends on material and method of fastening (usually Velcro® straps, but more expensive units have clamps). **Sources:** 5, 13, 75, 120, 130, 252, 290, 368, 370.

CARRYING

For shopping and other outings, you may attach a zippered purse to your wheelchair arm with Velcro® straps (Figure 7-8). **Manufacturers:** 14, 36, 103, 125. Cost is $14 and up from self-help firms. **Sources:** 13, 14, 36, 120, 125, 264, 290, 408.

A personal tote bag fits under the seat or on the side of the chair. Cost is about $12 from self-help firms. A wheelchair backpack is big enough to hold a light load of groceries. The straps fit any 14" to 20" chair with push handles; the top closes with Velcro®. **Manufacturers:** 14, 103, 125. Cost is $18 and up from self-help firms. **Sources:** 3, 14, 16, 120, 125, 264, 290, 408.

Use a reacher or long tongs to bring items within your grasp. See Chapter 2. You may keep your reacher or tongs on a chain or retractable dog leash to prevent dropping them.

Gloves with protective palms prevent injury to your hands when propelling long distances. **Sources:** 1, 252, 261, 290.

POWERED WHEELCHAIRS

Electrically powered wheelchairs and scooters help conserve your energy, especially if you have marked weakness, poor coordination, or arthritis in your arms and hands, or if you must cover long distances. Discuss the advantages, disadvantages, and possibilities of funding with your physician, therapist, or nurse.

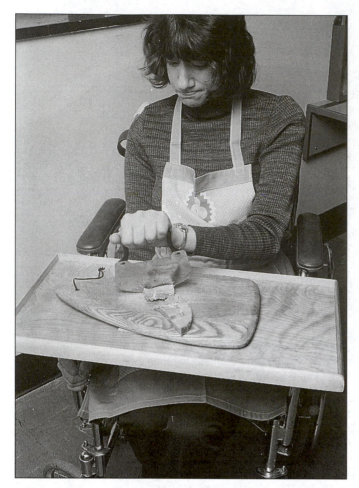

Figure 7-6. You may have a lapboard made to fit your wheelchair. (Photo courtesy of the O.T. Dept., Howard A. Rusk Institute of Rehabilitation Medicine.)

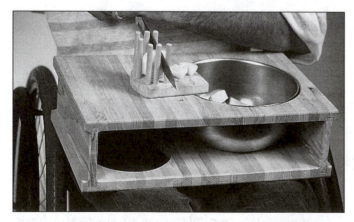

Figure 7-7. This laptop cutting board is designed to be used on your lap or placed in a drawer. (Photo courtesy of IDEA, Pewaukee, WI.)

If you have good trunk balance, a powered scooter can be useful at home and for shopping, work, or travel. Before purchasing one, talk with your therapist or nurse; then examine several models at a major durable medical equipment firm. Some considerations:

- Is it the correct length and width? Will it fit easily through narrow hallways and around sharp turns? Can you turn the scoot-

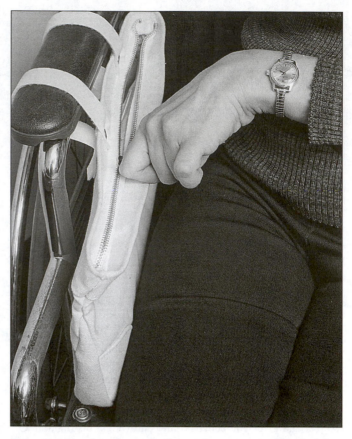

Figure 7-8. For shopping and other outings, you may attach a zippered purse to your wheelchair arm with Velcro® straps. (Photo courtesy of the O.T. Dept., Howard A. Rusk Institute of Rehabilitation Medicine.)

er around in the rooms of your residence?

- Is the seat adjustable? Can you raise or lower it? Does it swivel so you can easily approach a desk, counter, or sink? Does it lock while you are mounting or dismounting it?
- Is it easy to operate? Test drive it. Are the controls positioned so that you can rest your arms while driving? Does an automatic brake keep you from rolling if you stop the motor on an inclined surface?
- Does the unit dismantle? Will the parts fit into your car? Are the dismantled parts lightweight enough for you or a companion to handle?
- Can you independently operate the recharging mechanism?
- What is the guarantee and repair policy? Where is your nearest dealer? Will the firm pick up your scooter and provide a "loaner" should repairs be required?
- Will part of the cost of the scooter be covered by insurance? Make sure you have filled out all forms and have obtained the physician's signature before you agree to purchase a scooter.

A battery-powered scooter may be used inside and outside the home (Figure 7-9). Removable baskets permit carrying groceries and other items. **Manufacturers** of powered scooters and similar vehicles: 26, 44, 50B, 113, 302, 317. Cost is about $1,600 and up from self-help and hospital supply firms. Call manufacturer for names of local suppliers or visit your local durable medical supplier.

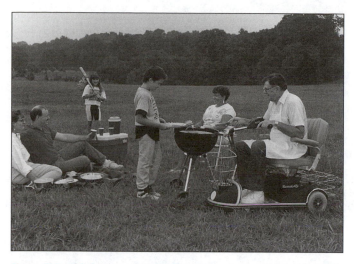

Figure 7-9. This battery-powered scooter may be used inside and outside the home. (Photo courtesy of Electric Mobility®, Inc., Sewell, NJ.)

If lifting a powered scooter into your vehicle is a problem, an electric lift is available. For further information contact 26, 44, 50B.

An electric wheelchair costs several thousand dollars (Figure 7-10). If you would benefit from a powered unit when going long distances, such as to work, school, or shopping, a removable power unit might be the answer. The power system attaches to your manual wheelchair and can be removed when not in use. **Manufacturers:** 86 (illustrated), 375. For further information and a demonstration, contact a local durable medical equipment supplier.

Portable ramps are for traveling and ascending a few steps (Figure 7-11). A solid, portable ramp is preferable if others must push your chair, because it provides a surface on which the helper can walk. Cost is $125 and up from self-help and specialized mail-order firms. **Manufacturers** include: 163, 168, 186, 316. **Sources:** 120, 125, 163, 168, 186, 261.

If you expect to push yourself up and down, the incline of the ramp should adhere to the following guidelines: The rule is 12" in length for every inch of rise. A ramp for two steps with a rise of 7" each (a total of 14") should be 14 feet long for you to wheel yourself comfortably and safely up and down. To save space, it may be built with a turn and have a platform for resting. The ramp must have railings and a non-skid surface. Consult a local contractor to build a ramp to suit your needs. The cost of a ramp is tax deductible as a medical expense.

If you have strong upper extremities or someone available to help you, a ramp may be designed so that half of it swivels to one side on Teflon glides when not in use.

If you live in a multi-story home and want to take advantage of the full living space, a variety of wheelchair and stair lifts are available to transport you from one level to another. Contact manufacturers for local distributors and cost. **Sources:** 2, 109, 140, 195, 286. See also Chapter 25. You may also install automatic or electric door openers to make handling your wheelchair more streamlined. **Sources:** 295, 315.

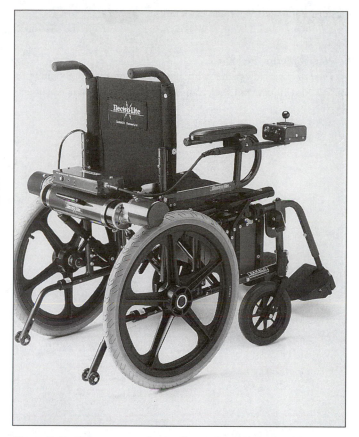

Figure 7-10. This power unit attaches to a manual wheelchair. (Photo courtesy of Damaco, Freedom on Wheels, Inc., Chatsworth, CA.)

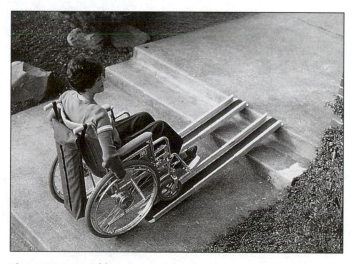

Figure 7-11. Portable ramps are for traveling and ascending a few steps. (Photo courtesy of Home Care Products, Inc., Kent, WA.)

GOING FURTHER

Addresses are listed in the Appendices.

PUBLICATIONS

Accent on Living. Periodical. **Source:** 3
Building Design Requirements for the Physically Handicapped.

Eastern Paralyzed Veterans Association.

Choosing and Using a Wheelchair. $.40 from the National Easter Seal Society.

New Mobility. Periodical.

Pushin' On. Newsletter with articles of interest to people with spinal cord injury and their families. Gives additional resources.

Free from Independent Living Research Utilization Project in *Prevention & Treatment of Secondary Complications of SCI.*

Ramps. Madison, WI: Access to Independence. **Source:** 4.

Salmen, J. P. S. (1988). *The DoAble ReNewable Home.* Free from the American Association of Retired Persons.

Spinal Network. Periodical.

If You Have Chronic Obstructive Pulmonary Disease

If you have chronic obstructive pulmonary disease (COPD), it is imperative that you respect your limits and follow a careful plan to eliminate overexertion and reduce stress. The less you do, however, the worse your condition will become. By pacing yourself and avoiding situations that increase your respiratory problems, you can have a productive life and do much that you desire. See Chapter 10 for some suggestions.

Your get-up-and-go depends on factors like the weather, air quality, the previous day's activities, and diet. Try not to take on more work than you can handle: If you do too much one day, you will pay the next.

Here are some helpful ideas:

- Organize your workplace so you can sit and reach everything you need without bending or lifting. A pair of reaching tongs can be helpful. See Chapter 2.
- If you use oxygen, for safety, you should replace your gas oven with an electric one. A microwave oven is an excellent choice because it does not produce the heat of a conventional oven. It usually has shorter cooking times, and the lightweight cooking utensils require less energy to lift.
- Check family service magazines and cookbooks for easy-to-prepare one-dish meals that can be made ahead of time. On your energetic days, bake and freeze meals for a day when you do not feel as well.
- Plan meals when you feel at your best and can take the time to ensure that they are nutritionally balanced.
- Try eating six smaller meals rather than three large meals a day. Smaller meals are easier to digest.
- Convenience foods save time and energy, but they often have high sugar and salt content.
- Keep on hand nutritious, natural, low-sugar, low-sodium "fast" foods like fruit, nonfat yogurt, low-fat ice cream, salt-free tuna, whole-grain bread, fruit juice, low-fat cheese, low-fat milk, and unsweetened cereals.
- Discuss diet planning with a registered dietitian recommended by your physician or hospital. Some foods are gas-forming and can bloat your stomach, making breathing difficult. If you are taking diuretics, you may need to eat more potassium-rich foods. If constipation is a problem, ask about increasing fiber or liquids. Being overweight adds to the burden of breathing, so request a safe weight-reduction program. A personal diet plan may be developed to overcome problems of fatigue, shortness of breath, difficulty swallowing, even poor appetite.
- If your stomach is upset, talk with your physician about your medication. Taking medication an hour ahead of meals may eliminate the upset. Never change your medication schedule without your physician's approval.
- Drink plenty of fruit juice and water. This is important to thin mucus, help prevent infection, and avoid constipation caused by inactivity.
- Be sure you have a well-ventilated work area while preparing foods. Use the exhaust fan when cooking at the range. Be sure you have plenty of fresh air.
- Use a small portable fan when you cook to keep air moving and blow away irritating odors.
- Avoid all aerosol spray products.
- Wear loose, comfortable clothing, but avoid long sleeves or folds that could catch fire.
- Slide, do not lift; wheel loads, do not carry them. Use a cart to pick up and drop off things that need to be put away around your house. Keep a cart on each floor of your home. See Chapter 16.
- Enlist help for kitchen cleanup. Let dishes air dry.
- Store equipment so you don't have to bend. Keep the most frequently used pans on the range. Instead of putting dishes away, reset the table for the next meal.
- Shop on days when the weather suits you and when a friend is available to carry the bags. Pick off-hours and weekdays to do your shopping. If you have an oxygen pack, place it in the cart while you shop. If shopping is too stressful, take the time at home to decide exactly what you need, then pay to have your groceries delivered. Many communities have volunteers will-

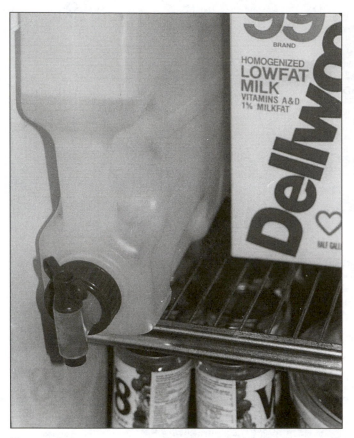

Figure 8-1. A narrow, space-saving beverage container keeps cool water or fruit juices right at hand and dispenses as much as you want from the dripless spout. (Photo by J.K.)

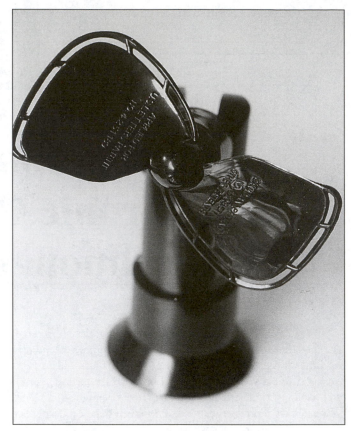

Figure 8-2. A lightweight, clip-on or battery-powered fan may be carried with you for where and when needed. (Caframo Ltd., Wiarton, ON, Canada. Photo by J.K.)

ing to help; call your church or Visiting Nurse Association.

- For light cleanup, use a small hand vacuum, but do not empty it yourself. If dusting, wear a mask. Dampen paper towels with water or lemon oil, then use them to dust.
- Let family members or friends help carry heavy items, especially up the stairs. If you must carry something, lift it while exhaling through pursed lips, rest, and then inhale through your nose. Repeat as necessary.
- If you are using oxygen, check out portable units that allow you to carry on favorite activities, from walking and swimming to traveling.
- If you feel you are not doing as well as you might, talk with your physician about programs that teach a person with COPD to control respiratory distress through exercise training, breathing techniques, stress management, and proper diet.
- Consider joining a support group, such as the Better Breathers. For location, call the American Lung Association, your hospital, or Visiting Nurse Association.

A narrow, space-saving beverage container keeps cool water or fruit juices right at hand and dispenses as much as you want from the dripless spout (Figure 8-1). The 2½" wide plastic jug fits against the refrigerator wall and holds one gallon. Cost is $7 and up from housewares stores and mail-order firms. **Sources:** 49, 171, 173, 369, 378, 387, 407.

Water filter pitchers and dispensers hold cooled water conve-

nient and ready. **Manufacturers:** 46, 388. Cost is about $15 and up from department stores.

Keeping air circulating will help you breathe easier, especially when the weather is humid or hot. Air conditioning may be indicated if you live in a humid, hot climate. Although most air conditioners are not portable, there are models that may be rolled from room to room. **Sources:** 87, 167. If you only require a fan to keep air moving, they are available from units that install on the ceiling to fans that fit double hung, slider, and casement windows, and portable units that stand on the floor or sit on a table. Some window fans are designed with speed settings as well as thermostatic controls to keep temperature at the desired level and a button to change air flow from intake to output. Vortex-design fans circulate air like a ceiling fan, rather than blowing in just one direction. Fan **manufacturers:** 305, 412. Cost ranges from $12 to more than $100 from department stores and mail-order firms. **Sources:** 50, 71, 87, 167, 176, 194, 319, 359, 369, 374, 407.

A lightweight, clip-on or battery-powered fan may be carried with you for where and when needed (Figure 8-2). Some models have adjustable stands. You may find it helpful to take a battery-powered unit for use outside your home, as in a warm car or office. **Manufacturer:** 55. Cost is $10 and up from housewares stores and mail-order firms. Unit shown is about $17. **Sources:** 49, 369. Other **sources:** small portable fans—71, 410; battery-powered—174, 211.

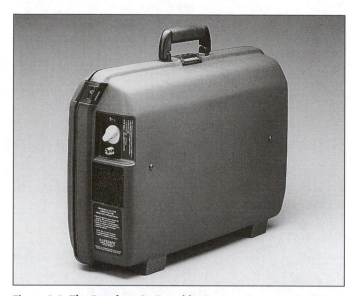

Figure 8-3. The Freedom O$_2$ Portable Oxygen Concentrator is packed as a suitcase, ready to travel. (Photo courtesy of Lifecare® International, Inc., Westminster, CO.)

Air filtration systems help clean air within your home of pollen, dust, bacteria, molds, yeast, and odors, and may be beneficial, especially if you use oxygen only part of the time. Discuss the best type of unit with your physician and respiratory therapist. **Manufacturers** include 288. **Sources:** 167, 194, 374. Filters that electrostatically clean the air may also be added to your furnace system. Consult your fuel contractor. Cost is about $60 and up. **Source:** 194.

New equipment has evolved that allows more independence when using respiratory aids. Lightweight canisters with shoulder holsters, wheeled tank holders that accompany you on a walk, and

smaller concentrators add up to greater freedom and involvement with life. The Freedom O$_2$ Portable Oxygen Concentrator is packed as a suitcase, ready to travel (Figure 8-3). At home or during domestic travel, it delivers 3 liters per minute flow from any 110V electrical outlet. **Source:** 237.

GOING FURTHER

Addresses are listed in the Appendices.

PUBLICATIONS

American Academy of Allergy and Immunology. Physician referrals and pollen information.

American Allergy Association. Information for people with food and chemical allergies.

American Lung Association. Publications, including the free, excellent *Help Yourself to Better Breathing*. Information, referrals, and support groups, including Better Breathing clubs.

Asthma and Allergy Foundation of America. Information, referrals for support groups, publications, equipment.

Haas, F., & Haas, S. (1990). *The Chronic Bronchitis and Emphysema Handbook*. New York: Wiley. **Source:** 426.

Moser, K. A., Archibald, C., et al. (1991). *Shortness of Breath: A Guide to Better Living and Breathing* (rev. ed.). St. Louis, MO: Mosby Year Book Pub. **Source:** 277B.

National Institute of Allergy and Infectious Disease. Information, publications.

National Jewish Center for Immunology and Respiratory Medicine. Referrals to local physicians.

Shayevitz, M. B., & Shayevitz, B. (1991). *Living Well with Chronic Asthma, Bronchitis, and Emphysema: A Complete Guide to Coping with Chronic Lung Disease*. Des Moines, IA: Consumer Reports® Books. **Source:** 75B.

If You Have Partial Loss of Vision or Are Blind

Eleven million Americans have partial or complete vision loss. This may be congenital or acquired. Once you reach age 65, visual losses related to age usually become more evident. Preventing damage and carefully monitoring any problems, including glaucoma and other diseases (such as diabetes) that might affect your eyes, are vital to maintaining your vision. An annual eye examination is the first step toward preserving your sight.

Adequate lighting is important. For each decade we age, the amount of light we need in order to see as well as we did 10 years earlier doubles! Ask your physician about high-intensity lights for close-up work.

If vision loss is new to you, contact the American Foundation for the Blind, your state Society for the Blind, the National Federation of the Blind, the National Society to Prevent Blindness, the National Association for the Visually Handicapped, or the U.S. Department of Agriculture Home Economics Extension Service for information on where to find a rehabilitation or training course. (Addresses in the Appendices.) Some programs send an individual to your home to show you how to manage daily activities with vision loss. Techniques include mobility training, space orientation, organization of your home, and use of other senses to compensate for lack of sight. Certain organizations provide funds for equipment and offer family counseling. It is important that your family understand what you are going through and offer help only if and when you desire it.

LOW VISION AIDS

If you have difficulty seeing but are not blind, lamps, large-print timers, broad-tip pens, digital watches, and other aids may help you perform daily tasks. This includes jobs you can no longer do wearing conventional glasses. Your physician can direct you to a low-vision service, an occupational therapist specializing in this area, or another specialist for testing and training.

Depending on the cause of your vision loss, a professional trained in low-vision techniques can teach you how to use a microscope for close work or a telescope for long-distance tasks, such as reading signs or identifying objects and people.

Hand-held magnifying glasses are available in many styles and strengths through opticians, department stores, and mail-order firms (Figure 9-1). They are helpful for reading small type on recipes, labels, and appliance controls. Some magnifiers have straps attached, so they can be worn around the neck to keep your hands free for preparing meals or doing needlework. Some magnifiers may be illuminated by either batteries or house current. **Manufacturer:** 37. Cost is $20 and up. Non-illuminating magnifiers cost $7 and up from optical suppliers, stationery stores, and mail-order firms. **Sources:** 50, 100, 120, 167, 169, 196, 240, 247, 258, 261, 290, 408.

An illuminated magnifier lamp on an adjustable base focuses light where you need it (Figure 9-2). It may be clamped in place or permanently mounted. The flexible arm covers a radius of 39". A lens cover reduces glare. The lamp shown magnifies 175%; other units let you add extra magnification. **Manufacturers:** 90, 251. Cost ranges from $30 to $200 or more from department and stationery stores or self-help and mail-order firms. **Sources:** 50, 87, 167, 196, 240, 247, 258, 261.

HANDLING RECIPES

Some basic and popular cookbooks are available in large-print and Braille editions or on audiotape. Cost is about $12 each and up. **Sources:** 23, 196, 240, 247, 261. The National Library Services for the Blind and Physically Handicapped distributes talking books, including cookbooks. This free library service is available if you are blind, unable to read printed material, or physically cannot handle a book. Ask your doctor, nurse, or therapist to send a form to the state division of your library.

Your favorite recipes can be transcribed onto audiotape by a friend, family member, 4-H member, Girl Scout, or Boy Scout (Figure 9-3). Ask the person to read slowly, pausing so that you can follow the steps as you later fix meals using your tape recorder.

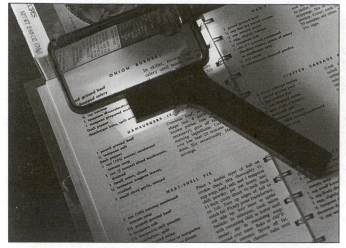

Figure 9-1. Hand-held magnifying glasses are available in many styles and strengths through opticians, department stores, and mail-order firms. (Photo by J.K.)

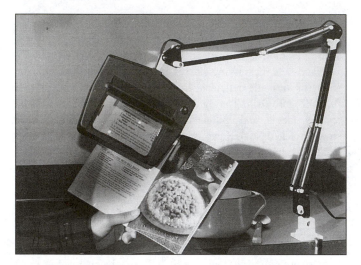

Figure 9-2. An illuminated magnifier lamp on an adjustable base focuses light where you need it. (Photo by J.K.)

A 7½" x 11 ¾" plastic magnifying sheet fits over a cookbook to enlarge the entire page and may be slipped inside when not in use. Support it about three to 4 inches above the page for enlargement up to four times. Cost is about $3 from variety stores and mail-order firms. **Sources:** 100, 175, 196, 270.

A magnifying recipe box increases print up to three times its size (Figure 9-4). The oversized, hand-crafted wood box holds more than 900 3" x 5" index cards. For information, contact **manufacturer:** 74. Cost is about $40 from gourmet stores and mail-order firms.

KITCHEN PLANNING

Use contrasting colors to define areas and equipment in your kitchen and home. Select solid colors rather than patterns. Brightly colored bowls contrast with a white counter, and light placemats are easier to see on a dark table top. Bright dishes make your food more visible and more appealing.

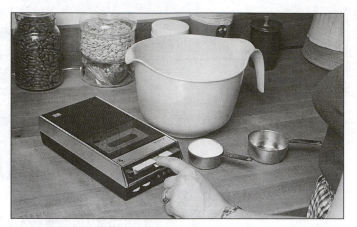

Figure 9-3. Your favorite recipes can be transcribed onto audio-tape by a friend, family member, 4-H member, Girl Scout, or Boy Scout. (Photo by J.K.)

Touch is your most vital sense; if you have a visual loss you must be in close physical contact with your surroundings. Your kitchen should be organized to ensure your safety and ease. Here are some helpful tips:

- Eliminate obstacles that you may bump into while walking.
- Do not use scatter rugs.
- Put a flat-edged rubber mat on the floor by your sink to help prevent slipping should water splash on the floor.
- Keep every utensil in a specific place; return tools to their places immediately after using them. Dividers keep items in drawers organized.
- Cover your stored knife blades. A countertop block or wall knife storage unit is safer than an in-drawer knife holder.
- Eliminate any utensils you do not use. They clutter drawers and may even be dangerous.
- Install a slightly raised front counter edge to prevent things from rolling onto the floor.
- Remove upper cabinet doors, or teach everyone in the family always to close them to prevent banging your head. If you are remodeling, install sliding doors, rather than swinging ones, on all cabinets.
- Use pullout shelves and drawers or lazy Susans to reduce the need to reach into the backs of cabinets. In-cabinet organizers let you pick up one item without moving others. Additional ideas and sources are given in Chapter 14.
- An electric range is safer than gas. A microwave is recommended.

TIMERS

A timer with raised numbers, tape, or glue-dot markings helps you time recipes. You may also use a low-vision or Braille watch. Cost is $15 and up from department stores and self-help firms. **Sources**: 120, 196, 240, 247, 261.

If you have partial loss of vision, a big timer with ½" or larger numbers may help (Figure 9-5). Cost is about $18 from department stores and self-help firms for this and other timers with raised numbers or marks. Most are spring-wound and have an adjustable bell duration. **Sources:** 120, 196, 240, 247, 261.

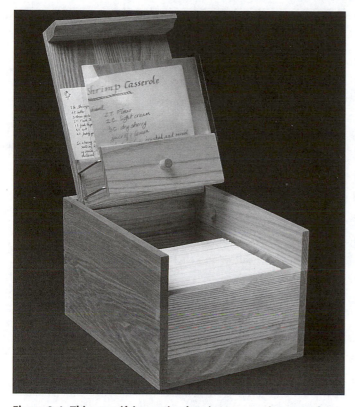

Figure 9-4. This magnifying recipe box increases print up to three times its size. (Photo courtesy of Concept Design, Inc., Saco, ME.)

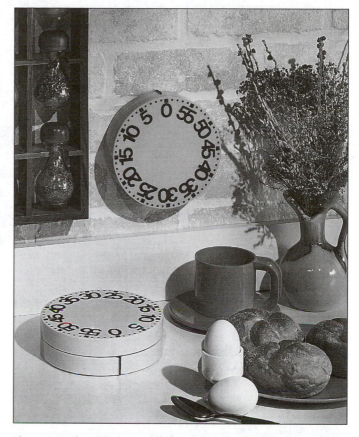

Figure 9-5. If you have partial loss of vision, a big timer with ½″ or larger numbers may help.

A tactile meat thermometer has large dots that register the temperature at 20° intervals from 120° to 200°. Cost is about $15 from self-help firms. **Source:** 247. A talking clock tells the time at the touch of a button. **Manufacturer:** 357. Cost is $25 and up from department stores and self-help firms. **Sources:** 120, 196, 240, 247, 290, 408.

LABELING

To keep track of your food inventory, store packaged foods in alphabetical order, or use another system that works for you. Many foods can be recognized by their smell, the sounds they make when shaken, or their weight. Rice is heavier than soap; corn oil sounds and feels different from vinegar when shaken. Spices and herbs have specific aromas.

If your vision is poor, make your own labels with wide white tape and a broad-tipped dark marker. If you have severe loss of vision, Braille marking kits and pressure-sensitive magnetic recording tape are available from self-help firms. **Sources:** 196, 240, 261.

MEASURING

The palm of your hand is the best small measuring device for dry ingredients, such as seasonings. With a little experience you can gauge how much is needed for all but the most critical measurements, such as baking powder.

A measuring spoon that lies flat on the counter is best for mea-suring small amounts of ingredients (Figure 9-6). Four different sized spoons are at both ends.

For large amounts, select measuring utensils with large numbers if you have partial loss of vision. Graduated measuring cups, which you can fill level to the top, are easy to use, even if you have complete loss of vision. For more tips on measuring, see Chapter 28.

A liquid-measuring cup with outside raised measurement indicators at every ¼ and ⅓ of a cup allows you to "feel" the correct amount (Figure 9-7). Position the tip of your thumb on the outside of the cup at the desired indicator and your index finger opposite it on the inside where you want the liquid to come. Stop pouring the liquid you are measuring when it touches your finger. Cost is about $1.50 from housewares stores. **Manufacturer:** 33.

A liquid level indicator is an electronic device that hangs over the lip of a cup, glass, or other container. It buzzes and vibrates when the liquid nears the top. Uses a 9V battery. Cost is about $14 from self-help firms. **Sources:** 196, 240, 261.

CUTTING

A reversible, low-vision cutting board is white on one side and black on the other to provide contrast with food being cut. A 9″ x 15″ plastic board is dishwasher safe. Cost is $20. **Sources:** 240, 261.

To protect your fingers when cutting, place the knife blade on the food to be cut, then check the thickness with the index finger

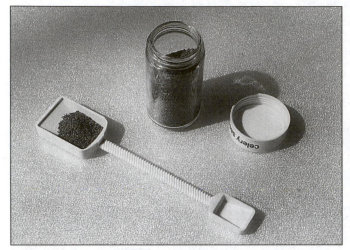

Figure 9-6. A measuring spoon that lies flat on the counter is best for measuring small amounts of ingredients. (Photo by J.K.)

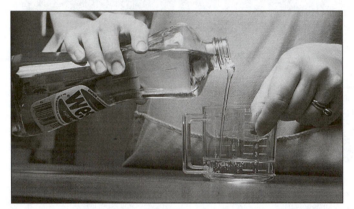

Figure 9-7. A liquid-measuring cup with outside raised measurement indicators at every ¼ and ⅓ of a cup allows you to "feel" the correct amount. (Photo courtesy of the O.T. Dept., Howard A. Rusk Institute of Rehabilitation Medicine.)

of your other hand. Remove hand, and if necessary stabilize food with a fork or use an adapted cutting board with holding nails.

A knife with a guide lets you select the thickness of the slice from ⅛" to ½" (Figure 9-8). The guide rests against the outer edge of the food, ensuring even slices as the serrated blade cuts. You determine the width of the slice by adjusting the space between the top of the knife and the guide edge. They are available in right- or left-handed models. **Manufacturers:** 162 (for bread); 278 (for general slicing). Cost is $18 and up for right- or left-handed models, from mail-order and self-help firms. Bread and bagel slicing aids are also described in Chapter 28. **Sources:** 196, 240, 247; for bread—162, 242, 270.

COOKING AND APPLIANCES

Some manufacturers provide aids, such as Braille overlays or controls, for their appliances. Instruction manuals in Braille, in large type, and on audiotape are available from Whirlpool Corporation. General Electric offers free Braille controls for many of their appliances. **Sources:** 156, 424. Sandpaper or brightly col-

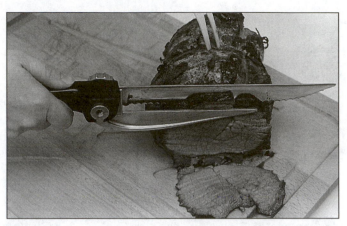

Figure 9-8. This knife with a guide lets you select the thickness of the slice from ⅛" to ½". (Photo courtesy of the O.T. Dept., Howard A. Rusk Institute of Rehabilitation Medicine.)

ored tape applied to the "off" positions on temperature controls assures you that an appliance is completely turned off. If you have partial loss of vision and find it difficult to match controls with burners on your stove, use different colors of tape or grades of sandpaper to code each burner with its control knob. Apply raised glue dots or symbols to help adjust controls on the back of a stove. If you have a hood over your range, trim the edge with a band of brightly colored tape to avoid accidentally hitting it.

Microwave cooking is safer than stove-top cooking. The ease of timing and operation, the lightweight dishes, and the lack of coils or flames make this the safest choice for cooking without looking.

Install a smoke alarm. Be sure to change the battery twice a year, when daylight savings time begins and ends. A talking smoke alarm is about $56 from self-help firms. **Source:** 247.

Use padded pot holders of fire-retardant materials. **Manufacturer:** 255. They are available through housewares and hardware stores as well as mail-order firms. **Source:** 256. Select pans with insulated handles and baking pans with handles for a surer grip. Additional safety tips are given in Chapter 12.

OTHER HELPFUL AIDS

A check-writing guide is a plastic template for filling in the information on a standard check. Cost is about $1 from self-help firms. **Sources:** 196, 240. Your bank can order large-print checks for you.

A telephone with an enlarged dial costs $40 and up from telephone stores and mail-order firms. **Sources:** 120, 177, 196, 240, 325.

An enlarged telephone dial fits over a rotary telephone dial. Cost is about $2 from mail-order and self-help firms. A version for touch-tone telephones costs $8 and up from mail-order and self-help firms. **Sources:** 120, 196, 240, 261.

A thermostat for people with loss of vision has raised numbers; it clicks for easy setting and temperature checking. **Manufacturers:** 188, 381. Cost is about $50. **Sources:** 196, 240.

Sound-activated lights for indoor and outdoor use eliminate groping in the dark for the switch. **Sources:** 196, 247.

Many communities have free radio reading services that broadcast the daily newspaper, including grocery and classified ads, over special radio frequencies. To find out if your town offers this service, call the Association of Radio Reading Services listed in the Appendix.

GOING FURTHER

Addresses are listed in the Appendices.

PUBLICATIONS

Aging and Vision: Making the Most of Impaired Vision. (1987). New York: American Foundation for the Blind with the American Association of Retired Persons. Large-print format; discusses causes of vision loss, using color contrast, devices for independence, travel, and communicating. **Source:** 22.

Carroll, T. J. (1961). *Blindness: What It Is, What It Does and How to Live With It* (rev. ed.). New York: Little Brown. Distributed by the American Foundation for the Blind, New York, 1987. Classic book on how blindness affects self-perception and social interaction, what can be done to restore basic skills and independence. For individuals, families, and trainers. **Source:** 22.

Dickman, I. R. (1983). *Making Life More Liveable.* New York: American Foundation for the Blind. $9.95. **Source:** 22.

Directory of Services for Blind and Visually Impaired Persons in the United States (23rd ed.). New York: American Foundation for the Blind. **Source:** 22.

List of Large Print Cookbooks. Available from the National Association for Visually Handicapped. **Source:** 284.

Reading Materials in Large Print. National Library Services for the Blind and Physically Handicapped.

Ringgold, N. P. (1991). *Out of the Corner of My Eye: Living with Vision Loss in Later Life.* New York: American Foundation for the Blind. Large print, $22.95; cassette, $22.95.

Seeing Clearly. Large-print newsletter, published at irregular intervals, with information of interest to people with partial vision. Free from the National Association for Visually Handicapped. **Source:** 284.

CHAPTER

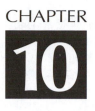

Conserving Energy and Handling Stress

The fatigue caused by a disability or aging can make you feel that a task is not worth the effort. But with a little organizing and a new perspective on the job, you can accomplish a lot. The trick is to eliminate non-essential chores and to focus on those that are most important to you and your health.

Before starting an activity, ask yourself these questions: Is this job necessary? If so, when should it be done? Who should do it? If I should do it, what is the best way to accomplish it?

As you go through your daily routines, look at the way you are working. Is your posture correct? Are your shoes comfortable? Does your chair offer proper support? Is your work surface the right height? Sometimes slight adjustments can produce big benefits.

Changing your work habits takes serious commitment and planning. It includes looking at your nutritional needs and—believe it or not—adding exercise to your schedule. Lack of specific nutrients can make you feel tired and irritable. Physical activity increases energy.

Help is available through local organizations. With your physician's recommendations, contact one or more of the following agencies or services: Visiting Nurse Association, an occupational or physical therapist, and support groups formed to handle your problem.

You will find more ideas for conserving energy throughout this book as well as in family service magazines and state university publications.

HOW TO PLAN YOUR TIME

By planning your activities in advance, you will accomplish more with greater efficiency while conserving your energy. Here is one plan for constructing a schedule that allows you to do less and enjoy it more.

- List your routines for each day of the week. Include chores you have to do, as well as recreational activities you would like to do.
- Cross out the jobs that are not essential, and delegate other jobs

to family members or home health workers. Discuss this reassignment of chores with your family, explaining the advantages they will gain from a more rested, happier you.

- Make a chart for each day of the week, with a box for each hour of the day. Write your chores and plans in the boxes. Slot your most essential jobs into the hours when your energy is at its peak. Save mindless tasks, like emptying the dishwasher, for low energy times. Keep some time boxes empty for unplanned leisure time. Allow 10 to 15 minutes for rest after each major task.
- Follow the plan for one week. Make note of where it did or did not work. Rethink and rearrange for the next week, allowing more rest or recreation as needed.

HANDLING STRESS

Stress affects everyone at one time or another. Stress can be useful when it motivates you to get a job done; it can be harmful when it keeps you from doing what you desire.

The effects of many diseases, such as arthritis, multiple sclerosis, chronic fatigue syndrome, Parkinson's, and heart disease, may be increased by stress. Learning ways to reduce tension can help you feel better. Here are some ideas to get started:

- Adjust your standards to meet your physical abilities.
- Sit down and worry for 5 minutes. Write down what is bothering you, then get back to the job at hand.
- Do not let your emotions affect your eating or sleeping habits. Good nutrition helps you overcome stress by supplying energy. Sleep and exercise are also important to your total well-being. If you are having problems eating or sleeping, talk with your doctor, nurse, or therapist. They can also provide an exercise plan to fit your abilities.
- Join a support group related to your problem or your disability. Churches, hospitals, and other organizations sponsor support groups on a vast array of topics. Check your community newspaper and telephone book. Call the social service department of the nearest hospital or your Visiting Nurse Association

for details. Information on support groups for people with chronic fatigue syndrome may be obtained through the Chronic Fatigue Immune Dysfunction Syndrome Society, the Chronic Fatigue and Immune Dysfunction Syndrome Association, and the National Chronic Fatigue Syndrome Society. Addresses are given under Agencies and Organizations in the Appendices.

GOING FURTHER

Addresses are listed in the Appendices.

PUBLICATIONS

Coleman, D., & Gurin, J. (1993). *Mind/Body Medicine: How to Use Your Mind for Better Health*. Yonkers, NY: Consumer Reports® Books. Discusses connection between stress and disease; examines approaches such as biofeedback, meditation, and psychotherapy; explores mind's role in specific diseases; and shows consumers how to become an active patient working with your health care practitioners. **Source:** 75B.

Davis, M., Escheman, E. R., & McKay, M. (1995). *The Relaxation and Stress Reduction Workbook*. Oakland, CA: New Harbinger, Ten Speed Press. Suggested exercises, self-assessment surveys, checklists, and fill-in-the-blanks. **Source:** 286B.

Feiden, K. (1990). *Hope and Help for Chronic Fatigue Syndrome*. New York: Simon & Schuster. Practical approach to overcoming CFS, including recognition of early symptoms, selection of a physician sensitive to your needs, treatment and medications, diet and exercise programs, dealing with the emotional impact, and additional resources. **Source:** 364B.

Mason, L. J. (1985). *Guide to Stress Reduction*. Berkeley, CA: Celestial Arts. Gives suggestions for relieving specific problems, including back pain, arthritis, chronic pain, headaches, and hypertension. Discusses types of stress reduction programs, including relaxation techniques. **Source:** 389B.

Mason, L. J. (1988). *Stress Passages: Surviving Life's Transitions Gracefully*. Berkeley, CA: Celestial Arts, Ten Speed Press, Berkeley. Relates stress to transitions in life; provides specific suggestions for handling the changes. **Source:** 389B.

Pacing Yourself. Bloomington, IL: Accent Books and Products. $3.95. **Source:** 3.

Also see Going Further in Chapter 11.

Tips for Aging Homemakers and Those Who Live Alone

It is no longer unusual to find an 83-year-old woman hiking in Nepal or an octogenarian teaching with the Peace Corps and choosing not to retire. As Alex Comfort writes in his book *A Good Age*, "Old people are simply young people who have been around a long time."

Your attitude is most important, even though your lifestyle or circumstances may be changing. You have a wealth of experience to draw on; use this wisdom to stay involved in your home, in useful paid or volunteer work, in your community, and in your personal relationships.

Although we tend to blame aging for our stiff joints, weak muscles, and tendency to huff and puff, the culprit is often inactivity. Regular exercise has been proven to not only extend our lifespan, but to reduce physical complaints and improve problem-solving ability, short-term memory, and concentration. Fear of falling, many seniors say, is their greatest fear. The best way to overcome this is to continue exercising, walking, even add some Tai Chi. This ancient Chinese gentle exercise routine can reduce the risk of falling and fractures by 47%!

Aging does bring on gradual physiological changes. Vision becomes less sharp, and some discrimination in hearing is lost. However, these can be overcome through safety precautions and technological aids. If you are experiencing visual problems and worry that you cannot afford treatment, contact the National Eye Care Project, which provides free eye care. Also, see the suggestions in Chapter 9.

Proper nutrition is essential for you now, just as it was when you were a youngster. Maintain your energy by eating a varied and balanced diet every day. Weight control, lower salt intake, increased fibrous foods, and lower fat consumption all help keep your body healthier. As we age, we need to consume fewer calories and provide high levels of vitamins C and D through diet. Ask your physician if you should also take Vitamin E.

Do not forget the benefits of fruits and vegetables. If you enjoy cooking in large amounts, make your favorite dishes, seal individual servings in plastic bags or small containers, then freeze for future use. See Chapter 15. Grow a pot or two of herbs on your window sill; they will help reduce salt intake by adding flavor and excitement to your meals.

Advances in food processing have put new products on pantry shelves. Rather than curb culinary creativity, convenience foods create more excitement in your meals. Look for foods in single- and double-portion packages. See also Chapter 23.

Everyone ages differently, and we each have our own concerns. You will find tips and techniques applicable to your own needs throughout this book.

SAFETY

Safety awareness becomes increasingly crucial as we age. If your balance is not always stable or your vision not as sharp, take extra precautions to avoid accidents.

- Use contrasting colors, light against dark, to help objects stand out. See the Reversible Cutting Board, Chapter 9.
- Add non-skid tape in white or bright colors to the edges of steps. This is especially important if you have loss of depth perception due to diminished eyesight, a stroke, or other factors.
- Mark your oven burners and their controls with strips of colored tape. Use a different color tape for each burner/control pair. Trim the edge of the range hood with a strip of bright yellow or red tape so you do not hit your head.
- Increase interior lighting to help you see more clearly. Interior battery-powered lights may be added to closets and cabinets. Cost is about $5 each and up from hardware stores and mail-order firms. **Sources:** 171, 173, 185, 270, 378.
- Eliminate all scatter rugs. Select light-colored carpeting that is dense, with a low pile, and no patterns.
- If you need help to install a smoke detector, replace electrical cords, repair unsteady steps, or add a railing, call your town hall, Office of the Aging, church, or Visiting Nurse Association. Community-supported home safety programs and free or low-cost chore services are available to help older citizens remain safe and independent at home.
- Wear suitable clothes while working in the kitchen and around

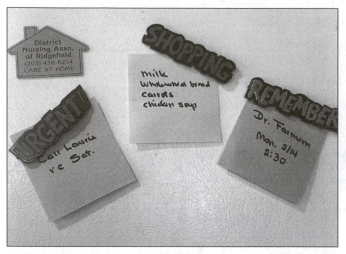

Figure 11-1. Refrigerator magnets with important notes attached are an excellent memory aid. (Photo by J.K.)

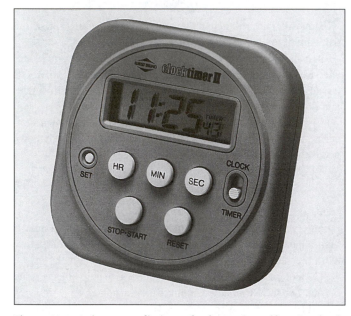

Figure 11-2. A timer can eliminate the frustration of burning food. (Photo courtesy of the West Bend Company®, West Bend, IL.)

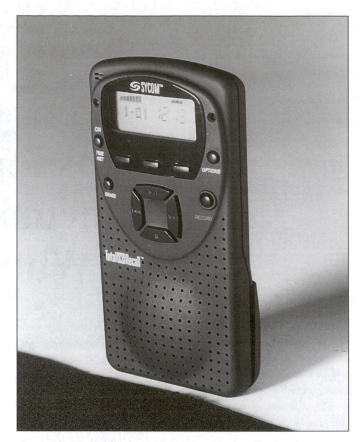

Figure 11-3. A small, electronic memo minder allows you to record immediately things you want to remember. (Photo courtesy of Hello Direct®, San Jose, CA.)

the house. Sturdy, well-fitting shoes reduce fatigue, improve posture, and provide more stable balance. Wear fitted or short sleeves when cooking. Long, loose sleeves can easily catch fire if you reach for a pan at the back of the range. Do not light a gas oven while wearing a flammable nightgown.

- Keep the range top clear of extraneous items.
- Stay in the kitchen while cooking on the stove.
- Turn off appliances immediately after use. Keep them clean and in good condition. Frayed cords should be replaced.
- Place a rubber mat in front of the sink to prevent slips, and wipe up all spills immediately. See Chapter 12.

MEMORY AIDS

Having a single place to list your scheduled appointments, hang your keys, or put your glasses reduces frustration. A large calendar filled in with events keeps you on schedule.

You may purchase an "everlasting" calendar to mount on your refrigerator through a stationery store or mail-order firm. Cost is about $13. **Source:** 364.

A pegboard with hooks and pockets puts everything within reach. A glasses cord or brooch holder places your extra eyes at your fingertips.

Refrigerator magnets with important notes attached are an excellent memory aid (Figure 11-1).

A timer can eliminate the frustration of burning food (Figure 11-2). Digital models are easy to read. **Manufacturers:** 131, 273, 422. Cost is about $15 and up from housewares stores and mail-order firms. **Sources:** 71, 240, 242, 427, 431. See Chapter 9.

A small, electronic memo minder allows you to record immediately things you want to remember, rather than finding a pencil and writing them down (Figure 11-3). Units the size of a small calculator or built into a talking watch cost about $15 and up from stationery, mail-order, and self-help firms. **Sources:** 167, 177.

If leaving a pan on the range top is a recurring problem, you might consider a microwave oven, which shuts off at a preset time. See Chapter 20.

If you have trouble remembering when and how to take your medicine, a timing device could be helpful. A medication holder is especially helpful when you have multiple medications (Figure 11-4). It notes the days of the week and times of the day you should take your pills. **Manufacturers:** 31, 174. Cost is about $9 and up

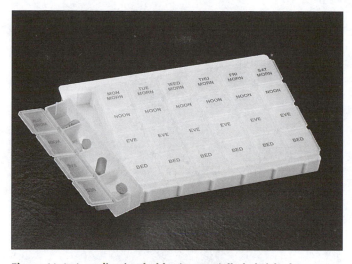

Figure 11-4. A medication holder is especially helpful when you have multiple medications. (Photo courtesy of Health Enterprises® Inc., North Attleboro, MA.)

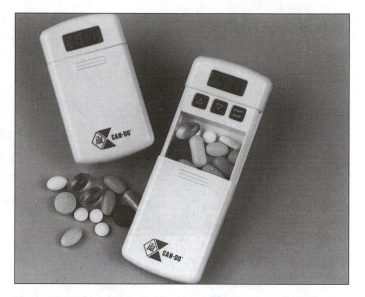

Figure 11-5. This pocket-sized, electronic pill box reminder has a digital timer that buzzes when it is time to take medicine. (Photo courtesy of Independent Living Aids, Inc., Plainview, NY.)

from pharmacies, self-help and mail-order firms, or ask your Visiting Nurse Association. **Sources:** 50, 100, 240, 261, 270, 378.

A pocket-sized, electronic pill box reminder has a digital timer that buzzes when it is time to take medicine (Figure 11-5). Once the alarm has sounded, it automatically resets itself, counting down from the previous time, and is compact for carrying. Cost is about $19 from pharmacies and mail-order firms. **Sources:** 50, 196, 240, 247, 261, 410.

A pill bottle opener, which pries up those frustrating child-proof tops, is about $1.50 from pharmacies and mail-order firms. **Source:** 270. You can also ask your pharmacist for easy-to-open bottles if there are no children in your home. Just keep them out of reach when grandchildren arrive.

Before crushing or splitting any pill, consult your physician or nurse. Many pills are timed-release or coated so that they do not dissolve until they reach the intestines; crushing them could result in stomach upset. Ask your doctor about alternative forms of your medication, such as gelatin-coated capsules or liquid.

A night light is an aid to orientation when waking during the night. Some turn on automatically when daylight fades; others turn on only when motion is sensed. One type, called the Limelite™, never has to have the bulb replaced and uses less than $.02 of electricity a year. The slim design fits flush against a wall. **Manufacturer:** 252B. Cost is about $9 each from house-wares stores and mail-order firms. **Sources** for Limelite™: 50, 194, 364, 407.

If getting out of the house is difficult, check with your town hall or office of aging about meals-on-wheels (Figure 11-6). Volunteers deliver hot meals on a regular basis, bringing good nutrition as well as friendship. You pay a weekly or monthly fee based on the number of meals you order.

TIPS IF YOU HAVE HEARING LOSS

Loss of hearing affects more than 16 million people in the U.S. A free check-up for hearing loss is offered by telephone. Call 1-

800-222-EARS between 9 A.M. and 6 P.M. E.S.T. An operator will explain the procedure, answer your questions, and give you a local telephone number for a recorded hearing test. After taking the test, you will be referred, if necessary, to a local hearing specialist for additional help.

A variety of aids and techniques are available to compensate for hearing loss. Do not buy a hearing aid through the mail—it must be custom-made for best results. Ask about follow-up care and a one-month trial. States regulate hearing aid sales. If you have a problem with a hearing aid, contact the Food and Drug Administration or the Federal Trade Commission.

A personal sound amplifier is not a hearing aid but a portable and lightweight device to help overcome mild hearing loss (Figure 11-7). It is battery powered and has a volume control. Cost varies widely from $20 to more than $70 and up from department stores and self-help and mail-order firms. Before ordering, make sure there is a money-back guarantee if the unit is not satisfactory for you. **Sources:** 50, 100, 415.

An amplifier handset and flashing light or loud signal may make using your telephone more reliable (Figure 11-8). **Sources:** 177, 248, 325.

A flashing light or loud signal for a doorbell is also available from your local telephone company or through mail-order firms. You may also purchase a wireless doorbell that installs instantly. The bell unit may be placed near where you are sitting or working. Cost is about $13 and up from mail-order firms. **Sources:** 59, 100, 173, 270, 374.

If you have severe hearing loss, a telecommunication device for the deaf (TDD) types incoming phone messages and allows you to type return messages. For further information, call your local telephone company or the Accessible Products Center. **Source:** 248. Lucent Technology also provides a unit for closed-caption television so you can continue to enjoy your favorite shows.

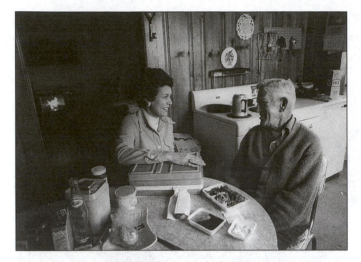

Figure 11-6. Volunteers deliver hot meals on a regular basis, bringing good nutrition as well as friendship. (Photo courtesy of ACTION, Washington, DC.)

If you enjoy the company of a pet, you might want to contact Dogs for the Deaf, Inc. for information on how a dog could help you handle your hearing loss. Address in Appendix B.

TIPS IF YOU LIVE ALONE

Many of us live alone for one reason or another, including personal preference. Some of us find ourselves suddenly alone when our partner dies, and we must deal with both grieving and day-to-day decisions. Some references at the end of this chapter give ideas that may make coping a little easier.

When you live alone, personal security, financial and health needs, and the ability to communicate determine your degree of independence and safety.

The telephone is your servant and major link to the outside world. It can bring groceries to your door and assistance during an emergency. It maintains contact with friends if your mobility is limited.

Many communities offer a reassurance service run by women's clubs, nursing services, town governments, or the residents of nursing homes. Each day, a person from the service telephones you at a specific time to make sure that everything is all right. If there is no answer, the service contacts a neighbor or person designated to stop by the house. To find out if this program is in your area, call your Visiting Nurse Association, town hall, Office of the Aging, or county health or fire department.

If you have difficulty managing your telephone, contact your local telephone office. Use your telephone to help you manage some of your errands (Figure 11-9). A flexible, 24" long, metal gooseneck arm holds the handset at a comfortable angle, leaving your hands free to take notes. The handset is held by a loop or clamp. A weighted "hang-up bar" or "flipper" on the cradle disconnects the circuit when the call is completed. The base clamp attaches to desk or table. Cost is about $60 for arm with clamp plus $10 for hang-up device from self-help firms. **Sources:** 13, 120, 252, 264, 393, 408.

If your fingers are weak or affected by arthritis, try a U-shaped

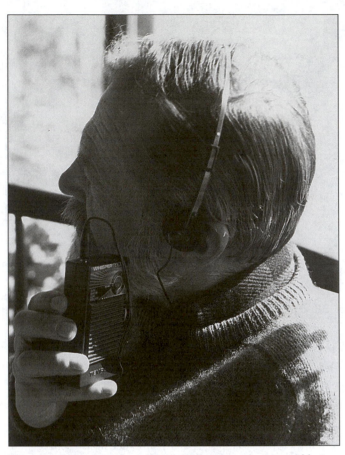

Figure 11-7. A personal sound amplifier is not a hearing aid but a portable and lightweight device to help overcome mild hearing loss. (Photo by J.K.)

phone handle that fits over the telephone receiver and fastens securely with a Velcro® closure. The frame bends to fit and rest on your hand, leaving fingers extended. Cost is about $7 from self-help firms. Sources: 120, 252, 290. If you use the phone a lot and your hands get tired, try a lightweight cordless phone headset.

Lucent Technology's Accessible Products Center provides detailed information on telephones. Products include big-button telephones that are easier to see and dial, amplifying handsets, flashing controls so you can see the telephone ring, headsets for hands-free communication, devices for the deaf that print incoming messages and let you type outgoing messages, artificial larynxes, and hands-free phones. Your local phone company may have many of these products available for you to try. **Source:** 248.

Sophisticated telephone equipment is also available from business or specialty stores and mail-order firms. These devices include cordless telephones that you can carry in a deep apron pocket, walker pouch, or wheelchair bag; memory telephones that store frequently called numbers so that you can dial them with the push of one button; answering machines; speaker phones; telephones that automatically record calls; and telephones that screen calls so you can know who's calling before you answer. Check out what features are most important to you, then study offers from business and specialty stores as well as mail-order firms. **Sources:** 87, 167, 176, 177, 325, 359.

If you have difficulty understanding what is being said, try a

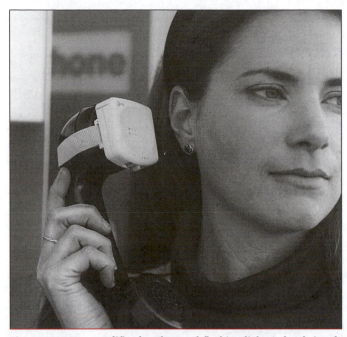

Figure 11-8. An amplifier handset and flashing light or loud signal may make using your telephone more reliable. (Photo courtesy of Hello Direct®, Inc., San Jose, CA.)

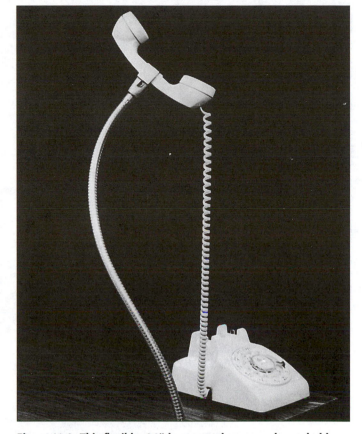

Figure 11-9. This flexible, 24″ long, metal gooseneck arm holds the handset at a comfortable angle, leaving your hands free to take notes. (Photo courtesy of Maddak®, Inc., Pequannock, NJ.)

Clarity® telephone (Figure 11-10). It amplifies only the high frequencies and has a sliding scale so that you adjust the sound to the best level for you. It has a large, lighted keypad. **Sources:** 50, 167, 177, 240.

Some push-button phones have big numbers that include three emergency buttons for the fire, police, and ambulance departments (Figure 11-11). This one has adjustable volume and can be programmed for up to 12 frequently called numbers. Cost is about $50. **Sources:** 50, 177, 240.

If you do not have a telephone outlet in a convenient place, such as near your bed, you might consider a wireless phone jack system. There are even legal devices that allow you to record a conversation to play back at your leisure. This is a great way to hear the grandchildren again or to help reinforce your memory and write down appointments.

A hook-on holster lets you carry a cordless telephone around your house (Figure 11-12). A padded clip slips over your shoulder or waistband, with Velcro® closures secure the telephone. Cost is about $15 from mail-order firms. **Sources:** 169, 177, 270, 415.

PERSONAL SECURITY

Personal emergency response systems are programs that provide a means of summoning help 24 hours a day (Figure 11-13). For a monthly fee, plus a nominal installation charge, you are connected to an answering service. The service provides a pendant that you wear around your neck. It has a button you push in case of an emergency, such as a fall or medical problem. If you cannot answer over the remote control unit or the telephone, help is sent. When you register for the service, you provide a list of people you wish called, such as your neighbor, a relative, nursing service, or fire department. **Source:** 198.

To find out about programs in your area, call your Visiting Nurse Association, office of the aging, fire department, or community relations/social service department of your nearest hospital. This program gives you and your loved ones peace of mind. Don't wait until you have an emergency to sign up.

Keeping your house secure is another concern. Always lock doors. For more security, an alarm system can alert you to smoke or fire, or detect if someone is attempting to force open a door or window. Vehicle alarm systems alert you if someone is coming in your driveway. Portable alarms may be taken with you if you move.

Alarm companies that install and maintain complete alarm systems are found throughout the country. Before buying an alarm, check the company's service record with neighbors, consumer magazines, the local police department, and the Better Business Bureau. **Manufacturers:** 198, 199, 291.

GOING FURTHER

Addresses are listed in the Appendices.

PUBLICATIONS
American Speech-Language-Hearing Association.

Berman, P. L. (Ed.). (1989). *The Courage to Grow Old*. New York: Ballantine, Random House. **Source:** 326.

Caine, L. (1990). *Being a Widow*.New York: Viking, Penguin. **Source:** 308B.

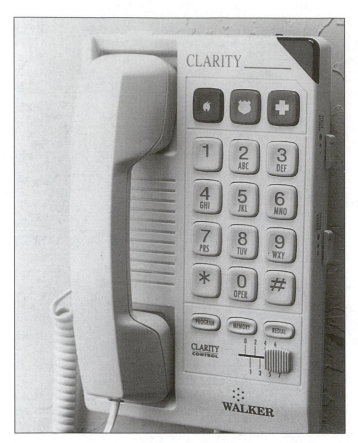

Figure 11-10. If you have difficulty understanding what is being said, try a Clarity® telephone. (Photo courtesy of Hello Direct®, San Jose, CA.)

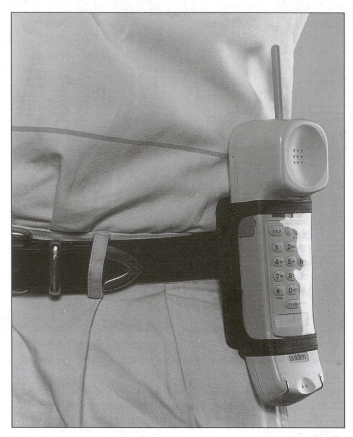

Figure 11-12. A hook-on holster lets you carry a cordless telephone around your house. (Photo courtesy of Hello Direct®, San Jose, CA.)

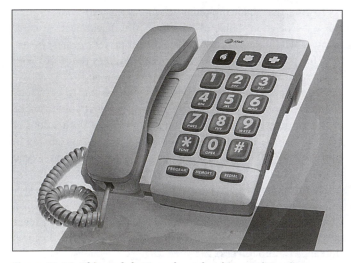

Figure 11-11. This push-button phone has big numbers that include three emergency buttons for the fire, police, and ambulance departments. (Photo courtesy of Hello Direct®, San Jose, CA.)

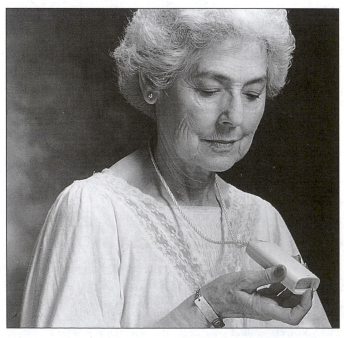

Figure 11-13. Personal emergency response systems are programs that provide a means of summoning help 24 hours a day. (Photo courtesy of Interactive Technologies, Inc., North Saint Paul, MN.)

Cirino, L. D. (1995). *On Your Own Terms: The Seniors' Guide to an Independent Life*. New York: Hearst Books. Offers strategies, tips, products, and resources for seniors, with the information you need to be more independent.

Have You Heard?, #D12219. Washington, DC: American Association of Retired Persons. Free from AARP.

How to Buy a Telephone: A Guide for Consumers. Free from the Consumer Information Center.

Loewinsohn, R. J. (1984). *Survival Handbook for Widows (and for relatives and friends who want to understand)*. Washington, DC: American Association of Retired Persons. $5.95 from AARP.

Meeting the Need for Security and Independence with Personal Emergency Response Systems, #D12905. Washington, DC: American Association of Retired Persons. Free from AARP.

National Hearing Aid Association.

National Institute on Deafness and Other Communication Disorders.

Resource Directory for Older People. #017-062-00143-0. Washington, DC: The National Institute on Aging. $10 from the Superintendent of Documents.

Rose, X. (1991). *Widow's Journey*. New York: Henry Holt. **Source:** 178B.

Salmen, J. P. S. (1985). *The DoAble ReNewable Home*. Washington, DC: American Association of Retired Persons. Free from AARP.

Scheller, M. D. (1992). *Growing Older, Feeling Better—In Body, Mind & Spirit*. Palo Alto, CA: Bull Publishing. Social worker-gerontologist addresses practical as well as spiritual matters that affect your quality of life: nutrition, exercises, stress management, and relaxation. **Source:** 51.

Self Help for Hard of Hearing People, Inc. Six pamphlets on Assistive Listening Devices and Systems (ALDS). $2.00.

Seskin, J. (1985). *Alone Not Lonely: Independent Living for Women Over Fifty*. Washington, DC: American Association of Retired Persons. $6.95 from AARP.

Singer, G. *Towards the Greater Enjoyment of Later Life*. (A workbook.); Singer, L. *Coping Exercise*. Pequannock, NJ: Maddak, Inc. **Source:** 252.

Solomon, D., et al. (1992). *A Consumer's Guide to Aging*. Baltimore: Johns Hopkins University Press. **Source:** 209B.

What You Should Know About Good Nutrition in Later Years. South Deerfield, MA: Channing L. Bete Co. $1.25 each. **Source:** 62.

Your Home: Your Choice—A Workbook for Older People and Their Families. (1991). Washington, DC: American Association of Retired Persons. Topics include staying in your home, changing your housing arrangements, supportive housing, and resources. Free from AARP.

Section Two

IN AND AROUND THE KITCHEN AND THE HOME

Safety

More accidents occur in the home than anywhere else. Most could be prevented with careful planning, correct use of equipment, and common sense. If your mobility, strength, coordination, energy, hearing, or vision are limited, it is even more important to take extra precautions.

DRESSING FOR SAFETY

- Wear nonflammable garments when working near the range.
- Wear fitted or short sleeves. Avoid long sleeves with frills that could get caught in an appliance or catch fire as you reach over the range.
- Wear shoes with non-skid soles and solid, low heels.
- Do not wear a plastic apron while cooking. Plastic aprons should be worn only when washing dishes or cleaning house.

WALKING SAFELY

- Secure all rugs and carpets, and eliminate all scatter rugs.
- Keep floors skid-proof.
- Use a cart with wheels, whenever possible, to avoid carrying.
- Store items so they are easy to retrieve. Use tongs, or ask for help to get things from high shelves.
- Wipe up all wet or dry spills immediately. Even small spills could cause you to slip and fall.

Woven mesh rug grippers, which can be cut to size, hold area rugs without gluing or tacking. Cost is $6 and up per pad, depending on size, from carpet stores, housewares stores, and mail-order firms. **Sources:** 15, 49, 173, 196, 270, 369, 410, 415.

Velcro® hold-down kits and double-sided carpet tape, such as the Lok-Lift® safety strips, may also be used to hold area rugs. **Manufacturer:** 295B. Cost is about $10 and up from hardware stores and mail-order firms. **Sources:** 185, 194, 270, 364, 374.

If your steps are slippery, installing low pile carpet or rubber treads could prevent a fall. Cost is about $15 per set for nylon carpet treads with foam backing and double-face adhesive tapes that stick to tile, wood, or concrete steps, from hardware stores and mail-order firms. **Sources:** 185, 270. Rubber treads are about $4 each from hardware stores and mail-order firms. **Source:** 410.

A long-handled dustpan and brush quickly clean up dry spills while you are standing or sitting (Figure 12-1). The extended handle stays upright for use with one hand. When you lift the handle, the pan closes, and dirt drops into the base until tipped over the waste container. Cost is $10 and up for dustpan only, or $12 and up for pan and brush from housewares stores, and self-help and mail-order firms. **Sources:** 5, 6, 21, 59, 71, 100, 108, 120, 155, 185, 238, 252, 264, 290, 369, 370, 408.

To clean wet spills without bending down, use a short-handled sponge mop. Cost is about $3 and up from housewares stores and mail-order firms.

Keep your hands dry and free of oil to prevent slippage of items from your grasp. A kitchen towel with an attached ring, Velcro® or snap fastener, or loop can hang on a nearby hook or knob for instant use. Make one yourself or purchase one from a housewares store or mail-order firm for $4 and up. **Source:** 270.

HANDLING HOT ITEMS

Safe, non-flammable pot holders are kitchen essentials. If you have any loss of sensation, you need full protection from heat.

To protect hands and forearms from hot oven walls, use flame-retardant silicone- or Teflon-treated, long oven mitts that extend to your elbows (Figure 12-2). **Manufacturer** of insulated hot mitts: 255. Cost is about $16 per pair for 17" long mitts from housewares stores, camping supply, self-help, and mail-order firms. **Sources:** 5, 13, 65, 71, 120, 185, 196, 256, 261, 270, 408.

Casserole paws, or two padded mitts joined by a wide quilted band, help protect your hands and forearms as you lift hot pans from the oven (Figure 12-3). **Manufacturer:** 143. Cost is $4 and up from housewares stores and gourmet firms.

Standard pot holders are often bulky and hard to use if your grasp is weak or uncoordinated. A mitt with a central thumb bends

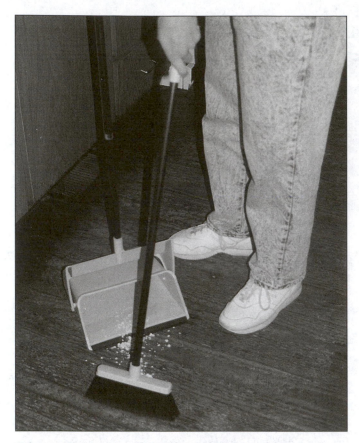

Figure 12-1. A long-handled dustpan and brush quickly clean up dry spills while you are standing or sitting. (Photo by J.K.)

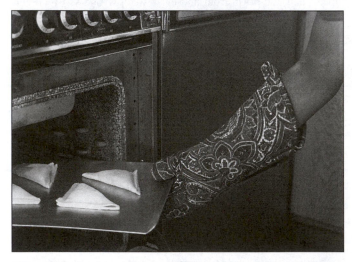

Figure 12-2. To protect hands and forearms from hot oven walls, use flame-retardant silicone- or Teflon-treated long oven mitts that extend to your elbows. (Photo by J.K.)

more easily and positions your thumb for the most secure grip (Figure 12-4). **Manufacturer:** 143. Cost is $3 each and up from housewares stores and mail-order firms.

When possible, slide, do not lift, to increase safety as you handle hot pans. Put a heat-proof countermat next to the range top for resting hot pots or skillets. **Manufacturers** include 343. Mats cost $2 and up from housewares stores. If you have difficulty remembering to turn off the oven or an appliance, a visual or audible

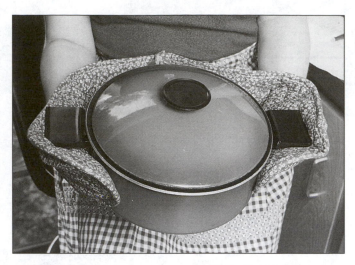

Figure 12-3. Casserole paws, or two padded mitts joined by a wide quilted band, help protect your hands and forearms. (Photo courtesy of the O.T. Dept., Howard A. Rusk Institute of Rehabilitation Medicine.)

timer is essential. For more memory aids, see Chapter 11.

TIPS FOR HOME FIRE PREVENTION

- Always stay in the kitchen while food is on the range.
- Keep the stove top clear.
- Never hang towels or window curtains close to the range.
- Do not use towels to remove hot pans from the oven.
- Do not use flammable liquids or sprays near a gas range. The pilot light can ignite vapors and cause an explosion.
- If you have small children, choose a range with controls out of their reach. Teach children to never touch the range.
- If you have a gas oven with no pilot light, do not turn on the gas until the match is lit. Otherwise, an accumulation of gas can cause an explosion. See also Chapter 19.
- Locate your gas range away from drafts that could extinguish the pilot light.
- Check that on/off indicator lights are working properly on your electric range to indicate when burners are operating.
- Use the proper size pans on burners. Do not place a small pan on a large burner as this could create enough heat to ignite clothing or overheat a pot handle.
- Repair faulty wiring, burner valves, and other hazards immediately.
- Plan a fire escape route with your family and by yourself. Have periodic fire drills.
- In case of fire, leave the house before calling the fire department.

Reduce the risk of a kitchen fire by wearing properly fitted clothing, cleaning up grease immediately, cooking over low heat, and covering pans to prevent grease from splattering. If grease should catch fire, smother the blaze with a pot lid. Alternatively, pour salt or baking soda on it; the carbon dioxide from the baking soda will snuff out a minor flame. If the fire is in the oven, immediately turn off the heat and keep the oven door closed to smother the flame. Never try to extinguish a grease fire with water. It causes the grease to splatter, and water conducts electricity, which may

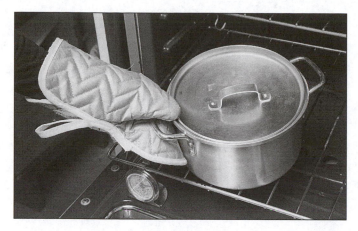

Figure 12-4. A mitt with a central thumb bends more easily and positions your thumb for the most secure grip. (Photo courtesy of the O.T. Dept., Howard A. Rusk Institute of Rehabilitation Medicine.)

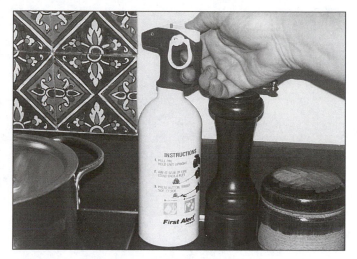

Figure 12-5. Keep a fire extinguisher on the counter or hanging on a kitchen wall so it is ready to use at a moment's notice. (Photo courtesy of the O.T. Dept., Howard A. Rusk Institute of Rehabilitation Medicine.)

produce a shock.

Keep a fire extinguisher on the counter or hanging on a kitchen wall so it is ready to use at a moment's notice (Figure 12-5). Before purchasing one, be sure you can operate it. Ask your occupational therapist or home economist to recommend units that are easiest to use. The extinguisher must be effective on grease, oil, gasoline, paint, and electrical fires. A safety seal will prevent accidental discharge and indicate the correct pressure. If the extinguisher is rechargeable, make sure it is serviced regularly. If you have a weak grasp, your therapist can make an adapted cuff that will facilitate handling an extinguisher. **Manufacturers** of lightweight extinguishers: 47, 199. Cost is $15 and up. **Sources:** 196, 312, 345, 369.

You should also have an immediate way of summoning help if a fire is the least bit out of control. See Chapter 11.

More than 80% of fire fatalities in the home are caused by smoke or toxic gases—not by the flames. A smoke detector gives you an early alert during the smoldering stage. The shrill alarm can pierce even your deepest sleep. If you are hard of hearing, a bed shaker attached to the smoke alarm will awaken you. You should have smoke alarms in three locations in your home: outside your bedroom, in the kitchen, and near the furnace. Many units now come with a button that allows you to silence a false alarm. Change the batteries twice a year—when daylight-savings time begins and ends. Consult your local fire department before purchasing one. **Manufacturers:** 41, 55, 199, 291. Cost is $15 and up. **Sources:** 50, 196, 261, 345, 359. A talking smoke alarm, which gives pre-recorded escape directions, is available from 247, 261. Cost is about $60.

See also Chapter 19 for information on security lights for use when power fails.

GOING FURTHER

Addresses are listed in the Appendices.

PUBLICATIONS

Burn Prevention Tips—Shriners Burns Institutes.

The Channing L. Bete Co. publishes several titles on home safety, including *Are There Fire Traps in Your Home?*; *Housekeeping for Fire Prevention*; *What Every Older Adult Should Know about Fire Safety in the Home*; *About Fire Escape Plans*; and *About Family Safety*. Cost of booklets is $1.25 each. **Source:** 62.

National Fire Protection Association. Send for list of publications.

A Safe Home is No Accident. (1991). Chicago: National Easter Seal Society. Checklist to help spot potential hazards. Brochure available from your local chapter.

Smoke Detectors. Free 6-page booklet from the Consumer Information Center.

Kitchen Planning

If a physical disability or age slows you down or affects your ability to reach, bend, lift, or carry, it may be time to remodel your kitchen to meet your needs.

The keys to working comfortably in your kitchen are an efficient floor plan and a smooth flow of activity. How much clear floor space is there? There should be a minimum 30" x 48" rectangle of floor space in front of all fixtures and appliances, especially if you are working from a wheelchair. A clearance of 40" is recommended between counters and opposing base cabinets, countertops, appliances, and walls.

Your kitchen doesn't have to be big or expensive. Be creative. How much do you have to lift and carry? How often do you have to move one thing to reach another? For more storage space, discard non-essentials, move things around, add in-cabinet organizers (see Chapter 14) and commandeer an unused bookcase from another room. Can you sit and rest while working? A pull-out work surface may be an easily added, welcome food preparation area.

HOW TO PLAN ALTERATIONS

1. Draw a floor plan of your kitchen as it is now.
2. Visit kitchen and appliance showrooms to see what is available in countertop cooking units, plumbing fixtures, seating, and kitchen designs.
3. Send for the free references at the end of this chapter. Check magazines and your library for more design ideas.
4. Check mail-order catalogs for ideas, such as specialized cabinets or pantries, to add to your present kitchen.
5. List the problems you have while handling appliances or working in your kitchen. Incorporate solutions to these problems in your new kitchen design.
6. In your plans, include an area where you can comfortably sit to work. Plan equipment and food storage areas so that what you use frequently is near at hand.
7. Brainstorm with family and friends before consulting with a contractor. Ask your therapist to sit with you and work out solutions that meet your physical needs.

BEFORE YOU REMODEL

1. Ask relatives and friends to recommend a reliable contractor or architect.
2. Get at least three written estimates—including cost of appliances and cabinets, duration of work, etc.
3. Before hiring, check with the Better Business Bureau to see if complaints have been filed against the contractor. Never offer work to a door-to-door solicitor without checking references very carefully.
4. Discuss with the contractor any problems you may encounter when changing the wiring and altering the height of pipes or appliances.
5. Plan to pay as the work is completed. Do not pay the full charge up front; do not pay the final amount until the job is satisfactorily completed.

FUNDING ALTERNATIVES

Talk with an occupational therapist, rehabilitation home economist, or architect about help with planning and funding. If you do not have money for kitchen changes, you may qualify for assistance under your state vocational rehabilitation program. Assistance can include counseling, diagnostic and physical restorative services, and the tools and equipment you need to continue your homemaking. Material and labor costs may be covered.

If you do not qualify for state assistance, check with local organizations set up to lend a hand, either physically or financially. Ask a tax consultant if costs for modifications made in your kitchen and in other parts of your home to accommodate your disability are tax deductible; or call your local Internal Revenue Office for information on Revised Ruling 87-106, IRB 1987-431.

The kitchen shown in Figure 13-1 is designed for efficient use by people with and without disabilities. There are standard-height counters as well as pull-out work surfaces. The cooktop is open underneath to accommodate a wheelchair. A mirror above the cooktop allows a seated cook to look inside the pans, even when

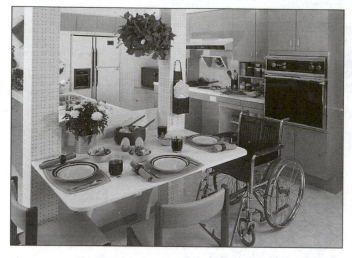

Figure 13-1. This kitchen is designed for efficient use by people with and without disabilities. (Horizon House, Howard A. Rusk Rusk Institute of Rehabilitation Medicine. Photo courtesy of Whirlpool® Corp., Benton Harbor, MI.)

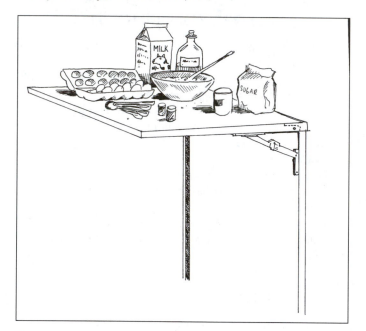

Figure 13-2. A drop-leaf table attached to the wall gives complete freedom of movement underneath and increases the available turning radius for a wheelchair. (Illustration by G.K.)

the pans are at the back of the range. Cabinets without doors provide quick access to utensils and condiments. Operating controls for the exhaust fan have been moved to the edge of the cooktop counter, within easy reach of the seated cook. The self-cleaning oven is built into a cabinet at a height convenient for use while standing or sitting.

The 31" high counter doubles as a dining table and sit-down work surface for meal preparation. **Source:** 424.

SITTING TO WORK

The best way to conserve your strength in the kitchen is to sit while you work. Select a comfortable chair that provides proper

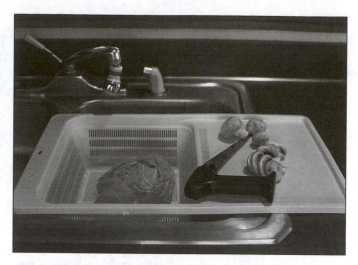

Figure 13-3. An over-the-sink cutting board provides an instant extra counter and cutting surface. (Photo by J.K.)

support. You will need a chair of standard height to work at a kitchen table and a higher chair or stool for sink and counter use. A foot rest adds support when you sit in a higher chair.

For a sit-to-work sink, a 5" to 5½" deep sink installed in a 31" high counter should enable you to sit, or to clear the arms of the chair if you are using a wheelchair. If you are very tall, you may want a higher work surface. See also Chapter 7.

Many swivel chairs have padded seats and half or full arms for comfort. Some seats adjust in height from 24" to 30". Stools should stand on self-leveling glides. If the foot rest ring does not provide adequate support for your feet, add a footstool. **Manufacturers** of chairs: 80, 347, 433. The cost of a chair ranges from about $60 and up from department stores and mail-order firms. **Sources:** 356, 359, 373, 433. Other sources for high swivel stools include business and office furniture stores, art supply firms, and bar stool companies. If you have normal trunk balance and good use of your upper extremities, a chair without arms may be sufficient. **Sources:** 52, 144, 158, 179, 293, 377. If you have arthritis, back pain, or trouble rising or sitting, special chairs are available. See Chapter 5.

A footstool to hold your feet at the correct position is especially important if you have weakness or arthritis in your legs. A long dowel or broom handle attached to the side of the footstool lets you move the stool under your feet without bending.

For added comfort, if you are working from a wheelchair or a stool, remove doors and floor molding of lower cabinets and decorative molding. This allows you to put your legs under the counter for a closer approach to work surface or sink.

A drop-leaf table attached to the wall gives complete freedom of movement underneath and increases the available turning radius for a wheelchair (Figure 13-2). Make sure the table is sturdy enough to support the weight of your arms and the cooking supplies. Folding wall-tables cost $50 and up from department stores and mail-order and self-help firms. **Source:** 13. Hardware for attaching a drop-leaf table is available from local building suppliers and is manufactured by **source** 376.

An over-the-sink cutting board provides an instant, extra counter and cutting surface (Figure 13-3). Portable units are avail-

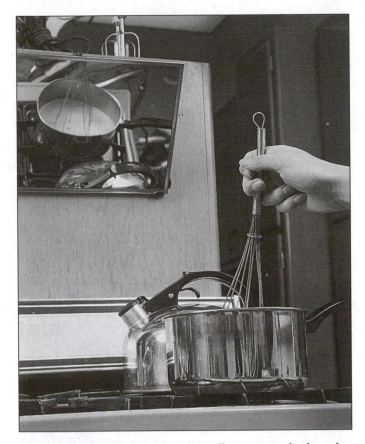

Figure 13-4. An over-the-range mirror allows you to check on the contents of pans without getting up. (Photo courtesy of the O.T. Dept., Howard A. Rusk Institute of Rehabilitation Medicine.)

able in wood or durable stain-resistant plastic. Some units feature both a cutting board and a colander that fit in a single or double sink. **Manufacturer:** 289. Cost is $10 and up from housewares stores and mail-order firms. **Sources:** 242, 407.

An over-the-range mirror allows you to check on the contents of pans without getting up (Figure 13-4). A carpenter can construct one that adjusts to your line of vision. Self-help firms also carry adjustable mirrors for about $25. **Sources:** 120, 408.

A computer desk may be used as the base of an efficient kitchen work area if you are operating from a wheelchair or a chair and cannot get into your kitchen (Figure 13-5). Double shelves hold utensils and small appliances while the pull-out board provides an added work surface. Cost starts at about $150, which is far lower than having a unit built to order. Check office supply and mail-order firms. **Sources:** 52, 99, 144, 153, 158, 179, 192, 293, 377. You can add undershelf lighting, and protect the surface with heat-proof counter mats.

Adjustable-height cabinets, which may be re-positioned, are available from kitchen specialty dealers. Cabinets for use from a wheelchair are manufactured by **source** 268.

For easy access, the Liftshelf lowers the cabinet contents with a single switch (Figures 13-6A and 13-6B). It is available in three sizes and is equipped with control switches, wiring harness, and 110V heavy-duty motor. Its tubular steel arms and white pine shelves may be installed in existing or new cabinets. The Liftshelf can be disassembled so that you can take it with you if you move. It is also available with chromed wire baskets or plastic shelves.

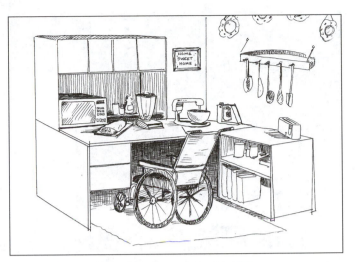

Figure 13-5. A computer desk may be used as the base of an efficient kitchen work area. (Illustration by G.K.)

Manufacturers: 7, 413. Cost is $530 and up.

APPLIANCES

Major appliances designed with increased adaptability for working from a wheelchair or seated position include a wall oven with a side-swing door, a 30" drop-in range for installation at sitting or wheelchair height, and smooth-top cooktops with top front-mounted controls. **Source:** 147. Slide-in dishwashers can be installed under 34" high counters; dishwashers with electronic controls require no turning of knobs. **Source:** 147. Front-loading clothes washers and dryers have front-mounted controls for easy access. **Sources:** 34, 147.

Compact dishwashers may be installed at any height (Figure 13-7). The shelves pull out for easy access without bending. The same company manufactures a clothes washer and a dryer that may be installed vertically or horizontally at any height. **Source:** 34.

PLUMBING

If turning faucets is difficult, a single-lever faucet may work for you. It operates with a push from your forearm or hand. If you have a spray attachment on your sink, you can fill pans on the counter and slide them to the range top without lifting. Single-lever faucets and spray attachments are available from faucet manufacturers and plumbing suppliers. **Manufacturers:** 24, 93, 115, 145, 223, 276.

Automatic faucets have no levers to push or pull. Place a pan under the faucet, and a sensor starts the water; when you remove the dish, the flow stops. Water temperature is adjustable with the turn of a knob. Models are available to fit most sinks. The faucet, called the Sensor Flo®, has a 30-second flow when your hands approach it. **Manufacturer:** 358. Ask your local plumbing suppliers for additional information.

The controls for this UltraFlo® push-button plumbing may be installed at the most accessible location (Figure 13-8). Both temperature and speed are controlled. **Source:** 406.

There is no need to carry pans of water from sink to range. An

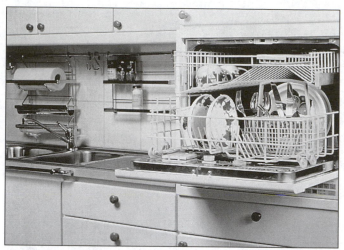

Figure 13-7. Compact dishwashers may be installed at any height. (Photo courtesy of Asko, Inc., Richardson, TX.)

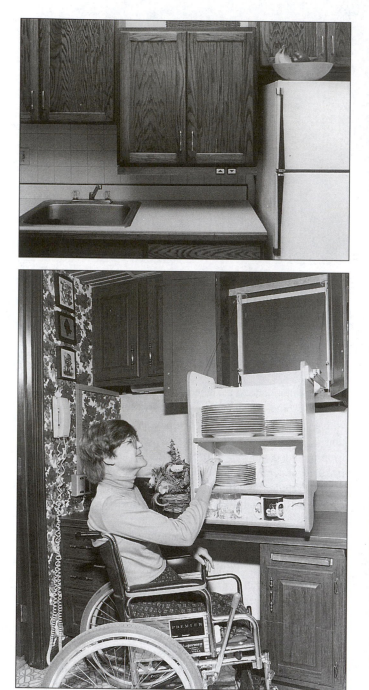

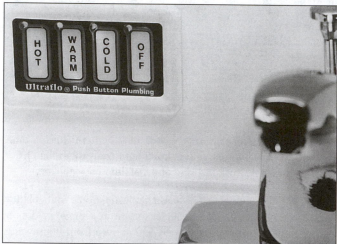

Figure 13-8. The controls for this UltraFlo® push-button plumbing may be installed at the most accessible location. (Photo courtesy of UltraFlo®, Sandusky, OH.)

for a filtering model from department stores. Non-filter units cost about $7 and up.

Figures 13-6A and 13-6B. For easy access, the Liftshelf lowers the cabinet contents with a single switch. (Photos courtesy of Accessible Work Systems, Inc., Bellevue, OH.)

instant hot water heater provides hot water at your sink for coffee, tea, instant soups, and cereals (Figure 13-9). The unit is available through builders, kitchen suppliers, and plumbing contractors. **Manufacturers:** 145, 197.

If it is not possible to remodel your kitchen to allow you to work at the sink, set up a comfortable work table with a water container (Figure 13-10). Some plastic containers filter and store two gallons of water. The container can be refilled by a family member as needed. Stored above the work area, it can dispense water at the press of a lever or button. **Manufacturer:** 388. Cost is about $25

DOORWAYS

If your grip is weak, an add-on lever or grooved handle that clamps onto the knob makes door opening easier (Figure 13-11). **Manufacturers:** 83, 324. Cost is $8 and up. **Sources:** 120, 264, 290, 408.

A permanent door lever handle, which may replace a doorknob, is available through building suppliers and hardware stores. **Manufacturers:** 225, 352.

A portable door knob turner lets you open doors with a push of your hand or forearm (Figure 13-12). Cost is about $10. **Source:** 290.

To add 2" more clearance in a doorway for easier wheelchair access, install swing-clear hinges (Figure 13-13). The door folds flat against the wall, rather than protruding into the passage as with

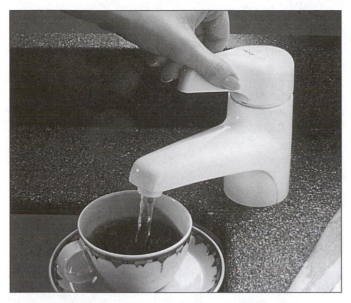

Figure 13-9. An instant hot water heater provides hot water at your sink for coffee, tea, instant soups, and cereals. (Photo courtesy of In-Sink-Erator®, Racine, WI.)

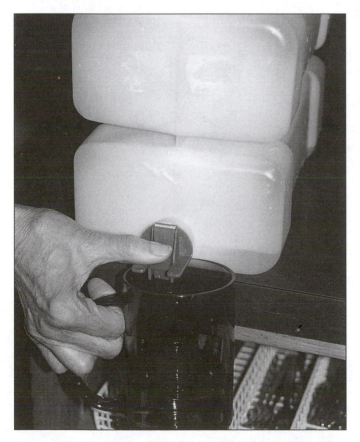

Figure 13-10. If it is not possible to remodel your kitchen to allow you to work at the sink, set up a comfortable work table with a water container. Some plastic containers filter and store two gallons of water. The container can be refilled by a family member as needed. Stored above the work area, it dispenses water at the press of a lever or button. (Photo by J.K.)

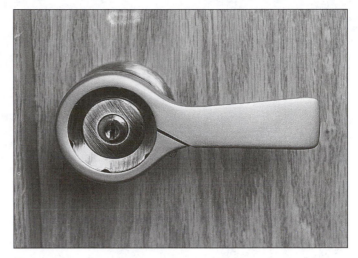

Figure 13-11. If your grip is weak, an add-on lever or grooved handle that clamps onto the knob makes door opening easier. (Photo courtesy of R & G Manufacturing, Moorhead, MN.)

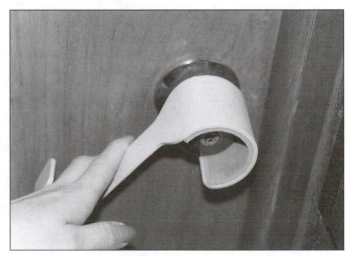

Figure 13-12. A portable door knob turner lets you open doors with a push of your hand or forearm. (Photo courtesy of North Coast Medical, Inc., San Jose, CA.)

ordinary hinges. Hinges fit into standard hinge holes and may be taken with you if you move. **Manufacturers:** 103, 376. Cost is about $18 per pair from hardware stores and self-help firms. **Sources:** 3, 120, 252, 264, 408.

LIGHTING

Proper lighting increases your safety and prevents eyestrain. When planning your kitchen, consider undercabinet lighting, which sheds extra light on countertop work areas. In addition, track lighting accommodates as many lights as you need to illuminate work spaces. **Manufacturers** of track and innovative kitchen lighting include 214, 241.

GOING FURTHER

Addresses are listed in the Appendices.

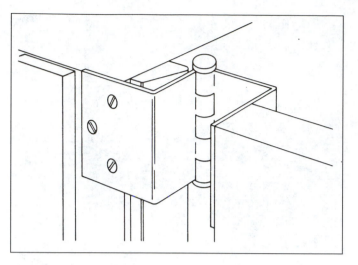

Figure 13-13. To add 2″ more clearance in a doorway for easier wheelchair access, install swing-clear hinges.

PUBLICATIONS

Cheever, R., & Goree, B. *An Accessible Home of Your Own.* Bloomington, IL: Accent Books and Products. $4.50. **Source:** 3.

Easy Access Housing. (1990). Chicago: National Easter Seal Society. 12-page brochure, available through your local chapter. Home adaptability and accessibility checklists, suggestions for solving common problems.

Kitchen Planning for the Physically Impaired. Louisville, KY: General Electric Consumer Affairs, General Electric Co. Free. **Source:** 156.

The Less Challenging Home. And *The Time Smart Kitchen.* Both illustrated booklets free from the Appliances Information Service, Whirlpool® Corporation. **Source:** 424.

A Place to Live: Independent Living. (1990). Bloomington, IL: Accent Books and Products. $4.95. **Source:** 3.

Salmen, J. P. S. (1988). *The DoAble ReNewable Home.* American Association of Retired Persons. Free from AARP.

Kitchen Storage

Making full use of available storage space is always important, but especially if you have weakness in your arms, use of one hand, incoordination, limited reach, or loss of vision. The first step in planning efficient kitchen storage is to look at how and where you use meal preparation tools and equipment.

ORGANIZING YOUR KITCHEN

Which items do you use most frequently?

- Group items according to their use, and store them near where you use them. Keep heavy pots and pans near the range or sink so you do not have to carry them very far. Collect baking utensils and ingredients in the same area; put vegetable peeling and cutting tools together.
- Keep duplicates of frequently used tools, such as measuring cups and spoons, in the places where they are used.
- Do you have to shuffle things around to find what you want? Get rid of clutter and equipment you never use.
- Keep frequently used tools, appliances, and foods where you can most easily reach them.
- Save top shelves and backs of shelves for seldom-used equipment. If necessary, ask for help in reaching seasonal or infrequently used items.
- Keep small appliances at the back of the counter. Slide them forward to use.
- Lightweight baskets and plastic food containers may be stored higher. Use a reaching device to retrieve them.

Once you have organized your kitchen utensils, pantry foods, and appliances according to their use, you are ready to put them in the drawers and cabinets. Before you do, however, consider using some of the helpful storage aids and ideas described in this chapter. More extensive kitchen reorganization is discussed in Chapter 13.

IN-CABINET STORAGE

If you have limited reach or difficulty picking up things, extension shelves, turn-tables, and pull-out units will maximize space and increase your efficiency.

Helper shelves are space-saving storage devices for foods and dishes. These adjustable, vinyl-coated, steel shelves come in several sizes: a smaller shelf unit expands up to 21", a larger unit up to 32". Other vinyl-coated, steel or plastic storage aids are specially designed for dishes, bakeware, cans, or food wraps. **Manufacturers:** 117, 161, 232, 343, 403, 417. Cost per unit is about $7 and up from housewares stores and mail-order firms. **Sources:** 59, 71, 76, 173, 185, 242, 270, 378, 387, 415.

If you are working with one hand or have marked weakness, a rack that stores plates vertically, rather than stacked, is easier to handle.

Lazy susans, or turntables, range in diameter and come in single- and double-tiered models. Single turntables are handy in the refrigerator for keeping small items together. **Manufacturers:** 319, 343. Cost is $5 and up from housewares stores.

Commercial storage aids are available to maximize cabinet space of any size, including rear and vertical areas (Figure 14-1). Vinyl-coated, steel units have ball-bearing slides for easy swiveling or gliding, even when fully loaded. **Manufacturer:** 69. Cost varies by unit from hardware stores, building supply firms, and housewares stores.

A three-level spice shelf lets you see the entire contents at a glance without moving containers (Figure 14-2). The Expand-A-Shelf™ is made of styrene; it measures 8" deep by 4" high and expands from 14" to 27". Cost is $15 and up in solid styrene or vinyl-coated steel from mail-order firms. **Sources:** 71, 171, 173, 242, 270, 387, 415.

Can racks have adjustable shelves to hold and dispense cans of different sizes (Figure 14-3). Shelves are tilted so, as you remove one can, another slides into its place. Made of vinyl-coated steel with removable shelves and sliding dividers, the 14" wide unit

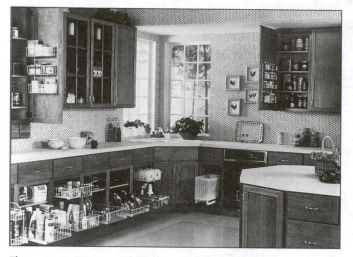

Figure 14-1. Commercial storage aids are available to maximize cabinet space of any size, including rear and vertical areas. (Photo courtesy of Clairson International, Ocala, FL.)

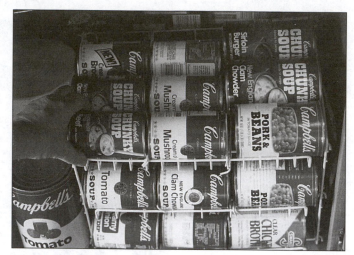

Figure 14-3. This can rack has adjustable shelves to hold and dispense cans of different sizes. (Photo by J.K.)

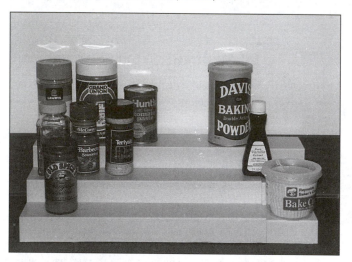

Figure 14-2. This three-level spice shelf lets you see the entire contents at a glance without moving containers. (Photo by J.K.)

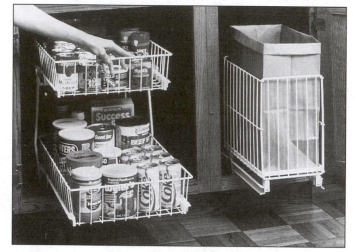

Figure 14-4. A two- or three-level under-cabinet or under-sink organizer for foods or cleaning supplies slides out for easy accessibility. (Photo courtesy of Clairson International, Ocala, FL.)

holds up to 60 cans. **Manufacturer:** 365. Cost is $10 and up from mail-order firms. **Sources:** 59, 270, 364, 387.

A two- or three-level under-cabinet or under-sink organizer for foods or cleaning supplies slides out for easy accessibility (Figure 14-4). **Manufacturers/**distributors: 61, 69. Cost is $13 and up from department and hardware stores or mail-order firms. **Sources:** 69, 171, 173, 270, 387.

Single-level slide-out trays let you utilize the full depth of a cabinet without struggling and bending. They come in several widths. **Manufacturers:** 117, 343. Cost is $15 and up from housewares stores and mail-order firms. **Sources:** 242, 364.

When shelves are far apart, you may install an under-shelf bin to utilize otherwise unused space. The basket clips to the upper shelf to hold small pans or food items. Some under-shelf bins are designed to store platters, plates, placemats, paper goods, and wine glasses. **Manufacturers:** 161, 365. Cost of chromed steel or vinyl-coated steel baskets is $5 and up from housewares stores and mail-order firms. **Sources:** 173, 192, 242, 270, 387.

A narrow broom closet may be converted into an efficient stor-

age unit (Figure 14-5). The one shown has been fitted with adjustable shelves, sliding drawer inserts, and pull-out units. These storage aids are available from building suppliers, housewares stores, and mail-order firms. The inside of cabinet doors is also a good place for storage. Hooks and holders for lids, bags, and food wraps can be installed on doors. **Manufacturers:** 161, 343. Cost is $5 and up from housewares stores and mail-order firms. **Sources:** 171, 173, 242, 270, 387, 415. A multi-pocketed plastic caddy for holding envelopes of dry and powdered mixes mounts quickly with self-adhesive tape on the back of a cabinet door. Cost is about $5 from mail-order firms. **Source:** 415.

DRAWERS

Loop handles on drawers, cabinets, or refrigerator doors are easier to operate than knobs if you have weak grasp or arthritis. When you have weakness or arthritis in your arms and hands, install gliders for drawers, which make pulling out and pushing in

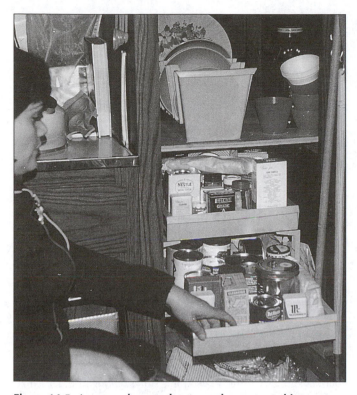

Figure 14-5. A narrow broom closet may be converted into an efficient storage unit. (Photo by J.K.)

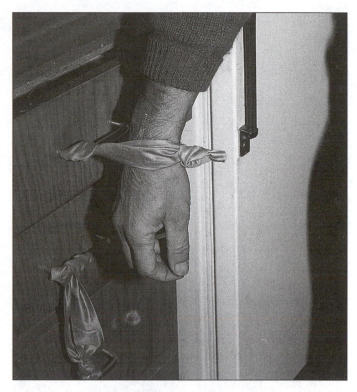

Figure 14-6. A loop of cloth around a drawer or refrigerator handle allows you to pull it open with your whole body. (Photo by J.K.)

easier. Gliders may be added to most existing drawers. **Manufacturer:** 376. Ask your hardware store or a local contractor for specific information.

If you have arthritis or weakness in your arms, a loop of cloth around a drawer or refrigerator handle allows you to pull it open with your whole body (Figure 14-6). This reduces stress on the wrists and hands.

Another way to reduce the stress of opening and closing drawers is to apply silicone spray or nylon tape along the drawer track. **Manufacturer** of spray: 419. It is available from hardware stores and mail-order firms.

If you have weak grasp or poor vision, keeping items separated is important. To avoid injury, use vertical dividers or small boxes in your drawers to store and organize utensils. Keep knives, blades down, in a holder apart from other items. Ready-made, modular drawer dividers or drawer-size trays eliminate stacking, making it easier to remove items with one hand or poor coordination. **Manufacturers:** 95, 343. Available from housewares stores and mail-order firms.

A piggyback sliding tray permits double-layer use of a drawer. **Manufacturers:** 343, 417. Cost is about $12 each and up from hardware and housewares stores.

Deep drawers may be converted to vertical storage with wood or masonite separators that are cut to size and installed with metal brads.

COUNTER AND MID-STORAGE AIDS

Make maximum use of the reachable space between your cabinets and countertop by adding extra shelves, a grid hanger, or pegboard to the wall at the rear of the counter. Pegboard may be cut to size, painted to match decor, and installed between cabinets and countertops. Purchase hooks and brackets to hang utensils in the most comfortable arrangement for you. They are available from hardware stores.

A Hide-Away™ organizer installs right under the cabinet to provide extra shelf space for spices and dry mixes that get lost easily in a cabinet. The plastic, two-shelf unit flips down when you need it and stays hidden when not in use. Cost is about $10 from mail-order firms. **Source:** 415.

A wall grid system is another space-saving way to store kitchen utensils. You may purchase a grid alone and use hooks to hang the utensils or buy a grid with shelves and hooks included. Grids must be periodically removed for washing. **Manufacturers:** 330, 353. Cost is about $15 and up for a single grid unit and $30 for a grid with shelves, from housewares stores and mail-order firms.

A kitchen utensil carousel and a spice storage carousel are examples of storage aids that hold frequently used tools and condiments neatly on your counter or in a cabinet (Figure 14-7). Several models are available in plastic, acrylic, or wood. **Manufacturers:** 215. Cost is $12 and up from housewares stores and mail-order firms. **Sources:** 82, 231, 270, 353, 373. A solution to cluttered drawers, the carousel places cooking utensils where they are easy to reach and grasp. For a carousel with compartments and hooks to hold utensils, cost is $15 and up from mail-order firms. **Source:** 171. For a carousel that holds herb and spice containers for easier access than reaching into a cabinet, cost is $12 and up from housewares stores and mail-order firms.

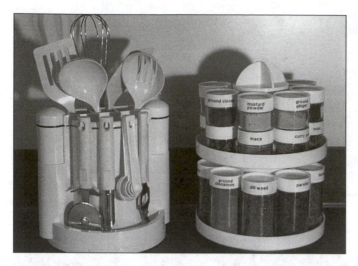

Figure 14-7. A kitchen utensil carousel and a spice storage carousel are examples of storage aids that hold frequently used tools and condiments neatly on your counter or in a cabinet. (Photo courtesy of M. Kaminstein. Photo by J.K.)

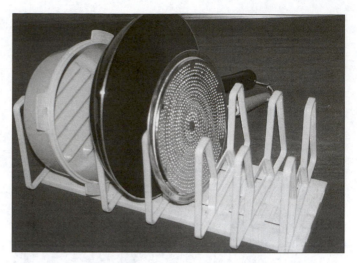

Figure 14-9. A bakeware organizer of plastic or vinyl-coated steel may be used on the counter or in a cabinet to store baking pans, cookie sheets, and serving trays. (Photo by J.K.)

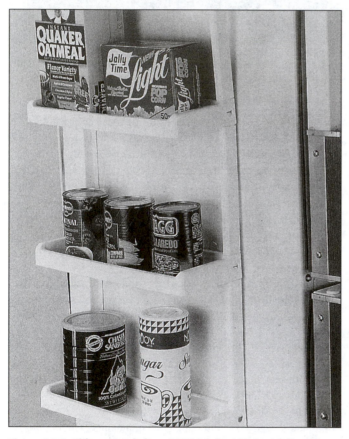

Figure 14-8. Side space shelves, 28" high by 13½" wide by 3" deep, mount on your refrigerator, washer, or other vertical surface to hold foods and supplies. (Photo courtesy of Jobar International, Los Angeles, CA.)

Manufacturer: 215. **Sources:** 82, 231, 270, 373.

A countertop shelf makes double use of the accessible space between the cabinets and countertop. A wooden sink rack utilizes otherwise unused space over the faucet area. **Manufacturer:** 134.

You may construct your own out of wood, or purchase a wood, vinyl-coated steel, or plastic shelf. Cost is about $15 and up from gourmet specialty firms, housewares stores, and mail-order firms. **Sources:** 173, 185, 192, 194, 270, 387, 415.

Side space shelves, 28" high by 13½" wide by 3" deep, mount on your refrigerator, washer, or other vertical surface to hold foods and supplies (Figure 14-8). Two suction cups at the top and two behind the second shelf secure the unit. Adhesive disks are included to increase seal if needed. **Manufacturer:** 209. Cost is about $10 per set from mail-order firms. **Sources:** 231, 387.

A bakeware organizer of plastic or vinyl-coated steel may be used on the counter or in a cabinet to store baking pans, cookie sheets, and serving trays (Figure 14-9). When working with one hand or weak arms, the file eliminates unstacking to retrieve one item. **Manufacturer:** 161. The cost is $6 and up from housewares stores and mail-order firms. **Sources:** 59, 242, 270, 415.

REFRIGERATOR STORAGE AIDS

Refrigerator door shelves are the easiest shelves to reach with weak or arthritic hands or from a wheelchair, so be sure to reserve this space for frequently used items. Bring your cart or wheelchair lapboard as close to the open refrigerator as possible for quick, safe transfer of items. Keep the heaviest packages on a shelf even with the height of the lapboard or cart so you can slide them to and from the refrigerator. Adding an extra shelf or pull-out shelves to your freezer does away with the need to shift items around. Several in-cabinet storage aids may also be used in a refrigerator. Check sizes and the design of your shelves to see what might work.

A beverage can dispenser uses gravity to bring cans to the front. It may also be used for storing other containers. Distributor: 61. Cost is $7 and up from mail-order firms. **Sources**: 171, 173, 270, 415. A freezer basket organizes frozen foods. Containers stack so that you can see foods. Made of vinyl-coated steel. **Manufacturer:** 161. Cost is $10 and up from mail-order firms. **Source:** 270.

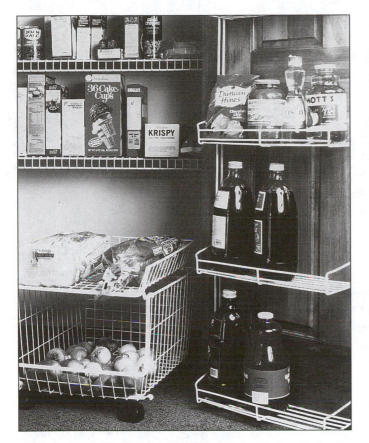

Figure 14-10. A skinny pantry organizer rack installed on the back of a door or free wall creates an instant pantry for canned or packaged foods. (Photo courtesy of Clairson International, Ocala, FL.)

OTHER STORAGE AIDS

Fruits, vegetables, even kitchen utensils can be stored in hanging tiered baskets. Baskets come as single, double, or triple units (three-basket unit is about 34" long) and can be hung in a convenient location. **Manufacturers: 142, 289.** Cost is $6 and up per set from department and variety stores or mail-order firms.

Stacking storage bins hold vegetables, fruits, cans, and equipment. They may be placed inside or outside a cabinet. **Manufacturers: 69, 343, 403.** Available from housewares and hardware stores, building suppliers, or mail-order firms. You can also decorate your walls with functional storage aids, such as baskets and small shelves. A wine rack can be turned into a handy storage container for table linen, silverware, and juice cans.

Hang a towel by the sink, a cane by the counter or a basket on the wall using a small strip of Velcro®. Also use hook-and-loop fasteners to keep long appliance cords neat. Look for adhesive-backed Velcro® products in variety, hardware, and sewing stores. Keep Velcro® products away from open flames. **Manufacturer: 409.**

A skinny pantry organizer rack installed on the back of a door or free wall creates an instant pantry for canned or packaged foods (Figure 14-10). Vinyl-coated wire or aluminum shelf kits adjust to door dimensions. **Manufacturers** include 69. Prices range from about $10 for a small, two-shelf unit to $33 and up for a four- to five-shelf, full-length door unit. The unit is available from building suppliers, hardware stores, and mail-order firms. **Sources: 71, 173, 270, 415.**

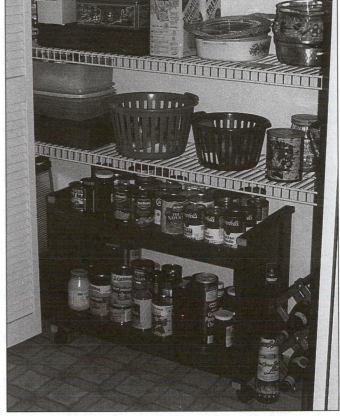

Figure 14-11. A converted television table provides rolling storage for in-closet storage of canned goods. (Designed by T.E. Lannefeld, Fort Myers, FL.)

A converted television table provides rolling storage for in-closet storage of canned goods (Figure 14-11). The entire closet has been fitted with vinyl-coated steel shelves, with lighter items stored on the higher shelves. Folding doors allow full access to contents.

Use the metal sides of your refrigerator or other appliances for magnetic storage aids (Figure 14-12). These include various-sized caddy pockets, paper towel holder, memo holder, utensils rack, towel bar, spice rack, and sets of individual hooks. **Manufacturer: 365.** Cost is $9 each and up from housewares stores and mail-order firms. **Sources: 231, 242, 270, 415.**

If you have good reach and strength in your arms, you might consider using some overhead space for a pot rack for storage of pots and pans (Figure 14-13). Racks of metal or wood construction are available in a variety of shapes and sizes from gourmet specialty and mail-order firms. **Manufacturer: 63. Sources: 65, 82.**

A wooden peg rack provides decorative storage on free wall space (Figure 14-14). Use this rack to hang mugs, pans, towels, extra pot holders, cookie cutters, and other utensils that have a loop or a hole in the handle. The rack mounts vertically or horizontally and expands to 60" or more. Cost is $12 and up from housewares stores and mail-order firms. **Sources: 59, 173, 242, 270.**

Keep extra plastic bags in a single dispenser. Unit mounts on wall door or inside cabinet. Push empty bags into top of dispenser, then pull from bottom when needed. **Manufacturer: 309.** Cost is about $6 and up from housewares stores and mail-order firms. **Source: 173.**

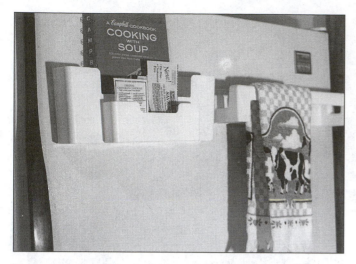

Figure 14-12. Use the metal sides of your refrigerator or other appliances for magnetic storage aids. (Photo by J.K.)

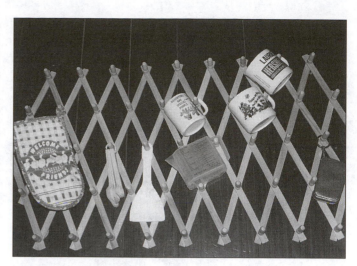

Figure 14-14. A wooden peg rack provides decorative storage on free wall space. (Photo by J.K.)

REACHERS

Tongs to pick up lightweight items come in many styles. If using a wheelchair, you may want a small pair that tucks next to you in your seat. If you have arthritis or back pain, a longer reacher saves added stress from bending. See Chapter 2.

Pick-up tongs are available in many styles to suit your needs. Some reachers have vinyl-covered or rubber-lined tongs or fingers to grip round or flat items. You must have enough strength to squeeze the trigger handle to maintain grasp on the object being lifted. Try out various reachers before purchasing; discuss the design features best for you with an occupational or physical therapist. Cost varies widely as does design. The most reliable reaching aids are available from self-help firms.

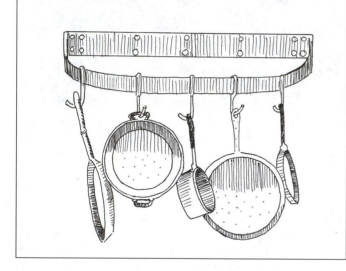

Figure 14-13. If you have good reach and strength in your arms, you might consider using some overhead space for a pot rack for storage of pots and pans. (Illustration by G.K.)

Food Storage

Storing food safely and correctly preserves its flavor, freshness, and nutrients. Leftovers should be refrigerated as soon as possible to prevent spoiling.

Keep your refrigerator at 40°F or below. Bacteria that cause food poisoning begin multiplying above 40°F. Most foods stored in the refrigerator should be covered tightly to prevent loss of moisture.

Check the labels on prepared foods to determine if they must be refrigerated after opening. Contents can usually be stored in their original containers if covered tightly. It is best, however, not to store leftovers in cans. If your home is very warm, you may want to refrigerate peanut butter, shelled nuts, and syrups.

Hot foods do not have to cool before being refrigerated. In fact, letting cooked foods stand at room temperature to cool is an invitation to food spoilage.

To keep your refrigerator clean, wipe up spills immediately. Baking soda mixed with warm water makes an excellent solution for washing the inside of your refrigerator; an open box of baking soda set inside the refrigerator will help reduce odors. Vacuum the back of and underneath your refrigerator at least twice a year; clean the drain pan underneath it every six months.

FREEZER STORAGE

For energy efficiency, keep your freezer at least three-quarters full. Freezer wrappings must be airtight, so that the food will not dry out or become "freezer burned." Foods wrapped in foil or paper should be put inside plastic bags for extra protection.

Label and date everything you freeze. Freezer labels cost about $3 per roll from housewares stores and mail-order firms. Cost of a freezer pen is about $1 from stationery stores and mail-order firms. **Source:** 270. It is also helpful to include the food's expiration date. Meat should be eaten within four months; baked goods within three months; casseroles within two to three months; and vegetables within eight to 12 months. An inventory chart on your freezer door helps you keep track of frozen foods. Cost is about $5 from housewares stores and mail-order firms. **Source:** 270.

Thaw food overnight in the refrigerator, or use your microwave, rather than leaving it on the counter to defrost.

Do not re-freeze foods after thawing. In case of power failure, do not open the freezer. Foods will stay frozen up to 24 hours before gradually thawing.

FOOD STORAGE TIPS

- Choose a cool, dry place to store pantry foods. Avoid storing food items under the kitchen sink or near the plumbing fixtures.
- Fresh meat, fish, fruits, and vegetables should not be washed before refrigerating. Wash them when you are ready to use them.
- Bananas, uncut melons, avocados, and pineapples are best stored at a cool room temperature and eaten as soon as they ripen. Berries should be kept dry and refrigerated until you are ready to use them. Other fruits may be stored in a crisper or, for easier retrieval, in perforated plastic bags on the refrigerator shelf.
- Before storing pantry foods, date them. Twice a year, check your pantry, rotating the older foods to the front.
- When storing canned goods, place new cans upside-down on the back of the shelf. Up-end those that were there so that you will use them first. Wash lids before opening. Throw away any dented, leaking, or bulging cans. If, when you open a can, liquid spurts out or contents look cloudy, discard the can and contents, without tasting.
- A bay leaf in dry foods, such as flour, cornmeal, oats, and rice will help keep bugs away. Bay leaves contain a harmless chemical that repels them.
- When handling meat, plastic or acrylic cutting boards are easier to clean than wooden boards. Prevent contamination from raw meat by using a separate board to cut fruits and vegetables.
- Wash your hands before starting a meal. Food is only as clean as the hands that prepare it.

A Foam Bin Liner helps keep fruits and vegetables fresher by

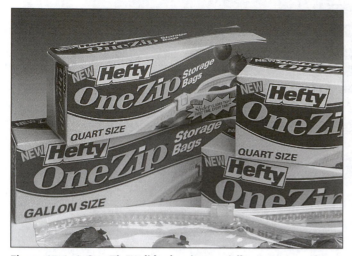

Figure 15-1. A One Zip™ slider bag is especially easy to use if you have limited vision or poor coordination but good pinch in one hand. (One Zip™ bags by Mobil Chemical Co., Pittsford, NY. Photo by J.K.)

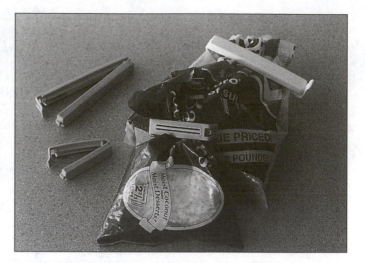

Figure 15-3. If twist ties and small plastic closures are difficult to use because of incoordination, use of one hand, or weakness, try Twixit™ Clips. (Twixit™ Clips by Larand International, Inc., St. Paul, MN. Photo by J.K.)

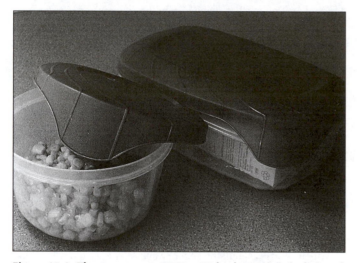

Figure 15-2. The cover on an EZ Topp™ food container is designed so that it releases with light pressure under the extended corner. (EZ Topp™ by Rubbermaid, Inc., Wooster, OH. Photo by J.K.)

preventing bruising and spoiling in your refrigerator crisper. The reticulated, or open-celled foam, the same used in supermarket produce refrigerators, allows air to circulate freely under and around food and prevents moisture from settling on the fruits and vegetables. To clean, wash with mild dishwashing liquid and water, rinse well, and let air dry. **Manufacturers:** 54, 255. Cost is about $4 for a large pad, which may be cut to size for smaller bins. Pads are available from housewares stores and mail-order firms. **Sources:** 71, 194, 270, 378, 410, 415.

FOOD WRAPS AND STORAGE CONTAINERS

Plastic bags and wraps are useful for refrigerator and pantry storage. If you are working with one hand, a zipper-top plastic bag may be easier to use than one that closes with a twist-tie. Put the bag edge on the counter, and press the grooves at the "zipper top" together for a tight seal.

A One Zip™ slider bag is especially easy to use if you have limited vision or poor coordination but good pinch in one hand (Figure 15-1). Rather than having to align grooves, a "slider" is moved across the top of the bag, sealing it securely. Available in varied sizes for short-term storage and for heavy-duty freezer use, you will find these bags in housewares stores and supermarkets. **Manufacturer:** 274.

Special plastic bags that "breathe" to absorb and remove the ethylene gas released by harvested produce decrease moisture and keep vegetables or fruits fresher longer. **Manufacturers** include 101. Cost is about $12 for 20 bags from housewares stores and mail-order firms. **Source:** 194.

Aluminum foil is practical for the freezer, since you can mold it around the food and exclude air. For freezer storage, use heavy-duty foil. Do not store tomatoes, tomato sauces, citrus fruits, barbecue sauces, and other high acid foods in aluminum foil wrap or containers. Store these foods in plastic or glass containers.

Non-breakable storage containers with tightly fitting lids can be used to store food in the freezer, refrigerator, and pantry. Before purchasing, make sure you are able to open and close the container lids.

The cover on an EZ Topp™ food container is designed so that it releases with light pressure under the extended corner (Figure 15-2). The microwavable, reheatable plastic containers are available in about 20 different styles. Cost is $1.50 and up from housewares stores. **Manufacturer:** 343.

Air-tight, shatterproof plastic canisters, which keep foods fresh and free from pests, are available with snap or flip-top locking lids. Snap-Ware® canisters of Flexiglas™ come as clear countertop or pantry canisters, each with a snap-lock lid that opens or closes with one hand. Cost is about $2.50 each and up from housewares stores and mail-order firms. **Manufacturer:** 141. **Sources:** 290, 359, 369.

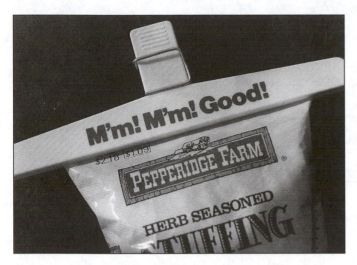

Figure 15-4. A large clip keeps bags of stuffing, crackers, and chips fresh. (Photo by J.K.)

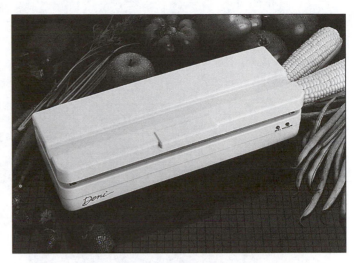

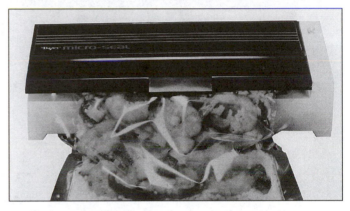

Figures 15-5A, 15-5B. Use an electric sealing unit to enclose single servings or large portions of food in durable plastic pouches for refrigeration or freezer storage. (Photos courtesy of Deni®, Keystone Manufacturing, Buffalo, NY, and Dazey® Corporation, Industrial Airport, KA.)

Disposable foil pans for baking and roasting in a conventional oven are available in many sizes and may also be used as freezer containers. If, however, you are working with one hand or have incoordination, these flexible foil containers are more dangerous to manage than a solid pan when filled with hot foods. They may not be used in a microwave.

A reusable, microwave plate cover eliminates the need for plastic wrap. The dishwasher safe plastic cover fits over a regular serving plate and is vented to release excess heat as well as to control moisture loss. Cost is about $8 for a set of two from housewares stores and mail-order firms. **Sources:** 270, 378, 410.

If twist ties and small plastic closures are difficult to use because of incoordination, use of one hand, or weakness, try Twixit™ Clips (Figure 15-3). These polypropylene reusable bag sealers snap shut with light pressure to tightly re-seal bread, freezer, cereal, pet, snack, and other foods. An extended edge makes the clip easy to open with one hand or weak hands. They may be labeled on the flat surface. Designed in Sweden, the hinged "kitchen close pins" are boil-, freezer-, microwave-, and dishwasher-safe. **Manufacturer:** 228. A set of 25 in assorted sizes (2¼", 4¼", and 5½") costs about $10 and up from variety stores and mail-order firms. **Sources:** 71, 185, 242, 270, 378, 410.

A large clip keeps bags of stuffing, crackers, and chips fresh (Figure 15-4). Cost is $1 and up from variety stores and mail-order firms. **Source:** 270. A spring-type plastic or wooden clothespin is also a handy aid for closing bags.

Use an electric sealing unit to enclose single servings or large portions of food in durable plastic pouches for refrigeration or freezer storage (Figures 15-5A and 15-5B). For easier filling, stand the bag in a bowl to stabilize it. A wide-based canning funnel will help. The appliance comes with pouches of assorted sizes or a roll of polyethylene to make a pouch of any size. When ready to use, immerse filled pouch in boiling water until the contents are heated. **Manufacturers:** 15-5-A, 94; 15- 5-B, 89. Cost is $40 and up from housewares stores. **Sources:** 176, 359, 407.

FOOD WRAP TIPS

- Freeze ground meat in patties. Wrap patties individually in foil or plastic wrap. Ground meat frozen in patties thaws faster and is easier to use as a burger or in a sauce or casserole.
- If meat or pastry browns too quickly while roasting or baking, cover the brown areas with pieces of foil.
- For easy freezing and reheating of foods, line casserole dish with foil or plastic wrap, fill, cover, and freeze. When frozen, remove contents from the dish and place in a plastic bag. When ready to use, peel off the wrapping, return the contents to the casserole dish to thaw, then heat.
- To reduce the need for scrubbing, line the bottom of your broiler pan with foil. Cover the top rack of the broiler pan with foil, but pierce the foil to allow fat to drip through to pan below.
- Marinate meat or poultry in a plastic bag. Shift the bag's position in the bowl periodically so the meat will marinate evenly.
- Mix meatloaf in a plastic bag. You can knead it with one hand just like bread, then put it into a pan.
- Roll pie crust between sheets of waxed paper. It will be easier to judge the size and to pick up, even with one hand.
- If you have weak grasp, here is a way to handle food wraps:

Place the box on the counter in front of you, hold the edge of the wrap between both hands. Gently shake out the amount you need. Hold the box in place with one arm. To tear off a piece of wrap, press down with your forearm along the "cutting" edge of the box.

GOING FURTHER

Addresses are given in the Appendices.

PUBLICATIONS

The Safe Food Book. Free from the Consumer Information Center.

CHAPTER

16

Getting Around

If your arms are weak, if you have arthritis, back pain, incoordination, or if you are working with one hand, a cart helps reduce stress on your joints and muscles. It is also a safe way to move several items at one time or to transport a heavy object.

Simple carrying aids, such as baskets and aprons with big pockets, also help increase the amount you can efficiently move from place to place.

WHEELED TABLES AND CARTS

A cart saves steps. It is not, however, a substitute for your prescribed walking aid; do not depend on it to support you. Push the cart forward, and use your cane, crutch, or walker for balance. When choosing a cart, consider the following:

- Select a unit for durability, not style.
- Make sure the cart will not tip if you lean on one side.
- Make sure the cart's height is comfortable. You should not have to lean over to push it.
- Raised handles help you to push more comfortably and efficiently. The top shelf should be high enough for you to set down and pick up items without bending.
- If you need more stability, select a heavier commercial cart. These carts are sold through office and restaurant supply firms. Alternatively, add stability by putting sandbags or canned goods (held in a box or pan) on the bottom shelf.
- Shelves with raised edges prevent items from slipping and falling off.
- Larger diameter casters move more smoothly.
- Microwave carts are not recommended for transporting items. They are normally too heavy and difficult to propel.

With a lightweight trolley, you can set the table in one trip, and then transfer hot items from the range to the dining area (Figure 16-1). The trolley moves easily on casters and can be pushed with your body while you use a walking aid or wheelchair. Raised edges on shelves keep things from rolling off. You could also use the shelves to store basic cooking supplies so you don't have to gather them each time you cook. **Manufacturer:** 69. Small trolleys, which cost $18 and up, are available from housewares stores and mail-order firms. **Sources**: 169, 242, 407.

Some carts can be used as work tables or even as a mobile eating place. The bottom shelf of the multi-use folding cart may be retracted so that you can sit at the cart without hitting your shins (Figure 16-2). The cart's high handles are designed to eliminate stooping while you push. It folds for storage. **Manufacturer:** 80. Cost is about $70 from housewares stores and self-help firms. **Sources:** 120, 408.

Library carts have large rubber casters for smooth movement and deep edges to keep items from sliding off the top or bottom shelf. Cost is about $135. **Source:** 153. A heavy-duty, molded, commercial busing cart has raised handles for maneuvering, textured shelves with rims on three sides, and one open side for easy loading and unloading. It is designed to move quietly and smoothly. Cart stands 36" high, or as tall as a standard countertop, so you can slide items from it rather than lift them. Containers that fit on the ends are available to hold flatware or trash. **Manufacturer:** 341.

A raised handle eliminates the need to bend while pushing (Figure 16-3). Stainless-steel carts used in business offices come in a variety of styles and sizes. The heavy-duty casters roll smoothly, and the weight provides stability. Raised edges and rubber bumpers safeguard walls and furnishings. Mail carts with removable deep wire baskets accommodate foods, dishes, and baking supplies. The front wheels swivel for precise maneuvering. Cost is $125 and up. **Manufacturer:** 43. Carts are available through office supply and durable medical firms. **Sources:** 16 (illustrated), 52, 158, 293.

AIDS FOR CARRYING LIGHT ITEMS

If you use a walker, attach a basket or bag to hold lightweight items. See Chapter 4. For wheelchair use, a lapboard with a raised rim can be used for safe carrying. See Chapter 7.

A sturdy basket with a single or double handle lets you carry lightweight things over your arm. A smock or apron with large

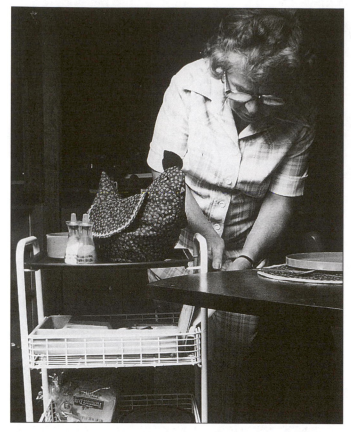

Figure 16-1. With a lightweight trolley, you can set the table in one trip and then transfer hot items from the range to the dining area. (Photo by J.K.)

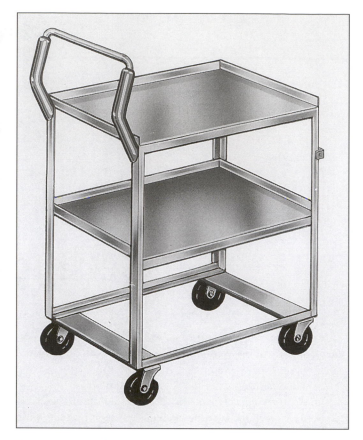

Figure 16-3. A raised handle eliminates the need to bend while pushing. (Photo courtesy of AliMed®, Inc., Dedham, MA.)

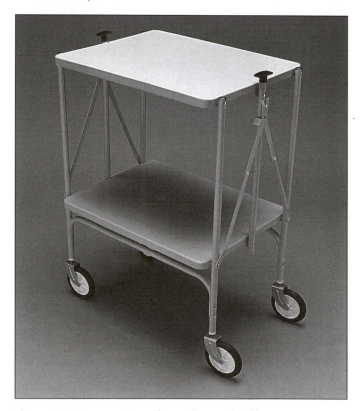

Figure 16-2. Some carts can be used as work tables or even a mobile eating place. (Photo courtesy of North Coast Medical, San Jose, CA.)

pockets does double duty, carrying small items while keeping clothes clean. A utility or cobbler's apron, which slips over your shoulders, distributes weight better than an apron that ties around your waist. Cost is $9 and up from department stores and mail-order firms. **Sources:** 42, 165, 173, 210. A wire basket with a wide handle and flat bottom is a convenient tote for carrying a snack or light meal. **Manufacturer:** 95. Cost is $6 and up from housewares stores. A buffet caddy basket stores and carries silverware and napkins in one trip. Cost is $5 and up in wicker, acrylic, or wood from housewares stores and mail-order firms. **Sources:** 71, 82, 173, 231, 242, 270, 378.

Non-slip trays for one- or two-handed use are available from self-help firms or restaurant suppliers (Figure 16-4). The Dycem® non-slip or other rubberized surface keeps objects from sliding. Tray is dishwasher safe. **Manufacturers** include 341. Cost is $20 and up.

MOVING LARGE ITEMS

Sometimes it is a large object that you wish to move, such as for cleaning, for better access to your wheelchair, or for a better view, as with a television cabinet. Adding casters or glides to the bottom of the item does makes the moving easier. If, however, you have weakness or back pain, enlist the help of someone else to do this heavy work.

It is recommended that you do not put wheels or gliders on

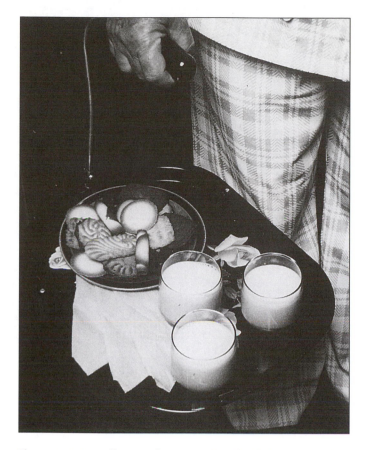

Figure 16-4. Non-slip trays for one- or two-handed use are available from self-help firms or restaurant suppliers. The Dycem® non-slip or other rubberized surface keeps objects from sliding. (Photo by J.K.)

chair legs as the chair may slip as you lower yourself into it or attempt to rise.

Self-stick wheels reduce stress and protect your back by turning storage units, bookcases, cabinets, clothes hampers, and trash

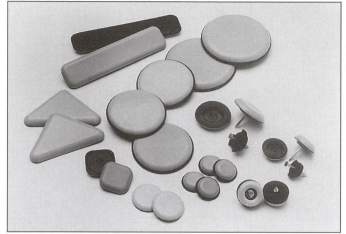

Figure 16-5. Magic Sliders® attach to the bottoms of the feet or base of furniture. Available in various sizes, these peel-and-stick Teflon/rubber disks prevent scratching of the flooring. (Photo courtesy of Magic Sliders®, White Plains, NY.)

containers into more easily movable items. A set of four Roll-Arounds™ comes with specially formulated peel-and-stick adhesive for permanent bonding. **Manufacturer:** 259. Cost is about $8 per set from variety stores and mail-order firms.

Magic Sliders® attach to the bottoms of the feet or base of furniture (Figure 16-5). Available in various sizes, these peel-and-stick Teflon/rubber disks prevent scratching of the flooring and will work with linoleum, ceramic tiles, wood, and carpeting. **Manufacturer:** 254. Cost is about $7 and up per set of four from variety stores and mail-order firms. **Sources:** 242, 304, 364, 369.

For outside moving of large loads, such as groceries in from the car or trash to the correct receptacles, ask for help. If necessary, you may use a wheeled unit designed for outdoor use. These include folding carts, which are available from housewares and boating stores or mail-order firms. **Sources:** 169, 312, 374.

Kitchen Cleanup

ENERGY-SAVING TECHNIQUES

- Use a wheeled cart or lapboard to carry your dishes from table to work area.
- Sit on a stool or tall chair when washing dishes; or add height to a standard kitchen chair with a cushion or leg extenders to make reaching less tiring. See Chapter 2.
- To sit closer to your sink, open the cabinet doors, and remove the base molding so you can extend your feet into the cabinet. Make sure the pipes are covered or wrapped to prevent burning your legs.
- Rinse dishes well; let them air dry in a dish drainer. Only silverplate, sterling, and cast iron need to be dried by hand.

TIPS FOR QUICK CLEANUP

- Line range-top drip pans with non-stick inserts so that you can wipe away spills and splatters more easily. **Manufacturers** include 142. Various sizes for electric or gas ranges cost about $4 each and up from housewares stores and mail-order firms. **Sources:** 59, 173, 270, 415.
- Mix ingredients right in a casserole. There is no extra bowl, and no transferring of ingredients.
- Cook with non-stick pans; use recommended utensils and recommended cleaning products to protect their finishes.
- Line bottoms of pans with foil when roasting or broiling meat or fish in standard oven.
- Use oven-to-table cookware, or serve directly from the pan.
- If you have prepared the meal, delegate the cleanup, or share it with family members.
- Soak pans immediately. Let residues soften while you eat. Fill pots used for starchy foods or eggs with cold water; use a little soap and hot water for greasy pots.
- Reduce cleanup with paper plates and cups. They may be used to heat food in the microwave oven.
- Use paper or foil muffin pan liners when making cupcakes or muffins.

Set up your work area for a coordinated flow of activity from right to left, or vice versa, with soiled dishes, wash water, rinse water (or spray), and drainer (Figure 17-1). If you are using only one hand, put the rinse water and drying rack next to the working hand.

If kitchen counter or sink space is at a premium, use a folding rack. Available in vinyl-coated steel or wood, a rack costs $9 and up from housewares stores and mail-order firms. **Sources:** 71, 82, 242, 270, 378, 427. Mini or half-size drainers and drains are made for small kitchens or for cooking for one. **Manufacturer:** 403. Cost is $3 and up from housewares stores.

Direct water back into the sink with a vinyl-coated steel, angled drainer tray. The tray slips under your regular dish rack. It comes in two sizes: 12" square or 12" x 16". Cost is $3 and up from housewares stores and mail-order firms. **Sources:** 171, 173, 415.

Make sure that your sink is a comfortable depth (Figure 17-2). Stretch your palms as far as you can toward the bottom of the sink. If you cannot reach the bottom, add a simple rack.

A rack may be built out of wood, which should be strong enough to support a filled dishpan. To prevent warping and splitting, the wood grain must run lengthwise; use two nails to fasten the ends of each slat to the upright pieces. Apply a water-resistant finish to keep the wood from getting water soaked. Alternatively, you can build up the sides of a commercially available vinyl-coated steel sink liner by attaching thick strips of wood.

Tap turners with extended handles increase leverage to help you operate faucets if your hands are weak or affected by arthritis (Figure 17-3). Some models resemble a wrench and may be left in place or removed when not in use. Cost is $24 and up from self-help firms. **Sources:** 5, 13, 120, 130, 264, 290, 370, 408.

An S-shaped closet hook on a dowel also makes a handy tool for turning handles. Single-handle, washerless faucets can be operated with a push of your hand. See Chapter 13.

A swivel sprayer aerator attached to your faucet lets you reach

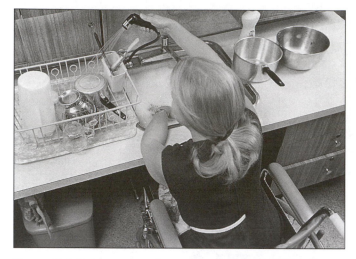

Figure 17-1. Set up your work area for a coordinated flow of activity from right to left, or vice versa, with soiled dishes, wash water, rinse water (or spray), and drainer. (Photo courtesy of the O.T. Dept., Howard A. Rusk Institute of Rehabilitation Medicine.)

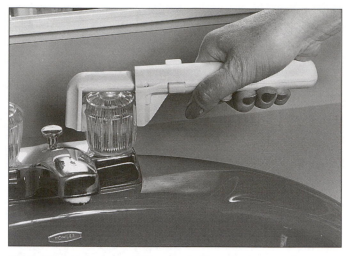

Figure 17-3. Tap turners with extended handles increase leverage to help you operate faucets if your hands are weak or affected by arthritis. (Photo courtesy of Sammons/Preston, a Bissell® Healthcare Co., Jackson, MI.)

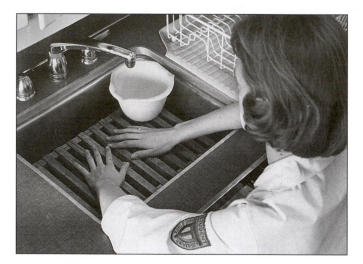

Figure 17-2. Make sure that your sink is a comfortable depth. (Photo courtesy of the O.T. Dept., Howard A. Rusk Institute of Rehabilitation Medicine.)

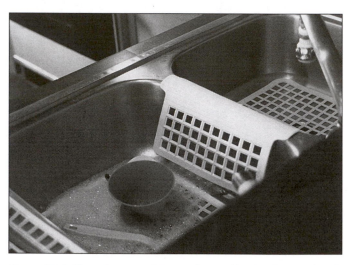

Figure 17-4. If you have weakness or incoordination in your hands or loss of vision, a sink guard or rubber mat cushions the bottom of the sink to help prevent breakage and to keep dishes from slipping while you scrub. (Photo by J.K.)

every corner. The unit fits standard faucets and is made to stay cool. Distributor: 149. Cost is $5 and up from hardware stores and mail-order firms. **Sources:** 270, 378, 415.

If you have weakness or incoordination in your hands or loss of vision, a sink guard or rubber mat cushions the bottom of the sink to help prevent breakage and to keep dishes from slipping while you scrub (Figure 17-4). Liners are also available to fit the sides of a sink. **Manufacturer:** 343. Vinyl-coated steel protectors, rubber mats for single or double sinks, and cut-to-fit-liners cost about $5 each and up. **Sources:** 59, 65, 185, 242. See Chapter 1.

Latex or neoprene gloves are especially helpful if your hands are weak, your coordination is poor, or you have loss of sensation (Figure 17-5). The neoprene helps insulate your hands against hot water. Look for latex gloves with raised rubber studs on the fingers and palms to help you grip wet dishes firmly. A knit cotton lining lets you slip them on easily. **Manufacturer:** 29. Cost is about $4

per pair in small, medium, or large sizes from housewares stores.

A plastic refillable dishwasher brush holds liquid detergent in its handle and has at one end a nylon bristle brush for scrubbing regular or non-stick pans. A second one could be helpful in the laundry for spot-treating shirt collars and stains. **Manufacturer:** 142. Cost is about $2 from department stores and mail-order firms.

A half-glove mitt covers your fingers and may be easier to slip on than a full glove (Figure 17-6). You can grasp a scouring pad with this flexible mitt. It does not, however, protect your hand against hot water. Cost is about $4 from housewares stores and mail-order firms.

To stabilize a pan for scrubbing, place a damp sponge cloth under it, or wedge the pan into a sink corner. A scrub sponge speeds cleanup and allows you to work with your fingers extended. **Manufacturers** include 102, 272. Cost is about $1 and up from housewares and grocery stores.

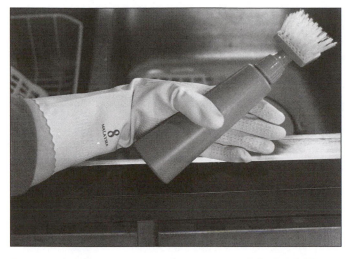

Figure 17-5. Latex or neoprene gloves are especially helpful if your hands are weak, your coordination is poor, or if you have loss of sensation. (Photo by J.K.)

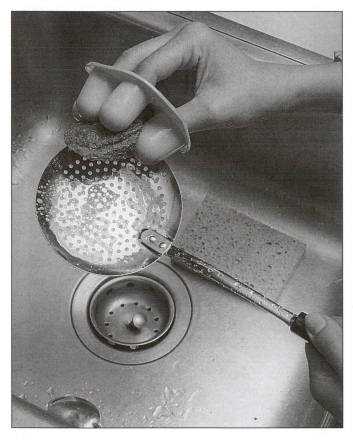

Figure 17-6. A half-glove mitt covers your fingers and may be easier to slip on than a full glove. (Photo courtesy of the O.T. Dept., Howard A. Rusk Institute of Rehabilitation Medicine.)

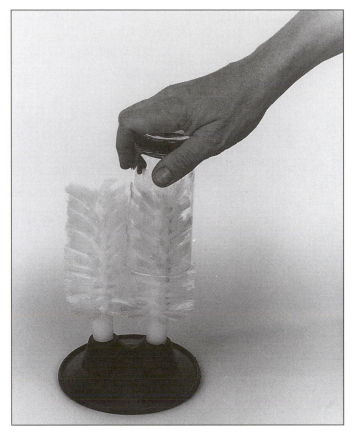

Figure 17-7. Suction-based brushes for washing glasses and dishes attach to the bottom or side of your sink. (Photo courtesy of Enrichments®, Sammons/Preston, a Bissell® Healthcare Co., Bolingbrook, IL.)

Suction-based brushes for washing glasses and dishes attach to the bottom or side of your sink (Figure 17-7). Cost is about $10 and up from restaurant suppliers, and self-help and mail-order firms. **Sources:** 120, 173.

A vinyl-coated steel dishwasher basket with a hinged top fits on the top rack of your dishwasher and holds small, hard-to-retrieve appliance parts and lids. **Manufacturer:** 343. Cost is $4 and up from mail-order firms. **Sources:** 270, 415.

18

Household Cleanup

Consider your limitations before cleaning your house. If you have arthritis or post-polio syndrome, sweeping, scrubbing, and vacuuming may be harmful unless you use joint protection techniques. If you have a pulmonary condition, select a time when you have both the most energy and the optimal weather. Wear a mask to avoid inhaling dust, and plan frequent rest periods. If you tire easily, create a realistic and flexible schedule that will leave you with strength for the more important aspects of life.

To clean without overdoing it, try these tips:

- Cut down on housecleaning. Remember the motto "This house is clean enough to be healthy and dirty enough to be happy."
- Clean when you feel energetic.
- Clean just one room each day.
- Do light, daily once-overs to avoid accumulating dirt and clutter. Rinse the sink or tub after use. Pre-dampened cloths and non-abrasive cleansers are among the convenient step-saving cleaning products available.
- Enlist your family's help for deep-cleaning jobs. Also, family members should be responsible for picking up after themselves. If necessary to conserve your own strength, hire outside cleaning help. Check with your local Visiting Nurse Association for housekeeping helpers.
- Use a wheeled cart to move items around the house. See Chapter 16.
- Reduce trips by stocking duplicate cleaning supplies in the bathroom and kitchen, and upstairs and downstairs.
- If chores seem overwhelming, rethink how much you really need to do. Set reasonable goals. Your well-being is far more important than a polished table or dusted chair rung.
- Before you become too tired, take time to rest and relax when you are in the middle of a job, as well as after cleaning is done.

To cut down on cleaning, eliminate tracked-in dirt. Keep a brush for shoes outside the entrance and a mat just inside the door. Both mats and brushes are sold by housewares stores and mail-order firms. Cost is about $15 and up. **Sources** for mats: 194, 270, 378; for brushes: 49, 169, 185, 270, 312, 367, 369, 374.

Quick cleanups following meal preparation or another activity reduce the need for heavy-duty cleaning. Choose tools equipped with features that make tidying up easier. A long-handled dustpan and brush eliminate bending and help keep your distance from the dust. See Chapter 12.

Bending may also be kept to a minimum by using a long-handled sponge to remove spills from the floor and a long-handled scrub brush or sponge to clean the tub or shower. Cost of sponge is about $4 and up from housewares stores and mail-order firms. **Sources** for sponge: 185, 238, 378. Cost of brush is about $6 from housewares stores and mail-order firms. **Sources** for brush: 71, 171, 270.

A long-handled, swivel-head brush has a universal ball joint that allows the head to turn in any direction, simplifying cleaning crevices and behind furniture or bathroom fixtures. **Manufacturer:** 183. Cost is about $15 and up from housewares stores and mail-order firms. **Sources:** 171, 185, 270.

Select the lightest possible cleaning aids to reduce the amount of energy you use. A foam mop is lighter than a string mop.

A lightweight foam broom statically attracts dust, pet hairs, and grit from carpets, bare floors, and moldings (Figure 18-1). Dirt removes with dry cloth. Cost is $7 and up from mail-order firms. **Sources:** 49, 71, 173, 185, 194, 242, 270, 345.

A mop with a control on the handle lets you wash floors without bending and without touching the water (Figure 18-2). If you stabilize the handle under your arm, you may squeeze the mop head with one hand. **Manufacturers:** 148, 262, 343. Cost is about $14 from housewares and hardware stores or mail-order firms. **Sources:** 148, 194.

A double-well bucket holds both wash and rinse water, eliminating the need to return to the sink for clean water. **Manufacturers:** 148, 343. Cost is about $7 from housewares stores and mail-order firms. **Source:** 185. You may also use cleansers that don't require rinsing.

Putting the bucket on a dolly makes it easier to move around (Figure 18-3). The cost of a dolly designed for pails or adapted from a multi-mover or from one for a plant is about $8 and up from hardware stores and mail-order firms. **Sources:** 169, 173, 185, 270, 364.

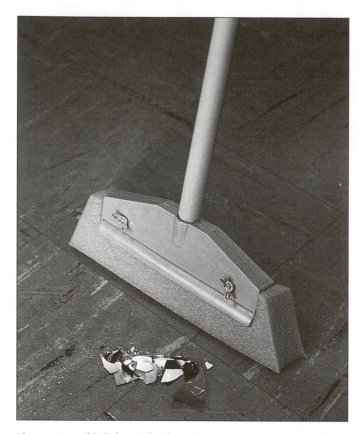

Figure 18-1. This lightweight, foam broom statically attracts dust, pet hairs, and grit from carpets, bare floors, and moldings. (Photo by J.K.)

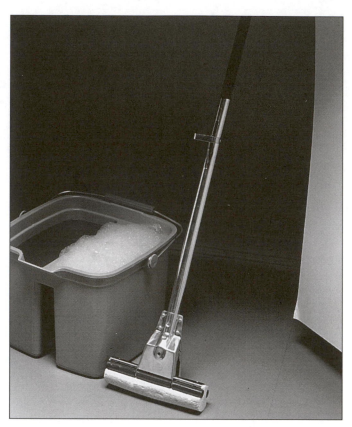

Figure 18-2. A mop with a control on the handle lets you wash floors without bending and without touching the water. (Photo courtesy of Fuller Brush® Company.)

Use a lightweight, hand-held vacuum to lift dirt from surfaces and upholstery. Rechargeable vacuums run eight to 10 minutes on a single charge; heavy-duty models run up to 15 minutes. If you have weakness, arthritis, or incoordination in your hands, use both hands to support and operate the appliance. **Manufacturers** include 41, 123, 189, 366. Cost is about $28 and up from housewares stores. **Sources:** 176, 356, 359, 373.

If you have arthritis, wear a dusting mitt to keep your fingers extended while dusting. If you have limited vision, weak grasp, or incoordination, the mitt permits better control than a cloth. Cost is about $3 from housewares stores and mail-order firms. **Source:** 270.

A telescoping duster of lambs wool or feathers will clean hard-to-reach places. **Manufacturer:** 142. Cost is about $13 each and up from housewares stores and mail-order forms. **Sources:** 49, 71, 167, 185, 312. Never climb on a chair or stool to reach; instead request help.

A flexible, fiberglass-handled dustmop bends when you clean under furniture, eliminating the need to get down on your knees. The acrylic mop head is machine-washable. Mop costs about $24 from mail-order firms. **Source:** 185.

CHOOSING A VACUUM CLEANER

When choosing a vacuum cleaner, consider the following:
• The types of floors and floor coverings you will be cleaning.

• The size of the area you will be cleaning.
• The amount of strength in your upper extremities.
• Whether you will be standing or using a glider chair or wheel-chair.

For light cleanup on non-carpeted floors, an electric broom may be easiest to maneuver (Figure 18-4). Dirt is collected in a cup, which is opened by a lever. **Manufacturers:** 41, 123, 189, 296, 332, 366. Cost is about $45 and up, depending on size and power. **Sources:** 167, 204, 356, 359, 373.

A lightweight carpet sweeper can be used on carpets and bare floors. As you push and pull it, rotating bristles adjust to floor surface. Dirt collects in a pan or two bins. The sweeper has wrap-around rubber bumpers to protect walls and furniture. **Manufacturers:** 148, 183, 189, 296. Cost is about $30 and up from housewares stores and mail-order firms. **Sources:** 71, 120, 148, 185, 296, 359, 369, 407, 410.

If you have carpets and are able to do general cleaning while standing, an upright vacuum cleaner is usually the best choice, because you can maintain good posture. If you have back pain or weakness in your arms and legs that makes pulling a weight stressful, choose a vacuum with a power drive. This type of vacuum moves by itself—all you do is guide it. Some machines include headlights, edge cleaners, and flexible joints for cleaning under furniture. Comparison-shop at reputable housewares and appliance dealers. **Manufacturers:** 114, 123, 189, 296, 366. Prices range from $80 and up. **Sources:** 87, 167, 185, 204, 296,

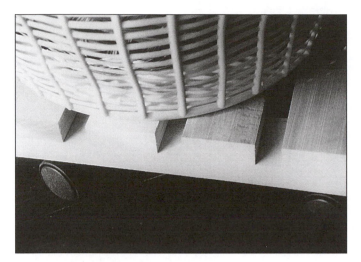

Figure 18-3. Putting a bucket or basket on a dolly makes it easier to move around. (Photo by J.K.)

356, 359, 373.

If you sit in a glider chair or wheelchair to clean, a canister vacuum cleaner is preferred. Select the lightest unit with adequate power to do the job you need. Before you purchase one, check whether it is light enough for you to pull around, whether it rolls smoothly from surface to surface, and whether the controls are easy to operate. **Manufacturers:** 114, 123, 189, 366. Cost is about $100 and up. **Sources:** 71, 204, 356, 359, 373.

For light cleaning while sitting, you might try an over-the-shoulder or hand-held vacuum that you hold in your lap. **Manufacturers:** 189, 296. Cost is $60 and up. **Sources:** 204, 356, 359, 373.

If you are planning extensive remodeling, consider installing a central vacuum cleaning system. The automatic on/off vacuum controls are installed directly into the walls. You only have to manage the hose and attachments. A caddy holds cleaning attachments. The system takes the dirt to a central collector, and it is vented outside to prevent re-circulation of dust during cleaning. Write to manufacturer for details and cost. **Source:** 291.

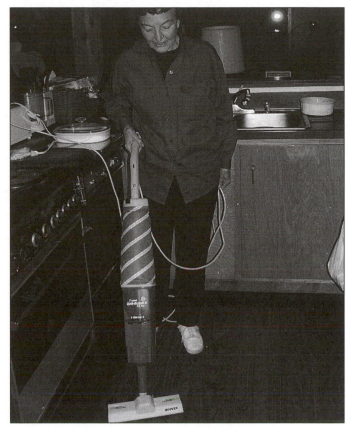

Figure 18-4. For light cleanup on non-carpeted floors, an electric broom may be easiest to maneuver. (Photo by J.K.)

GOING FURTHER

Addresses are given in the Appendices.

PUBLICATIONS

Aslet, D. (1992). Is There Life After Housework? Cincinnatti, OH: Writer's Digest Books. **Source:** 431C.

Campbell, J. (1992). *Clutter Control*. New York: Bantam Doubleday, Dell Publishing.

Felton, S. (1984). *The Messies Manual: The Procrastinator's Guide to Good Housekeeping*. Old Tappan, NJ: Fleming H. Ravell Co.

Section Three

KITCHEN UTILITIES, TOOLS, AND APPLIANCES

CHAPTER

19

Using Gas and Electricity

During the past 30 years, the number of home appliances requiring electricity has increased from 40 to more than 200. Each new appliance puts a drain on your household power supply. It is estimated that more than half of all houses in the United States need to be rewired. If you depend on electricity to handle meal preparation tasks, it is wise to check your household's electrical capacity. Look for these signs of inadequate wiring:

- Lights dim when appliances are being used.
- Fuses blow or circuit breakers frequently trip off.
- You need several two- and three-way plugs in sockets to accommodate lights and appliances.
- You have to disconnect appliances before you are able to use others.

If you note any of these problems, have your wiring checked. Appliances won't work at peak efficiency; motors will burn out sooner. Your electrician may recommend that you add an additional circuit to accommodate increased usage.

Appliances are classified as "heating" and "non-heating" units. Heating appliances, such as toasters, microwave ovens, electric skillets, or broilers, require a lot of power and should be used one at a time. Non-heating appliances, such as can openers and mixers, require less power and may generally be used simultaneously.

When you select an electrical appliance, make sure that it has a label stating that it has been approved by Underwriters' Laboratories (UL), a non-profit organization that tests products for safety.

Grounded three-pronged plugs and outlets are safest, but not always available. Whenever there is a choice, select a grounded unit to protect yourself against electrical shock. If you need an extension cord, use a heavy-duty, #16 approved heating cord.

If you are having your kitchen remodeled, electrical outlet strips may be built into facings on the back of the counter or under cabinets. These strips allow you to leave appliances with separate on/off controls (can openers, food processors, mixers) plugged in and ready. Electrical outlet strips are available through electrical contractors and supply stores. **Manufacturer:** 156.

If you are not remodeling, but can only reach a limited space

and need extra outlets for appliances used one at a time, a grounded multi-plug or a lateral outlet will accommodate four to six plugs in a sideways position (Figure 19-1). It allows use at the back of a counter. This six-outlet surge protector gives you front access to the plugs; a lateral plug may also be used behind furniture and increases safety by eliminating bent wires. UL approved. Cost of either type is about $6 and up from hardware stores and mail-order firms. **Sources:** 169, 345, 378.

When an electric appliance lacks an on/off switch, a line switch spliced into the cord lets you operate the machine without plugging and unplugging it. Make sure the switch is UL approved. **Manufacturers** include 156. Cost is about $2 each from hardware and housewares stores.

If plugging and unplugging cords is difficult for you, a small plug-in switch may help (Figure 19-2). It inserts directly into the socket; you can operate it with your thumb or the back of your hand. Note that this switch control is not powerful enough to use with a heating appliance. If your vision is limited, put a small piece of tape or other material you can feel with your hand on the "off" side of the switch so you can tell by feel whether an appliance is on or off. **Manufacturer:** 156. Cost is about $2 from hardware stores and electrical supply firms.

An outlet power strip with a circuit breaker makes more outlets conveniently available to you. It is especially helpful when sockets are not reachable. Pushing down on a plug is easier than trying to insert it sideways into a socket. Depending on the model, a strip accommodates three to six appliances and has a built-in shut-off should you use more power than the circuit can handle. The strip can be reset by eliminating overload and pressing the circuit breaker button. Some units include a surge protector. Check that the one you choose is UL listed. Manufacturers include 156. Cost is about $9 and up from hardware and housewares stores or mail-order firms. **Sources:** 169, 242, 369, 387, 407, 415.

If you cannot get plugs into and out of a socket or handle a specific control, a plug-in unit may be constructed for you (Figure 19-3). Consider having a rocker switch, which operates with light

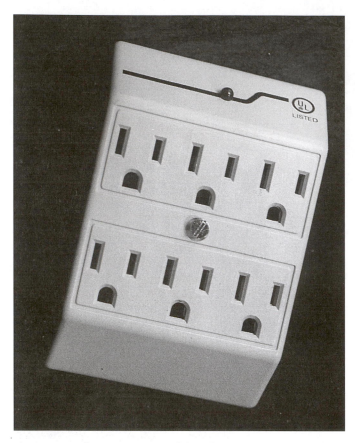

Figure 19-1. If you are not remodeling, but can only reach a limited space and need extra outlets for appliances used one at a time, a grounded multi-plug or a lateral outlet will accommodate four to six plugs in a sideways position. (Photo by J.K.)

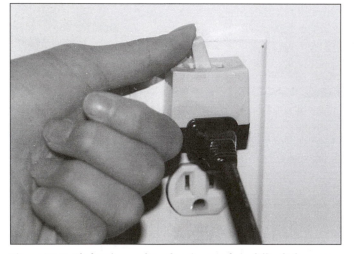

Figure 19-2. If plugging and unplugging cords is difficult for you, a small plug-in switch may help. (Photo courtesy of the O.T. Dept., Howard A. Rusk Institute of Rehabilitation Medicine.)

pressure from the heel of your hand. A signal light indicates when the current is on. A local electrician will be able to construct this type of unit for you.

A plug adapted with a built-in wooden knob provides an easier grip to insert the plug and to pull it out (Figure 19-4). The plug is fixed to the wood with epoxy adhesive.

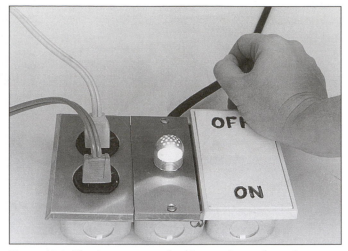

Figure 19-3. If you cannot get plugs into and out of a socket or handle a specific control, a plug-in unit may be constructed for you. (Photo courtesy of the Electro-Engineering Department, Howard A. Rusk Institute of Rehabilitation Medicine.)

Another answer for pulling a plug out is a plug ejector. This unit replaces the conventional wall plate and has a lever that removes plugs with a single push. Cost is about $8 each. **Sources:** 238, 261.

If you are using a wheelchair, have back problems, or limited reach, a vertical outlet extension will raise the level of present outlets 20", eliminating bending and stretching. Cost is about $20 from manufacturer and **source:** 7.

LIGHTING

Good lighting increases safety. It is easy to add more lights to avoid working in a shadow. Here are some suggestions:

A fluorescent light, about 2 feet long, easily installs under an upper cabinet to give direct light on your work area (Figure 19-5). It comes with a plug-in cord and line switch. **Manufacturer:** 156. Cost is about $13 from housewares and hardware stores.

If you need an occasional light to find items in a cabinet or closet, under the kitchen sink, or even on parts of the kitchen counter where a socket is not handy, a battery-powered fluorescent light may do the trick. It runs on four AA batteries. The lightweight, 7" or 12" long unit has an adhesive Velcro® fastener so you can stick it up where needed. Cost is about $9 and up from mail-order firms. **Sources:** 169, 173, 270, 378, 387, 415. Other larger battery powered lights for dark halls, closets, and stairwells are available from housewares stores and mail-order firms. **Source:** 173.

Touch-sensitive lights turn on or off when you touch any metal part of a lamp (Figure 19-6). You may buy a whole touch-lamp for about $25 and up from department stores or a plug-in or screw-in adaptor to allow use of your present lamps for about $18 from self-help firms. **Sources:** 13, 120, 238.

ELECTRICAL SAFETY AIDS

A power failure light goes on automatically if the electricity goes off (Figure 19-7). It plugs into any wall socket and is kept

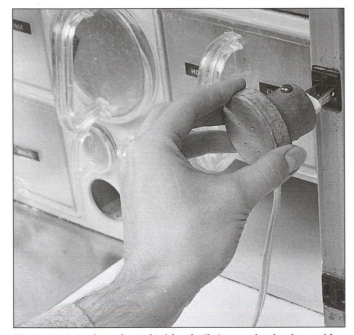

Figure 19-4. A plug adapted with a built-in wooden knob provides an easier grip to insert the plug and to pull it out. (Photo courtesy of the Electro-Engineering Department, Howard A. Rusk Institute of Rehabilitation Medicine.)

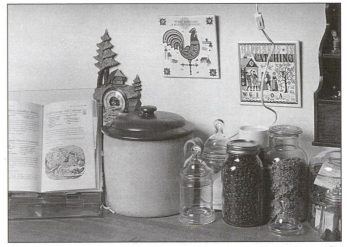

Figure 19-5. A fluorescent light, about two feet long, easily installs under an upper cabinet to give direct light on your work area. (Light by General Electric® Appliances, Louisville, KY. Photo by J.K.)

recharged by house current. You may also use it as a portable flashlight or night light. **Manufacturers** include 41, 156, 188, 349. Cost is about $17 and up from housewares and hardware stores or mail-order firms. **Sources:** 15, 50, 71, 196, 345, 359.

Outlets conveniently located for you may be at an inquisitive position for your toddler. A safety outlet cover keeps your child's fingers out of electrical sockets. See Chapter 26.

For additional information on lighting, electrical aids, and safety, see Chapter 9, Chapter 11, Chapter 12, and Chapter 13.

COOKING WITH GAS

Many homemakers like the quick response of a gas range when cooking. If you have severe loss of coordination or loss of vision, or if you have trouble remembering to turn a burner off, you should consider a safer alternative, such as a microwave oven. See Chapter 20.

If you are using an older model gas range, contemplate the fact that new gas ranges cost almost 50% less to operate than an older model. As of 1990, all new ranges including gas ovens were required to have pilotless electronic ignitions. This means with a new range you no longer have to handle matches. On newer models, also look for easy-to-use controls located at the front of the stove, rather than at the back. Bending is also reduced, because the broiler is usually in the upper part of the oven.

On the other hand, if you have difficulty using your hands and have an older stove with no automatic pilot, a few simple techniques may help you more safely light the burners and oven range.

If you have use of only one hand or poor coordination, this method keeps your fingers out of the way and does not allow gas to accumulate. To safely light a burner, strike the match to light it; then lay the match across the gas jets. Finally, turn on the gas.

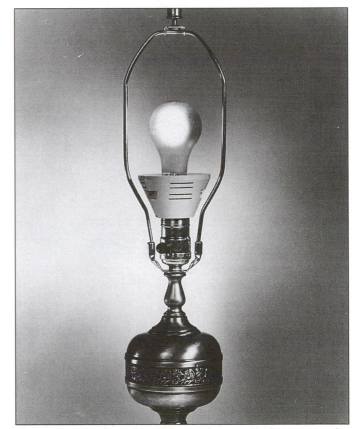

Figure 19-6. Touch-sensitive lights turn on or off when you touch any metal part of a lamp.

When you have finished cooking and the range is cool, remove the burned match.

A small piece of sandpaper taped to the side of the range is a handy match-striking surface.

A stove valve turner helps handle controls if you have marked weakness or arthritis in your hands. Turners come in 5" or 9" long lengths. Of formed steel wire, the plastic-coated triangular grip

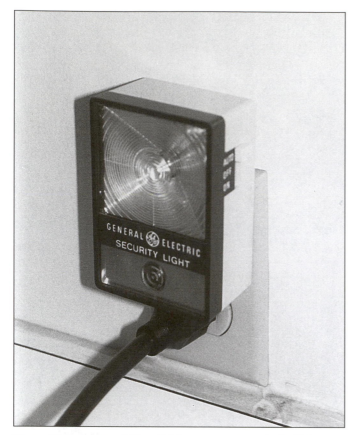

Figure 19-7. A power failure light goes on automatically if the electricity goes off. (Light by General Electric® Appliances, Louisville, KY. Photo by J.K.)

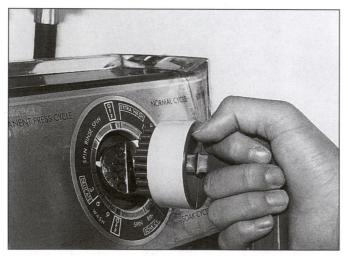

Figure 19-8. This universal handle will turn various sizes and shapes of stove and appliance controls. (Universal handle by Etac USA, Inc., Waukesha, WI. Photo by J.K.)

fits various sizes of stove valves and has a molded plastic handle with grip rings and a hang-up tab. Cost is about $12 and up from self-help firms. **Sources:** 252, 261, 264.

A universal handle will turn various sizes and shapes of stove and appliance controls (Figure 19-8). Retractable rods conform to the shape of the control so that you may turn it easily, even with

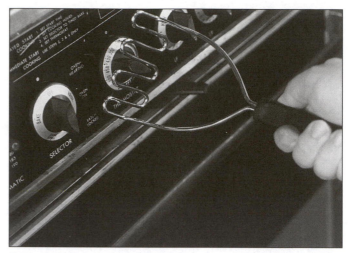

Figure 19-9. A potato masher may become a control turner when fingers are weak. (Photo by J.K.)

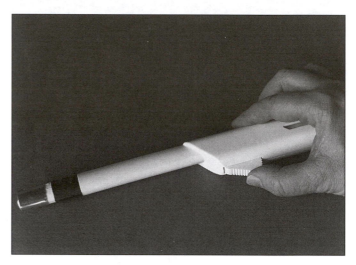

Figure 19-10. Use a gas match lighter to light the burner or an outside grill with one hand, if you have good grasp. (Lighter by Scripto-Tokai. Photo by J.K.)

marked weakness in your hands. **Manufacturer:** 122. Cost is about $20 from self-help firms. **Sources:** 5, 13, 122, 252, 290, 408.

A potato masher may become a control turner when fingers are weak (Figure 19-9).

Use a gas match lighter to light the burner or an outside grill with one hand, if you have good grasp (Figure 19-10). **Manufacturers** include 142, 181, 278, 355. Cost is about $3 to $15 from housewares stores and mail-order firms. **Sources:** 270, 378.

OVEN BROILER

Lighting the gas broiler and oven when there is no pilot light requires little or no bending if you use long fireplace matches. A 12" long match should reach most gas jets. Turn on the gas only after you have lit the match and put it in place. Long matches are sold by department stores and mail-order and self-help firms.

Manufacturer: 142. Cost is about $3 per box, and each match may be used several times. **Source:** 270.

If bending is hard for you, use long-handled barbecue tools for the broiler. With a long fork, you can turn foods from a seated or standing position. See Chapter 29.

If lifting is difficult, use a lightweight or foil broiler pan, remove cooked food with tongs, then leave the foil pan in the broiler until it cools. Take out the pan with its congealed grease with a pair of tongs or long spatula. **Manufacturers** of tongs: 112, 142, 289. Cost is about $3 and up from housewares stores and mail-order firms. Another solution is to eliminate use of your low broiler and invest in a new countertop broiler. See Chapter 20.

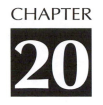

CHAPTER

20

Selecting
Small Appliances

Portable electrical appliances make quick work of time-consuming tasks like chopping, whipping, mixing, pureeing, and slicing. You can choose inexpensive, basic devices like hand mixers and can openers or multi-purpose units that grind, crush and mix, extract juice, broil and bake, even make bread or ice cream from scratch.

Small appliances may be moved to your most comfortable workplace—on a counter, lowered surface, or even the dining room table. If architectural barriers prevent you from using your kitchen and remodeling is not feasible, careful selection of portable appliances can put an efficient kitchen within your reach. Basic appliances like countertop ovens, microwave ovens, broilers, broiler ovens, and electric skillets are great helps if you cannot manage a large range and are unable to exchange it for a more suitable one.

GENERAL PRINCIPLES

The following sections deal with popular appliances, noting special features to check when purchasing a particular kind of appliance. Ways to adapt controls and other design elements are illustrated should you have hand limitations. The examples given here are only a guide. You are responsible for considering your own safety, for determining whether a certain appliance is right for you, and studying, then following, the directions that come with the appliance.

Before purchasing any appliance, evaluate your needs.
- What types of cooking do you do?
- How will the particular appliance help you?
- Is it versatile enough to meet your needs, or will it soon gather dust?
- Can you pick up the appliance, if necessary, and move it around?
- Does it have built-in safety features?
- Can you adjust or handle the controls quickly?

- Will you be able to assemble and disassemble it to clean it?
- Is it versatile enough to fill more than one need, or is the single function enough to warrant its purchase?

When you select any small appliance, apply the same criteria that you use in selecting major kitchen equipment. If considering two or more portable appliances, check Chapter 19, which discusses power requirements and aids in handling plugs.

PRE-SHOPPING ADVICE

Before you head for the stores, do some homework:
- Clip and compare ads.
- Check reports in consumer testing magazines.
- Talk with friends and neighbors about the appliances they use and how they like them. When visiting, ask to try your friends' appliances and see how functional these units are for you.
- Determine how much room you have for an appliance. If space is tight, write down the measurements.
- At the store, be prepared with a list of the features you want in your appliance.
- Read all the hang tags and guarantees.
- Look at the appliance. Pick it up, and try the controls. If all the appliances are boxed, ask a salesperson for permission to open and handle the models in which you are interested.
- Examine the construction to make sure there are no rough edges or loose parts.
- Read the control markings. Are they easy to read and durable so they won't be scrubbed off?
- Check the brand. Is it made by a reputable manufacturer?
- Find out what the servicing arrangements are.
- Make sure that the appliance is UL listed and that the UL label does not only refer to the cord.

If all the factors check out and you like and know you will use the appliance, take it home. Now read the instruction book, and enjoy!

WARRANTIES AND GUARANTEES

When you buy an appliance, you expect it to be free of defects or problems. Occasionally, however, a defective unit may reach the market. This is why manufacturers usually stand behind their products with some kind of guarantee or warranty.

The terms guarantee and warranty are interchangeable. Both vary in the services they promise. An appliance may be guaranteed for a 10-day, home-trial period or for the lifetime of the product. However, there is usually a time limit of 1 to 5 years.

Most guarantees and warranties have certain requirements that you as the purchaser must fulfill in order to be eligible. First, you may be asked to send in a registration card within a specified time period. If you fail to do this, your appliance will not be protected or covered for service.

Second, your guarantee or warranty can be voided if you misuse, damage, tamper with, or have your appliance repaired by an unauthorized service dealer. To keep your guarantee in effect, you must go to an authorized dealer. When purchasing an appliance, check the list of approved dealers. Is there one near you? Are you buying an appliance that can be sent through the mail without undue expense? Check to see who will make good on the guarantee—the manufacturer or the store that sells the item. Make sure that the address of the manufacturer is given. What does the agreement cover? Parts only or parts and labor? Who pays for the servicing? Is the entire product covered or only specific parts? Are parts readily available or is this the last of the particular model? Brand-name units are usually easier to have repaired. Read all tags and instructions carefully. Mark them with the date of purchase; if possible, clip the receipts to the tags. Save them in a convenient place, like one folder for all appliances. They are your record and guarantee of service. If you misplace the terms and place of contact, it is often hard to trace the responsible party.

CAN OPENERS

A good can opener should completely cut the lid out, leaving a smooth rim. For safer removal, the lid should be raised by a magnet. An electric opener should support the can while it's being cut so you don't have to hold it. Check the following factors in making your selection:

Will you be using the opener with one or two hands? If you work with one hand, choose a unit that does not require you to hold the can while opening it, or one that lets you set the can on one or more damp sponges while you manipulate the controls. You may be able to use your present opener if it has a vertically straight cutting blade.

Do the controls move easily? If you have weakness or arthritis in both hands, you need controls that require minimal pressure to operate. An electric can opener with a power-piercing or mechanically linked cutting blade and gear wheel is easier to use because the motor activates the cutting blade. When manual pressure is required, you may have difficulty making the initial cut. Long levers or extended controls that work with downward pressure are usually the easiest to manage.

If your hands are affected by arthritis, select a unit that lets the heel of your hand or your full palm do the pressing. If necessary, ask someone to attach a wider bar to the top of the lever so the weight is distributed more evenly and does not put pressure on just one part of your hand.

Can you move the opener if necessary? Not all of us have enough room at our food preparation place to keep a can opener always accessible. You may wish to slide the opener to the front of the counter for greater control when using it. If you have poor coordination, choose a sturdy unit with a wide or stable base and more weight to prevent tipping.

Is the cutting blade easy to see, yet protected so you can't cut yourself? When learning to use a new opener, you may want to remove the magnet until you have a feel for positioning the can under the cutting blade.

Is the opener easy to wipe clean? Does the blade remove for washing?

Added features on some electric can openers include knife sharpeners and plastic bag openers.

Finally, try out your selection in the store before you buy it. Take along an empty can. If testing is not possible, make sure you can return the opener after trying it at home. Check with the salesperson as well as with your guarantee.

If you use only one hand or need a lightweight unit you can move from place to place, see also the one-handed rechargeable electric can opener in Chapter 1. Easy-to-operate manual can openers are shown in Chapter 27.

An electric can opener with a vertically straight cutting blade works with one hand if you support the can on damp sponges (Figure 20-1). An adjustable height can opener has a power-piercing blade. It stops automatically when the can is fully opened and has a knife/scissors sharpener on the back. The handle/blade and magnet remove for cleaning. A knob in the front turns with one hand to set the opener in two positions: a high position for tall cans or a compact one for regular and small cans. It comes with a three-year warranty for repair of any parts if the opener is returned to an authorized service location. **Manufacturer:** 381. Cost is about $15 and up. UL listed. Similar openers with straight vertical blades by other **manufacturers** also work well with the "sponge" method: 41, 131, 166, 299, 329, 334.

A one-handed can opener is held over the can, power pierces, and lifts the cover when the cut is complete (Figure 20-2). Cost is about $25 from housewares stores. **Manufacturer:** 94.

A non-rechargeable, electric can opener works with one hand by depressing a single lever (Figure 20-3). It removes the whole top of the can with its edge, leaving a non-sharp rim. **Manufacturers:** 224, 399. Cost is about $35 from housewares stores and mail-order firms. **Sources:** 65, 167, 345.

ELECTRIC SKILLETS AND COOKERS

An electric skillet is the most versatile appliance. Many homemakers rely on this one appliance to do most of the cooking. If you can only make minimal kitchen changes, an electric skillet will let you fix full meals for your family and yourself. If you are a handicapped student living on your own, an electric skillet can be used to prepare breakfast as well as dinner. Before using your skillet, read the instruction book carefully. You'll be surprised at how much you can do.

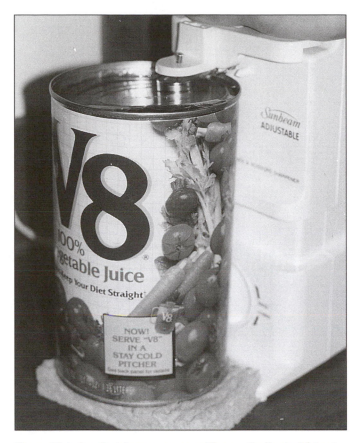

Figure 20-1. An electric can opener with a vertically straight cutting blade works with one hand if you support the can on damp sponges. (Can opener by Sunbeam® Appliance Co., Laurel, MS. Photo by J.K.)

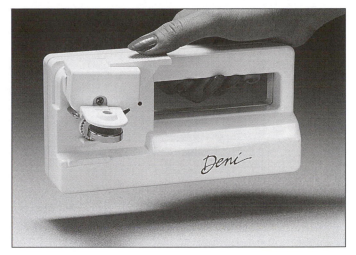

Figure 20-2. This one-handed can opener is held over the can. It power pierces, then lifts the cover when cut is complete. (Photo courtesy of Deni, Keystone Manufacturing Co., Inc. Buffalo, NY.)

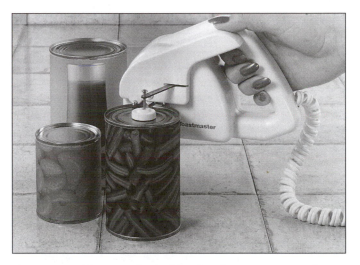

Figure 20-3. This non-rechargeable, electric can opener works with one hand by depressing a single lever. (Photo courtesy of Toastmaster®, Inc., Columbia, MO.)

Features to consider in selecting an electric skillet include the following:

- Handle design: construction must be of non-heat conducting material. Placement of the handles is important. A single handle is preferred if you are working with one hand. Double handles are best if you have weakness, arthritis, or incoordination in your arms and hands. Look for handles that are large enough for you to grasp without touching the hot sides of the skillet. Even so, always wear pot holders when lifting or moving the skillet.

- Control: The temperature control should be located so that you can insert and turn it easily. As most controls are now placed under the handle, this may be hard to manage, so try it in the store before buying. At home, let the skillet cool completely before removing the control. The control knob should be big enough to grasp and have molded or ridged edges. A baffle in back of the control prevents you from accidentally touching the hot metal and burning your fingers. If your fingers are very weak, you may need to adapt the control. The controls should be large enough for you to read easily and have a signal light to tell when the correct temperature is reached. Note: Always plug the control into the skillet before you place it in the wall socket, and turn it off completely before unplugging it from wall. Also unplug it from the wall before removing the control from the skillet. Let pan cool

before removing the control.

- Cover: The cover knob should be high enough for you to pick it up without touching the metal with your fingers or forearm. A vent allows browning of foods without their becoming soggy. A high-domed skillet lets you use it for baking or cooking large roasts and poultry.

A lightweight 11" x 11" double-handled electric skillet of aluminum for even heating has a non-stick interior for easy cleaning (Figure 20-4). It is dishwasher safe and immersible when the heat control is removed. The handles are set out from the pan so you can pick it up without touching the metal. If you have arthritis in your hands, try using your full palms to lift it. The control extends beyond the handle for easier turning. **Manufacturers** of this and similar skillets include 285, 381, 422 (illustrated). Cost is about $25 and up from housewares stores. Use a wooden utensil to prevent scratching the non-stick finish. See Chapter 21.

If you have marked loss of coordination, look for a deep-sided skillet. The wide legs and low profile make it an ideal cooking

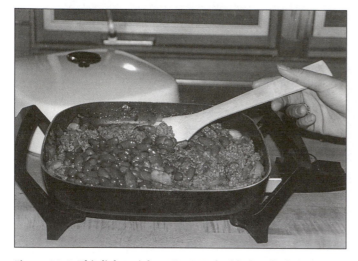

Figure 20-4. This lightweight 11″ x 11″ double-handled electric skillet of aluminum for even heating has a non-stick interior for easy cleaning. (Skillet by The West Bend® Company, West Bend, WI. Photo by J.K.)

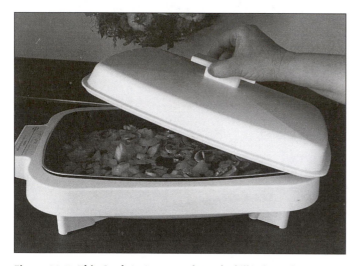

Figure 20-5. This Cook 'n Serve cool-touch skillet has a low pro-file for easy handling. (Skillet by The West Bend® Company, West Bend, WI. Photo by J.K.)

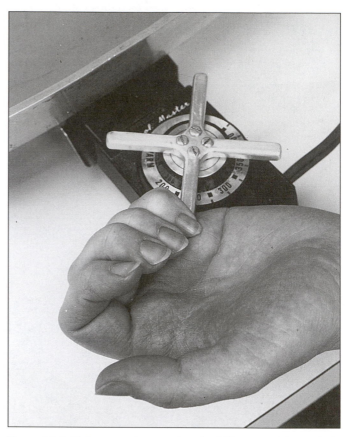

Figure 20-6. If the control on an electric skillet, casserole, or simi-lar appliance is difficult to turn because your hands are weak, incoordinated, or affected by arthritis, adapt it with a dowel or spoked handle. (Photo courtesy of the O.T. Dept., Howard A. Rusk Institute of Rehabilitation Medicine.)

appliance. For even more stability, place the unit on a rubber counter mat to keep it from sliding. A deep skillet can cook whole roasts or poultry. The higher sides help reduce spilling. **Manufacturers:** 41, 285, 422. Cost is about $30 and up from housewares stores.

This Cook 'n Serve cool-touch skillet has a low profile for easy handling (Figure 20-5). The white thermo-plastic and aluminum base is designed so the outer surface stays cool while cooking. A release lever detaches the non-stick lined pan for quick cleaning. When detached from the adjustable temperature control, the skil-let is dishwasher safe. The T-handle top may be lifted by hand or with a large fork if you have weak grasp. **Manufacturer:** 422. Cost is about $52 from housewares stores and mail-order firms. **Source:** 359.

A single-handed skillet is easier to maneuver if you are work-ing with one hand. **Manufacturer:** 131. Cost is about $60 from housewares stores. **Source:** 359.

If picking up the cover of a skillet threatens to burn your fin-gers, the tines of a large fork will keep your hand away from the hot cover.

The cover knob on an electric skillet may be replaced with an open wooden handle so you may lift the cover more safely. Most skillet knobs are attached with a single screw that removes easily. A new, non-heat conducting handle may be made at home or pur-chased from a hardware store.

If the control on an electric skillet, casserole, or similar appli-ance is difficult to turn because your hands are weak, incoordi-nated, or affected by arthritis, adapt it with a dowel or spoked han-dle (Figure 20-6). If you turn the control on this skillet with the back of your hand, it adjusts temperature. The dowel is attached to the center of the standard skillet control.

If you find that your energy is high in the morning and gone by evening, you might consider a slow cooker (Figure 20-7). This allows you to start cooking the meal in the morning and let it sim-mer all day. A dishwasher safe, four- or six-quart, oblong con-tainer cooks casseroles and stews and will hold a chicken or roast. It is separate from the base so you can lift it for serving or storage in the refrigerator. The base may be used as a griddle for French toast, pancakes, eggs, and other foods. If you have poor use of your fingers, you may want to add a dowel to the single control knob. **Manufacturer:** 422. Cost is about $23 and up from house-

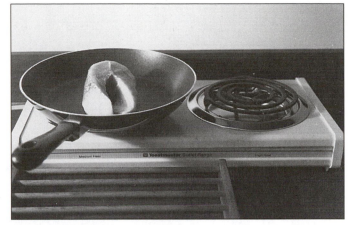

Figure 20-8. This self-cleaning, double buffet range has one 550 watt and one 1,000 watt burner. (Buffet range by Toastmaster®, Inc., Columbia, MO. Photo by J.K.)

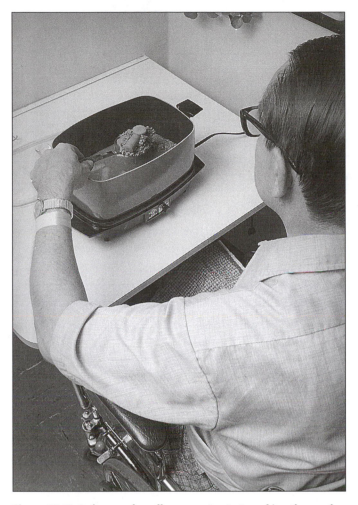

Figure 20-7. A slow cooker allows you to start cooking the meal in the morning and let it simmer all day. (Photo courtesy of the O.T. Dept., Howard A. Rusk Institute of Rehabilitation Medicine.)

wares stores. **Sources:** 135, 359. Although it comes with a glass top, a plastic replacement cover is about $7 and up from authorized appliance repair stores.

If you are using a wheelchair or must work at a lowered surface but extensive kitchen remodeling is not possible, a portable electric range may be an inexpensive solution. Consider it carefully, because the combination of other appliances may do all that you need. A microwave oven and electric skillet, for example, allow great versatility. Putting a trivet or raised, heat-proof pad in front of the portable range lets you slide pans to and from the burners.

A two-burner, countertop range may be placed on any convenient work surface, such as a counter or table. As a safety precaution and for easier cleanup, put a counter mat under it. Note: If you prefer to have a microwave oven with a browning unit, it will allow you to do everything that a table range will, plus almost all that an oven will. See microwave ovens later in this chapter.

If cost is a major consideration or you do very little cooking or have use of an oven with assistance when needed, then a table top range is a possible substitute.

Features to consider in selecting a tabletop range include the following:

- Low-to-the-counter styling: this eliminates the need for you to lift pans up and down.
- Tubular-type cooking elements: these lift up and are easy to clean. Some models have solid surfaces, which are even better.
- Large, easy-to-turn control knobs: these must be located at the front of the unit for convenient, safe use.
- Infinite heat controls: controls should range from high to medium to low as well as off so you may quickly adjust heating temperatures.

This self-cleaning, double buffet range has one 550 watt and one 1,000 watt burner (Figure 20-8). The controls have ridged knobs for turning easily. **Manufacturer:** 399. Cost is about $50 and up from housewares stores. Elements tilt up to clean. A single-burner range is about $30. A similar double-burner range is made by **source** 89.

With table ranges, electric skillets, and other small appliances, you may prepare meals at the table. The convenient height lets you sit to work. When the meal is cooked, there are no hot dishes to carry.

Other electric cooking units you might consider, based on your style of food preparation, include woks (see Chapter 30), steamers, combination sandwich/waffle makers, even a rice cooker. Electric steamers come with a lightweight plastic base, basket, vented tray, and lid for cooking a variety of foods, including vegetables, fruits, rice, seafood, cabbage rolls, stuffed peppers, and cereals. A steamer cooks quickly and gets hot so you have to handle it with care and pot holders. If you have marked weakness, incoordination, or poor vision, this unit is not recommended. **Manufacturers:** 41, 299, 303, 334, 381, 401 (rice cooker). Cost is about $35 and up from housewares stores and gourmet firms. **Sources:** 71, 359. For other cooking units, see the Handi® Electric Skillet in Chapter 11 and the electric wok and fondue pot in Chapter 30. An electric, single-hamburger maker is **manufactured** by 89.

LIQUID HEATERS

Instant soups, coffee, tea, cocoa, and other hot beverages are prepared easily with a liquid heater. It is designed to bring water

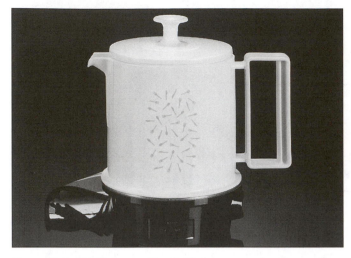

Figure 20-9. This hot pot with a baffle keeps your hand away from the hot pot. (Photo courtesy of Regal® Ware, Inc., Kewaskum, WI.)

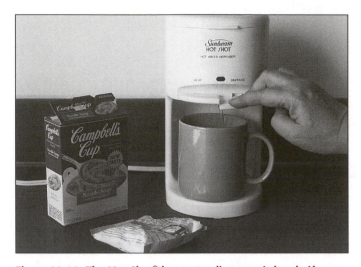

Figure 20-10. The Hot Shot® hot water dispenser is handy if you have marked weakness in your hands and arms, loss of vision, or poor coordination. (Hot Shot® by Sunbeam Appliance Co., Laurel, MS. Photo by J.K.)

to a boil faster than a stove or microwave. The heater may be a pitcher that you pick up and pour from or a container into which you pour the water and then release the hot liquid into a cup below. For heating greater amounts of water, there are electric kettles.

Features to consider when selecting a liquid heater include the following:

- Does the unit have a temperature control? Look for settings from warm to boil. See that you can turn the control lever quickly to prevent liquids from boiling over.
- Can you pick up the container without your hand coming in contact with the pot? Look for a non-heat-conducting handle set out from the side so you can grasp it without touching the surface of the pot or with a baffle along the inner side.
- Does it have a cover to increase safety?
- Does the base stay cool when the liquids heat up? Make sure that the heater is UL listed.
- Can you handle the plug? Most units require that you unplug them when not in use.
- If heating liquids other than water, make sure that the interior is non-stick for easy cleaning. Most heaters cannot be immersed.

A hot pot with a baffle keeps your hand away from the hot pot (Figure 20-9). You can slip your hand through the handle and use a hook grasp. Of lightweight polypropylene, it may be used for heating soups, stews, and sauces, as well as water. Cover locks on for safety and has a non-drip spout. Cord removes when not in use. UL listed. **Manufacturers:** 329, 334. Cost is about $15 and up from housewares stores.

The Hot Shot® hot water dispenser is handy if you have marked weakness in your hands and arms, loss of vision, or poor coordination (Figure 20-10). Pour up to two cups of cold water in the top, close the cover, press a lever. Place your cup underneath with the instant soup, cocoa mix, tea bag, or other ingredients. In about 90 seconds, a signal light announces the water is hot. If you have marked loss of vision, you can count. Water pours down into cup when you push a second lever. The dispenser eliminates the

need to lift or handle hot pans or kettles, but can only be used for water. Levers may be extended if you have minimal use of your hands. Automatic shut-off turns unit off when water has reached boiling point. Exterior stays cool; interior is stainless steel. For maximum safety when not in use, unplug unit. See Chapter 19 for line switch and alternate methods. UL listed. **Manufacturers:** 288, 381. Cost is about $20 and up from housewares stores and mail-order firms. **Sources:** 196, 247, 261, 359.

Avoid lifting a tea kettle if you have weak wrists and hands or tremors by placing it on a tipping platform (Figure 20-11). Wooden posts adjust to hold any kettle from 6" to 8" in diameter. A local carpenter could make one for you, or you may purchase it from a self-help firm. Cost is about $60. **Sources:** 5, 120, 252, 264, 408.

An electric kettle may be filled right from the kitchen spray hose without removing it from the tipping base. An energy-saving, shut-off device cuts power when water reaches the boiling point. A safety device turns the kettle off if the water level is insufficient. The handle does not heat. Cord is detachable. **Manufacturers** include 41, 84, 334, 399. Cost is about $55 and up from housewares stores and mail-order firms. **Sources:** 71, 73, 345, 427.

If you drink or eat slowly, an electric cup warmer keeps your beverage hot and ready at hand (Figure 20-12). **Manufacturers:** 89, 346. Cost is about $10 and up from housewares stores and mail-order firms. **Sources:** 364, 410.

COUNTERTOP OVENS AND BROILERS

A good, countertop oven-broiler may substitute for a regular oven when major kitchen remodeling is not possible. You may place it on a countertop at the most convenient level. Leave a space for resting pans in front of the oven door, especially if you have weak arms or find carrying difficult.

Features to look for include the following:

- Easily accessible on/off controls.
- Temperature controls that you can read easily and turn without

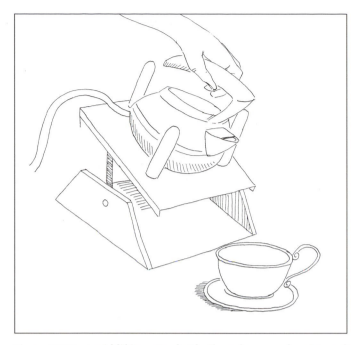

Figure 20-11. Avoid lifting a tea kettle if you have weak wrists and hands or tremors by placing it on a tipping platform. (Illustration by G.K.)

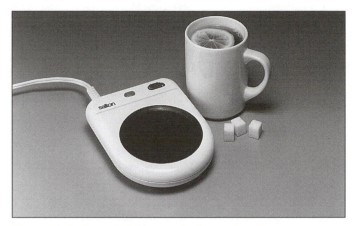

Figure 20-12. If you drink or eat slowly, an electric cup warmer keeps your beverage hot and ready at hand. (Photo courtesy of Salton/Maxim, Inc., Mt. Prospect, IL.)

touching the metal. On combination broiler-ovens, there should be a thermostatic control from about 250° to 450°.

- An automatic timer that turns the unit off after pre-set time has elapsed—an excellent idea if you tend to forget. Also look for a signal light that tells when correct temperature is reached and stays on to tell you to turn it off.
- Stable shelves that remain flat and do not tip when you pull them two-thirds of the way out. If the oven slides when you pull the rack out, set it on a rubber counter mat.
- Several rack positions on larger models to accommodate different kinds of food and cooking.
- Broiler pans heavy enough that they do not warp when heated. They must be deep enough to hold a substantial amount of fat without spilling when you remove the pan from the oven. Slotted racks reduce the chance of grease flaring up.
- Doors that operate safely and do not come off. Handles should be of non-heat-conducting material and large enough for you to grasp without touching the hot surface. (Most doors are made of glass so you have to be aware of not dropping or placing pans on them.)
- Bake and broil elements located at the top and bottom of your oven. Tubular elements are more durable than wire or coil types. For best distribution of heat, an element should not go around in a rectangle but be formed to cross over the center of the area. Removable elements make it easier to clean the interior.
- Self-cleaning interiors and easy-to-clean shelves. Some units come with non-stick finished pans.
- Insulation. Oven walls should have some insulation if you plan to use the appliance for baking. Snug-fitting doors help keep the temperature at an even level.
- Power requirements. Make sure you have wiring equal to the demands a broiler-oven will put on it. As with other heat-pro-

ducing appliances, only one heating appliance can normally be used on a circuit at one time.

Consider what you want to cook with the appliance. Are you going to use it as a daily substitute for your oven or mainly for reheating and broiling? The extra cost of a good portable oven, one with convection or combination cooking, is worth the expense if you plan to use the unit for a majority of your cooking and baking tasks. Also consider the merits of a microwave oven, which are discussed later in this chapter.

Portable electric ovens and broilers vary in their abilities to reach and maintain specific temperatures. Read the instruction book carefully, and begin with simple dishes that do not require exact temperatures. It is wise to test your new appliance with an oven thermometer and to vary the rack height the first few times you cook until you have determined the best arrangement.

Some convection ovens have a side-opening door with a long handle for safer and more convenient handling of pans (Figure 20-13). Most have four cooking systems: convection bake, broil, slow cook, plus regular baking. The air in a convection oven circulates around the food, cooking up to one-third faster than a conventional oven. It has a continuous cleaning interior and is large enough to handle a 10-pound turkey. It broils on all sides without turning. The outside of the oven stays cool. Door removes for cleaning. UL approved. **Manufacturers** of convection ovens: 92, 131, 399, 421. Cost is about $200 from housewares stores. **Sources:** 65, 204, 356, 359, 373.

A smaller, toaster-broiler-oven with automatic thermostat, automatic shut-off, and temperature indicator light also has continuous cleaning (Figure 20-14). The door opens down for full access, resting on the handle, and large knobs turn easily. An accessory hook-on handle lets you pull the rack or shelf out without touching metal. Heavy-gauge broiler pan may be used as a casserole dish. It comes with a limited warranty for all repairs for one year, with an optional extension possible. **Manufacturer:** 92. Cost is about $80 and up from housewares stores. **Source:** 167. Other toaster-broiler ovens are made by 41, 131, 334, 399, 421.

A toaster oven for baking and toasting works well if you want a unit to toast and heat foods (Figure 20-15). Make sure you read the directions before heating any prepared foods. Some packaging

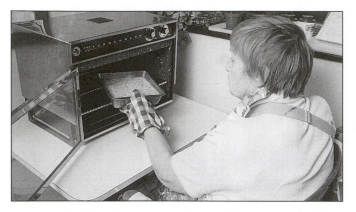

Figure 20-13. This convection oven has a side-opening door with a long handle for safer and more convenient handling of pans. (Convection Oven by Farberware® Inc., Bronx, NY. Photo courtesy of the O.T. Dept., Howard A. Rusk Institute of Rehabilitation Medicine.)

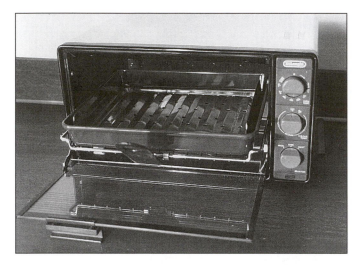

Figure 20-14. A smaller toaster-broiler oven with automatic thermostat, automatic shut-off, and temperature indicator light also has continuous cleaning. (Oven by DeLonghi America, Inc., Carlstadt, NJ. Photo by J.K.)

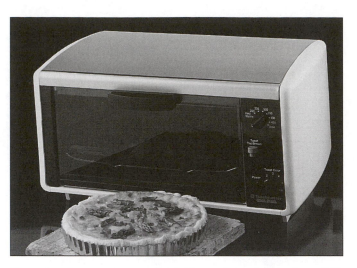

Figure 20-15. A toaster oven for baking and toasting works well if you want a unit to toast and heat foods. Make sure you read the directions before heating any prepared foods. Some packaging cannot be heated in a toaster oven, so must be transferred to another container. This oven has a signal bell, automatic shut-off, and top browner. (Photo courtesy of Toastmaster®, Inc., Columbia, MO.)

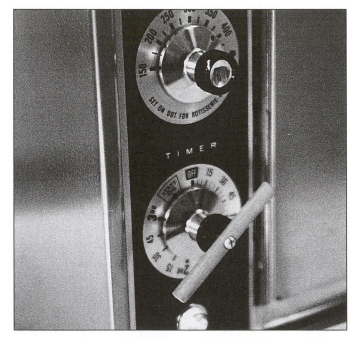

Figure 20-16. If a control is too small for you to grasp or is hard to turn, it can be adapted with a short dowel attached to the knob with a screw. (Photo courtesy of the O.T. Dept., Howard A. Rusk Institute of Rehabilitation Medicine.)

cannot be heated in a toaster oven, so food must be transferred to another container. **Manufacturers** include 41, 92, 166, 399, 421. Cost is about $50 and up from housewares stores.

If a control is too small for you to grasp or is hard to turn, it can be adapted with a short dowel attached to the knob with a screw (Figure 20-16).

Cookware for toaster ovens costs about $4 and up per pan from toaster oven manufacturers and mail-order firms. **Sources:** 283, 378, 410.

BROILERS

If you have limited arm function, an open grill is easier to use because it eliminates the handling of doors, pans, and racks. Food is placed on a rack over a tubular broiling element. It does not splatter or smoke, because the drippings do not hit a hot surface. The drip tray may be foil-lined for easy cleaning.

Some electric broilers have a cooling zone to keep them free from smoke and splatter (Figure 20-17A). **Manufacturers:** 131 (also available with a rotisserie), 166 (dishwasher safe), 260, 346. Cost is about $35 and up from housewares stores.

The counter top electric grill in Figure 20-17B has two heat zones with an enclosed heating element. Safety features include cool-touch handles and a splatter guard. Entire unit is dishwasher safe.

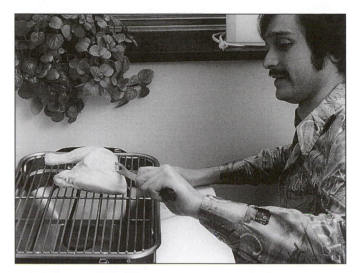

Figure 20-17A. This stainless-steel electric broiler has a cooling zone to keep it free from smoke and splatter. (Broiler by Farberware®, Inc., Bronx, NY. Photo courtesy of the O.T. Dept., Howard A. Rusk Institute of Rehabilitation Medicine.)

MICROWAVE OVENS AND ACCESSORIES

Microwave ovens are now used in more than 80% of the kitchens in America. This form of cooking has many advantages that increase safety and save energy:

- If you have weak arms and hands, most utensils designed for microwave use are very lightweight.
- If you have poor coordination, vision, or sensation, a microwave oven is safer, because there is no open flame. Note: You should always use a potholder when removing items from the microwave oven, because heat from the food does travel to the container.
- There is no forgetting to turn off a burner; you set the microwave control to the desired time, and it turns off automatically.
- Microwave cooking can reduce your fat intake. Most foods micro-cook in moist heat without added oil, margarine, or butter. The speed of the microwave also means less time in the kitchen, which gives fewer opportunities to nibble.
- A microwave oven lets you make sauces with minimal stirring and even preserves or dries foods.

Ask yourself the following questions before purchasing a first or new microwave:

- What size do I want? What do I want to use it for?

Microwave ovens come in three basic sizes: compact, mid-size, and full-size. The compact is most economical and is adequate if you will only use the oven for light cooking and basic heating. The mid-size and family units have additional features that allow defrosting and browning and eliminate the need to rotate foods while cooking.

- Is the oven wattage as high as I need? Compact ovens are usually 500 watts, which means that recipe times may need to be adjusted, because cooking takes a little longer than with a larger microwave. Mid-size and full-size units are 600 to 850 watts, which allow you to cook more types of foods and to cook them faster.

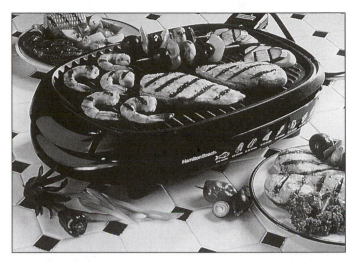

Figure 20-17B. This countertop electric grill has two heat zones with an enclosed heating element. (Health Smart™ Indoor Gourmet Grill. Photo courtesy of Hamilton Beach/Proctor-Silex, Inc., Washington, DC.)

- Will I need to re-wire for installation? Most units work on 110V power, which means you use a regular wall socket. You may not, however, be able to use the circuit for other heating appliances at the same time.
- Will the interior accommodate the size pans and types of foods I want to cook? Compact units take a dinner plate or 9" casserole. Mid-size and family units hold 9" x 13" pans and are high enough for roasts and other foods.
- Does the unit sit on the counter? Can it be hung under a cabinet? Placement of the oven depends on its overall dimensions, how much space is required for the air vents, and the strength and coordination in your arms. Most countertop units are the same depth as standard upper cabinets, leaving a space in front to slide pans in and out.
- Which way does the door open? Do you have space to set foods on the side that is open? This may take some planning and clearing on your part.
- Can I operate and understand the control panel? Most microwave ovens have push-button panels with digital timing. If you are not used to digital numbers, look for a unit with push-buttons and recipe guides on the front. If you can learn to set times digitally, you have a bigger choice. The simplest type of control, found on compact units, is a rotating dial, which you set to the number of minutes or fraction of minutes.
- Do the foods heat evenly? Heat is not even within a microwave oven unless additional features, such as a rotating cooking base or fan, are incorporated. The interior is hotter near the sides of the oven. As a result, you will have to rotate foods in a compact oven or older model of a larger microwave. Some have built-in turntables; for one that does not, a portable turntable will solve this problem.
- How many power levels do I need? The number of power levels ranges from five in smaller units to 99 in more elaborate ones. With added levels, cooking will be more precise and the finished product can be pre-programmed.
- What other features would I like? These might include automat-

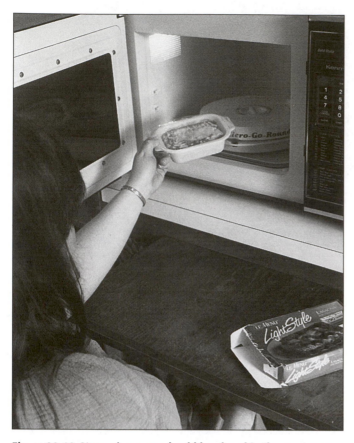

Figure 20-18. Your microwave should be placed in the most convenient location, so that getting items out with one hand or two weak arms is safe and easy. (Oven by Sears Roebuck®, Chicago, IL. Kitchen at Ballard Green Housing, Ridgefield, CT. Photo by J.K.)

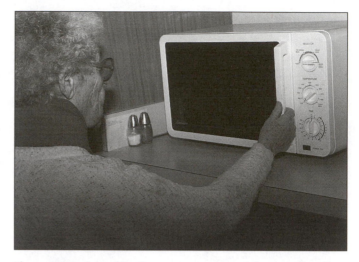

Figure 20-19. A combination oven serves more than one function in your kitchen. (Photo courtesy of Ballard Green Housing, Ridgefield, CT.)

ic defrosting, a sensor, or temperature probe to tell when food is ready, delay start for putting food in to cook later, memory reheat, slow cooking, an oven shelf, or a browning unit.

Study consumer testing magazines and family service and cooking publications. Look at the features on various models in stores or through catalogs from the companies. Try the latches and controls. **Manufacturers:** 20, 147, 150, 156, 159, 253, 275, 303, 348, 349, 356, 361, 381, 385, 401, 424. Single-dial microwave ovens are **manufactured** by 156, 159, 303, 356.

The cost of a microwave oven ranges from less than $90 for a compact oven to more than $400 for a programmable combination oven. Check warranties and guarantees carefully before you purchase. See the discussion in an earlier section of this chapter. Housewares and appliance stores offer a variety of microwave ovens for hands-on testing.

Your microwave should be placed in the most convenient location so that getting items out with one hand or two weak arms is safe and easy (Figure 20-18). Oven by 356.

The need to rotate pans may be eliminated by use of a spring-wound turntable. About 7" in diameter, it turns for up to 15 minutes, holds five pounds, and is top rack dishwasher safe. **Manufacturer:** 287. Cost is about $12 and up from housewares stores and mail-order firms. **Sources:** 359, 364, 407.

A combination oven serves more than one function in your kitchen (Figure 20-19). Look for a two-way cooking system that

has both microwave and convection cooking. **Manufacturers** include 147, 159, 303, 361, 381, 401. Cost is about $150 and up from housewares stores.

Braille numbers and letters are available free of charge from several appliance manufacturers. If you have severe loss of vision, these can be affixed to the control panel of any microwave oven. Operating instructions may be brailled for you by the National Braille Association for $.12 per brailled page, with a $5 minimum. The *Sharp Carousel Microwave Cookbook* is available in braille from the National Braille Association. See Appendix B.

If finding a suitable location for your microwave is a problem, you might consider a microwave cart. It can be left in one place or rolled into position. Carts are available in wood or laminate construction with enclosed cabinets or open fixed or adjustable shelves. Check the dimensions carefully before purchasing, and make sure the height is even with your countertop for safest transfer of foods. Cost is about $45 and up from housewares stores and mail-order firms. **Sources:** 65, 356, 359, 373.

Microwave carts are not meant to be rolled from place to place as a transporting aid. See suitable carts for this in Chapter 16.

SAFETY TIPS

- Read your operating manual carefully before beginning to use your new microwave oven. Study and follow the instructions in order to get best results. Microwave cooking requires an adjustment to new procedures.
- Learn your oven's personality, or cooking pattern, by watching as food cooks. You may find your oven cooks more quickly on one side than the other so that the dish has to be rotated.
- Put your cooking dish in the center of the oven for more even cooking.
- Always use a potholder to remove heated foods from the microwave. Although only foods, not the containers, heat in the microwave, the heat is transferred to the pan or cup.
- Lift covers and wraps off foods on the far side so that steam escapes away from your face. You may use a long-handled fork to lift the plastic or lid and release the steam.

- Use microwave-safe, clear plastic wrap to cover foods, and turn back a corner to vent or allow steam to escape. Avoid contact of plastic wrap with food while heating. Wax paper and plain white microwavable paper towels are excellent coverings when defrosting or cooking foods.
- Use only microwave-safe utensils in your microwave oven. These include glassware, such as that made by Anchor Hocking and Corning, and plastic containers by 29, 79, 121, 287, 343, 404.
- Mark microwave-safe cookware with a large "M" using a permanent marker, indicating that it can be used for the microwave. This is especially helpful if you tend to forget or have children. Most flexible plastic tops are only for storage and cannot be put in microwave. Hand washing may also be recommended for the covers.
- Do not use plastic containers, such as margarine, yogurt, and deli food containers, for heating. These are not made for microwaves and may chemically break down when heated at high temperatures.
- Do not recycle plastic dishes in which frozen microwave foods come; they are not made for multiple use.
- Limit trays designed for both microwave and conventional ovens to the microwave, because chemicals in the packaging can migrate at conventional oven temperatures.
- Do not use Melamine, because it may char and become brittle.
- Do not use plastic bags provided for fruit and vegetables or to wrap breads and other foods. They cannot withstand high temperature use.
- Do not use styrofoam to heat foods. It may melt.
- Microwaving an egg in its shell is not recommended. The internal pressure builds up, and the egg may explode. Use microwave recipes that poach or scramble eggs.
- Use rubber spatulas or plastic-coated or wooden utensils with microwave dishes to avoid scratching. Do not cut on microwave dishes with a knife.

The following utensils and containers will make use of your microwave oven easier and safer.

Plastic containers for microwave ovens come in many styles and sizes (Figure 20-20).

A microwave steamer holds foods like vegetables or fish above a small amount of water while steam rises through the vents. **Manufacturers:** 121, 142, 287, 404. Cost is $7 and up. **Sources:** 71, 270, 378, 387. An adjustable steamer for fresh, frozen, or canned vegetables and other foods fits inside various sized microwave-safe dishes. See Chapter 29.

Microwave mugs hold 8 to 16 ounces, have large handles for safe grasping, usually stack for storage, and are dishwasher safe. **Manufacturers**: 121, 343, 404. Cost is about $2 each and up from housewares stores and mail-order firms.

A set of two plastic cook and serve cups are for heating single servings of soup or desserts (Figure 20-21). Each cup holds 15 ounces and comes with a cover. The long handle makes the cup easy to grasp with one hand. Dishwasher safe. Distributor: 61. Cost is about $4 per set and $3 for a similar microwavable covered skillet from housewares stores and mail-order firms. **Sources:** 231, 270, 378.

A divided tray holds one large or two small servings of an

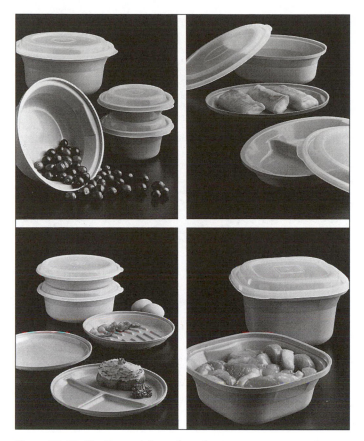

Figure 20-20. Plastic containers for microwave ovens come in many styles and sizes. (Photo courtesy of Nordic Ware®, Minneapolis, MN.)

entire meal. The bottoms are microwave-, but not browning-safe; tops cannot go in the microwave or dishwasher. **Manufacturers:** 343, 404. Cost is about $3 each and up from housewares stores and mail-order firms. **Sources:** 169, 359, 378.

A spud ring or baked potato holder keeps pierced potatoes securely in the right position for cooking, then lets you pick up all four at one time (Figure 20-22A).

A microwave burger maker lets you form, cook, and serve in the same dish (Figure 20-22B). The single-serving unit may be used for beef, turkey, veal, or fish burgers. Fat drips down into lower pan. Top rack dishwasher safe. **Distributor:** 61. Cost is about $3 from housewares stores and mail-order firms. **Sources:** 270, 378.

A thermoplastic splatter lid keeps liquids and grease in the pan so oven interior remains clean. It lets excess moisture escape, yet prevents drying out (Figure 20-23). It fits various sized containers, reduces the use of plastic wrap or paper, and is dishwasher safe. **Manufacturers:** 112 (the grid lid), 121 (the slotted lid), 287 (not shown—with adjustable vent to lock steam and heat inside). Cost is about $3 each for splatter lids and plate covers from housewares stores and mail-order firms. **Sources:** 71, 173, 270, 364, 378, 407, 410. For heating more than one plate at a time, splatter covers come with stacking lids or holders. Cost is about $10 and up per set from housewares stores and mail-order firms. **Sources:** 364, 410.

Other microwave accessories include coffeemaker; popcorn

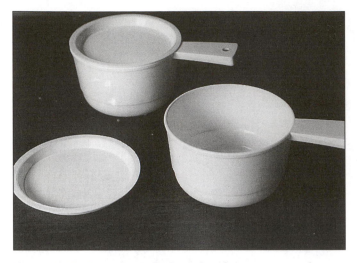

Figure 20-21. A set of two plastic cook and serve cups are for heating single servings of soup or desserts. (Distributed by Chadwick-Miller, Inc., Canton, MA. Photo by J.K.)

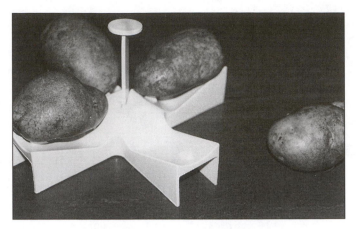

Figure 20-22A. A spud ring or baked potato holder keeps pierced potatoes securely in the right position for cooking, then lets you pick up all four at one time. (Holder by Ekco® Housewares, Inc., Franklin Park, IL. Photo by J.K.)

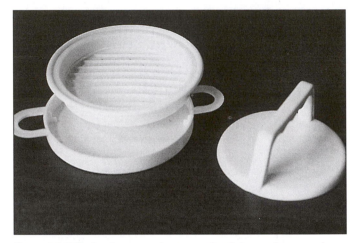

Figure 20-22B. A microwave burger maker lets you form, cook, and serve in the same dish. Distributed by Chadwick-Miller, Inc., Canton, MA. Photo by J.K.)

maker; measuring cups; poultry roaster; muffin and cakepans, including bundt, ring, and spring-form; roast and bacon pans or racks; micro-kettles for soup, tea, or coffee; and omelette/poacher pans. Browning and seasoning condiments for microwave use, including salt-free varieties, are available from grocery and gourmet stores as well as mail-order firms.

HANDY MICRO TIPS

- When reheating single portions, microwave on medium (50% power) for a longer time. This permits more uniform heating.
- When heating a casserole or large amount of food, stir it once or twice during cooking to ensure an even temperature throughout. Food must be heated to at least 165°F to kill illness-carrying micro-organisms.
- To get more juice from a lemon with greater ease, microwave on high for 45 seconds; remove fruit. Pierce with a fork and squeeze out the juice.
- To drain fat easily, use a microwave-safe colander, with a microwavable dish underneath, to cook ground beef. Grease will drip to bottom.
- When making a main dish, double or triple the amount, cook the food 90% of the way, then package and freeze.

TOASTERS

Most toasters are slot-type units that hold slices in a vertical position. If you use a wide variety of thicker breads and rolls, a wide slot toaster or a countertop toaster oven with a horizontal rack may be easier to handle. See toaster ovens earlier in this chapter.

Slot-type toasters come with either a wide single slot, or two or four regular slice designs, but will toast only one slice if desired. Models vary in price and quality; before purchasing, check the construction, safety features, and controls.

Features to consider in selecting a toaster include the following:

- Timing mechanism. Does the thermostat heat up and cool off quickly? It should automatically compensate for any voltage fluctuations in your home.
- Controls. Can you easily reach and operate both the lever that presses down the toast and the color-control dial? Can you do this without touching the hot metal? Some toasters are made with stay-cool sides. Ask if the toast-color control is accurate.
- Some toasters automatically lower and raise the bread, eliminating the need to handle levers. Make sure that there is a release button so that, if necessary, you can interrupt the toasting cycle.
- Toaster slots. Are they large enough for the types of breads, rolls, or muffins you eat most regularly? Some units have wide slots for English muffins, bagels, or thick bread. Are the coils set so that you will not come in contact with them? Does the toasted food come up high enough for you to get it out easily?
- Crumb tray. Is it hinged or does it slide out easily for cleaning?
- Handles. Are they of a stay-cool or non-heat-conducting material and large enough for you to grasp firmly?
- Switch. Does it have a two-pole safety switch so that the toaster is shockproof when not working, even though plugged into an outlet?

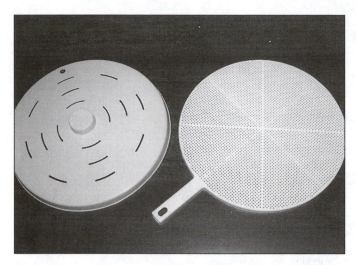

Figure 20-23. A thermoplastic splatter lid keeps liquids and grease in the pan so oven interior remains clean. (Grid lid by Ekco® Housewares, Inc., Franklin Park, IL. Slotted lid by Ensar Corp., Wheeling, IL. Photo by J.K.)

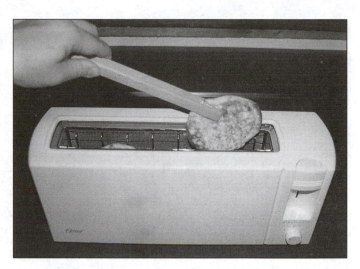

Figure 20-24. This toaster has a centering device for thin breads and an automatic pop-up. (Toaster by Oster®, Milwaukee, WI. Photo by J.K.)

- Base. Is the base solid so that it will not tip?
- Current conductors. For added safety, is the current carried by steel bars or heating tape rather than wires, as the latter tend to flex and wear thin?

A cool-sided, long slot toaster takes thin or thick breads, muffins, and bagels (Figure 20-24). The lever and browning control operate with a light touch. **Manufacturers** of cool side models: 224, 299, 318, 334, 346, 381, 399, 416. Cost is about $35 and up from appliance and housewares stores. If you have incoordination or loss of sensation in your hands, you might try a pair of toaster tongs for safer removal of hot breads and muffins. **Manufacturer:** 142. Cost is about $4 and up from mail-order firms and housewares stores. **Source:** 410.

ELECTRIC KNIVES

The design of electric knives may vary, but basically they all operate in the same way. Twin blades are hooked together and inserted into a motorized handle. The handle may be rechargeable and cordless, allowing you to use it anywhere. Or it may have a cord, in which case the handle is usually lighter. With both types, fingertip controls start the blades sliding back and forth against each other. Releasing the pressure stops the blades.

If you are preparing food for a large family, you may wish to consider an electric knife. It is especially helpful for slicing meat. You should have good grasp in one hand or partial use of both hands. You should not have any problems with your sight, perception, or coordination if you are planning to use an electric knife. If you have arthritis, you may find that a lightweight, electric knife eliminates a lot of the stress involved in cutting. Consider an electric knife in relation to tasks that could be done by a food processor. The major difference is that it slices larger pieces of food. For shredding and dicing tasks, the processor is easier.

Features to consider in selecting an electric knife include the following:

- Weight and balance. Pick up the knife, and hold it as though you were cutting. Maintain this position for several minutes; see how the weight feels. Try several brands to get an idea of the differences in balance. When cutting, you can stop to rest and may put your forearms on the arms of a chair to provide additional support.
- Length and handle design. Smaller grip-sized handles are good if you have normal grasp in one hand. Open handles have been used by homemakers with almost complete loss of grasp in both hands: Slipping one hand under the handle supports the knife while the other hand applies pressure to the control that activates the blades. Check that the length of the handle is not unwieldy for you.
- Controls. You should be able to handle the controls easily, including the safety lock that turns the knife off so that it cannot be started accidentally and the button that starts the blades. Check the blade-release mechanism. You must be able to release the blades without hitting the switch control. When releasing the blades, unplug the knife from the outlet if it has a cord. Hold the knife slanting down, push the release button, and shake the blades until they slip part way out.

Always handle the blades on the smooth side, keeping your fingers away from the cutting edge. The plastic sheath on the blades hooks them together until they are inserted and further protects your hands.

An electric knife may be used for many jobs. It can carve all kinds of meats, slice vegetables and fruits, cut cheese, cakes, sandwiches, and ice cream. It should not be used to cut through frozen foods or bones, because this dulls the blades and shortens their life and usefulness. When slicing raw meat, place the meat in the freezer for about 1 hour until it is partially frozen.

Blades should be washed well and dried after each use. Wipe handle clean with a sponge. Plastic grease-guards prevent meat juices or fat from getting inside the handle.

Do all cutting on a wood or plastic board to protect the blades. A textured surface holds the meat stable even when you're cutting

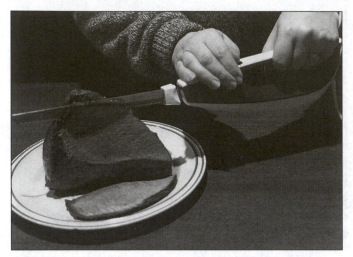

Figure 20-25. This electric carving knife comes with a 10-foot cord and carves everything from cakes to hard salami. (Sunbeam® Appliance Co., Laurel, MS. Photo by J.K.)

with one hand. Some electric carving knives have open handles for one- or two-handed use (Figure 20-25). A thumb-tip safety switch turns power off when released. **Manufacturers:** 166, 334, 381, 399. Cost is about $22 and up from housewares stores.

ELECTRIC MIXERS

Electric mixers are available in three basic styles:
- A lightweight, portable model with a cord.
- A heavier stand or counter model.
- A rechargeable, light-duty mixer.

Your choice will depend on two factors: the amount and type of mixing you wish to use the appliance for, and the extent of weakness or incoordination in your hands and arms.
- If you only want to mix very light mixtures and find that using a spoon is tiring, then a rechargeable unit may be satisfactory.
- If you bake occasionally and want to save time and energy, then a portable mixer will do. To use a portable mixer, you should have good grasp in one hand or be able to hold the mixer handle securely in both hands. If you are in a wheelchair, a hand mixer is helpful, because you can put the bowl on a lapboard or in your lap to work.

If you do a lot of baking, have poor coordination, or weak arms, you may prefer a standard mixer, which requires no holding. You must add the ingredients and scrape with a spatula. The base may be heavy to move.

PORTABLE HAND MIXERS: CORDED AND RECHARGEABLE

Features to consider in selecting a hand mixer include the following:
- Weight and handle design. Choose a handle that is comfortable for you. If you have weak grasp, a handle that circles your hand is less apt to slip out of your grasp. Very lightweight models have less power, so you will have to compromise between weight and power. Hold the mixer in your hand for several minutes to see how it balances.

- Heel rest. Put the beaters in the mixer, then set the mixer down on its end to see if the heel rest is stable.
- Controls. See that you can turn the motor on and off without difficulty. Make sure that you can eject the beaters without too much force. If you have arthritis in your hands, choose a model that allows you to manipulate the controls with the side of your hand, rather than putting too much pressure on the end of your thumb.
- Beaters. Those that do not have a center shaft are easier to scrape and clean.

Some mixer hints:
- To insert beaters if your grasp is weak, hold the mixer upside-down on your lap or another surface. Press down on the beaters with the palms of your hands.
- Place a damp sponge cloth under the bowl to keep it from sliding while you're mixing.
- Thin rubber spatulas are useful in helping you clean beaters as they slip between the blades. Be sure your mixer is totally off before putting a spatula near the blades of the beaters.
- Spin off excess batter by setting your mixer at its lowest speed and lifting the beaters just above the mixture in the bowl.

The rechargeable mixer shown in Figure 20-26 hangs on the wall and comes with two or five speeds and four attachments. It is handy for whipping up eggs, light batters like pancake batter, puddings, and beverages, but is not designed for cake or heavy cookie dough. **Manufacturers** of rechargeable units: 41, 416. Cost is about $28 and up for the set from housewares stores and mail-order firms.

If you find holding a portable hand mixer tiring, try different ways to rest it while beating (Figure 20-27). Balance the mixer in the corner of a dish drainer. This way the bowl cannot tip. **Manufacturers** of hand mixers: 41, 84, 166, 299, 334, 381, 399. Cost is about $20 and up from housewares stores.

STANDARD MIXERS

When buying a standard mixer, check the features listed for hand mixers, such as beater design and the ease with which you can manage the controls and beater ejection.
- Design and weight. Is the unit compact enough to be stored on your counter where it is ready for use? Can you slide it out of the way when it's not needed? Most standard mixers have motor and beater units that detach from the stand for use as a hand mixer. These are usually much heavier than a portable hand mixer.
- Bowls. Stainless-steel or plastic bowls are much easier to handle than glass. Be sure to ask about the bowls, because unbreakable ones are usually optional equipment and much more expensive when bought separately.
- Speed control. Make sure that you can handle the control lever. There are usually nine to 12 speeds on a standard mixer. Look for an easy-to-read guide that tells you what speed is best for specific mixtures.
- Motor and hinge. Make sure you can tilt the motor-beater handle back to lift the beaters from the bowl while adding ingredients or scraping the bowl and beaters.

Optional accessories for some standard mixers include a fruit juicer, food grinder, vegetable slicer, coffee bean grinder, knife

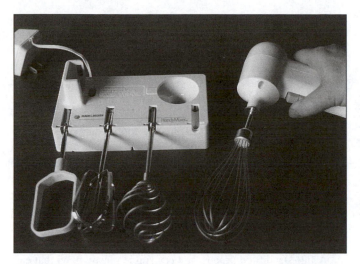

Figure 20-26. This rechargeable mixer hangs on the wall and comes with two or five speeds and four attachments. (Photo courtesy of Black and Decker® [U.S.] Co., Shelton, CT.)

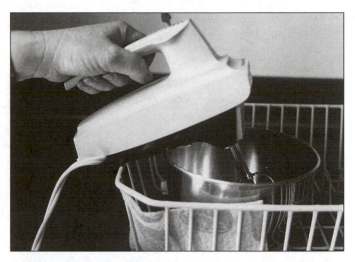

Figure 20-27. If you find holding a portable hand mixer tiring, try different ways to rest it while beating. Balance the mixer in the corner of a dish drainer. (Photo courtesy of the O.T. Dept., Howard A. Rusk Institute of Rehabilitation Medicine.)

sharpener, and dough-hook attachment (on the most powerful units). Cost varies with the number of accessories you purchase, so you must decide on the value of the additions in relation to your own cooking patterns. Standard heavier mixers with stainless-steel bowls cost about $50 and up. **Manufacturers:** 166, 222, 299, 381. **Sources:** 65, 71, 427.

You may also want to check out the possibilities of a food processor, which can do almost everything a mixer does and more. See food processors later in this chapter.

European-style standard mixers combine the portability of a hand mixer with a standard counter base (Figure 20-28). Most have an oscillating power arm and plastic mixing bowl. **Manufacturers:** 224, 329, 334. Cost is about $60 and up from housewares stores and mail-order firms.

One answer to lifting a standard mixer is a pop-up shelf under your countertop. The hardware for shelves is carried by building suppliers. **Manufacturer:** 417. Another answer is a sliding shelf that lets you pull it forward when needed. Your home economist or occupational therapist can design such a unit for you.

ELECTRIC BLENDERS

An electric blender accomplishes in a few seconds what might take a half hour or more to do by hand. The blades blend, mix, chop, grate, puree, liquefy, and shred. If you have marked weakness, incoordination, or arthritis in your hands, a blender could be helpful, even healthful, especially if you use a lot of fresh foods.

Before buying a blender, however, make careful comparisons with a food processor. A blender is better at whipping up beverages and soups. A processor, on the other hand, does heavier jobs than a blender but is not always as good at mixing liquids.

Features to consider in selecting a blender include the following:
- Base height. The lower the base, the easier it is to add ingredients through the top of the blender container and to lift it on and off the base. Some bases are only 3½" high. A base is usually heavy, so if your arms are weak it is hard to move from place to place.

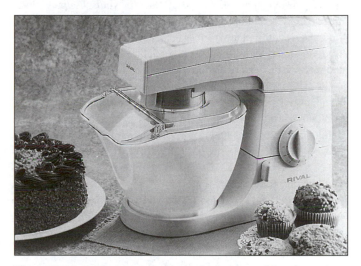

Figure 20-28. European-style standard mixers combine the portability of a hand mixer with a standard counter base. (Photo courtesy of the Rival® Company, Kansas City, MO.)

- Container. Blender containers of high-impact, heat-resistant plastic are lighter to lift and safer than glass. If you have use of only one hand or loss of function in both hands, a handle on the side of the container lets you lift it with a hook grasp.

Most containers hold between 32 and 56 ounces. Measuring marks on the side help when adding ingredients. Make sure you can lift off the cover to add ingredients; if your fingers are weak, attach a loop to the container cover.
- Assembly. Take the container apart. You have to be able to remove the bottom to scrape out food that collects there. Most base assemblies unscrew. Tightening or loosening is easier if you put the emptied container in the base and turn against the sprockets just until loosened.
- Controls. Most are push-button or sliding controls. A few have dials that require moderate grasp in one hand to turn. Blenders have a variety of speed settings. You can get by with two speeds: high and low. The most you will need is four or five.

- Options. Some blenders come with half-pint jars in which you can chop herbs or blend and store small amounts of foods like salad dressing or sauces.

You can buy a blender for $17 and up from housewares stores. **Manufacturers:** 41, 84, 166, 222, 299, 381.

If you live alone or only wish to use a food processor for small amounts of food, a food processor/drink blender is a compact, two-in-one appliance. The combination appliance means you need only one base for two appliances. These liquefier blenders have several speeds and plastic containers for both the processor and blender. **Manufacturers:** 299, 381. Cost is about $50 and up from housewares stores.

FOOD PROCESSORS

If you have weak arms, arthritis in your hands, poor coordination, limited vision, or do a lot of cooking from scratch, a food processor could be a great help. This kitchen helper does in seconds what might take you an hour. It is not an appliance to keep in a closet and pull out; it is one to use in place of your chopping block, knives, graters, and other cutting or mixing aids. You must, however, make a central place for it at the area where you prepare meals. To use a processor to its fullest potential, read the instruction book, and invest in at least one good food processor cookbook.

Processors come in a variety of styles and sizes. There are compact units that will chop an onion, mince herbs and vegetables, puree fruits or vegetables for a sauce, and work well for doing small jobs. For larger jobs, like making coleslaw or bread, you need a full-sized processor. Most full-sized processors consist of a motor base, see-through container, a variety of stainless-steel blades for cutting, mincing, slicing, pureeing, shredding, and a plastic blade for mixing, as well as a food pusher to keep your fingers away from spinning blades. Additional accessories include a spatula that fits the contours of the bowl and a whipper-blender attachment for recipes that require whipped cream, egg whites, or mayonnaise.

Features to consider in selecting a food processor include the following:

- What do you want your food processor to do? Small jobs or heavy mixing like cakes, cookie doughs, and breads?
- How much space do you have to put a food processor in a central location? Some units locate the mixing bowls on top of the motor bases, others beside it. The former take about the space of a blender, the latter the space of a toaster.
- Can you handle the assembling and disassembling of the unit? This includes putting the bowl on, adding the proper blade or disk, locking each part into place, and reversing the procedure. Each machine has safeguards to prevent accidental opening or injury; be sure you can handle these interlocks and other safety mechanisms. The blades on a processor are very sharp; read and follow the manufacturer's instructions.
- Can you manipulate the controls? If working with one hand, check to make sure the unit stays in place while you turn the controls. A damp sponge cloth helps stabilize a small processor. Larger ones usually have rubber feet.
- How much pre-cutting will you have to do? Processors do not

completely eliminate cutting. Most smaller processors require that foods be cut into 1" pieces. Check out the latest reports in consumer testing and family service magazines. Compare the versatility of one processor against another.

In the store, look at the design. Is it durable? Will it clean easily? The cost of a food processor ranges from $20 to more than $200.

A compact food processor minces, chops, dices, and blends food like full-sized units (Figure 20-29). However, it does small amounts, not more than one cup. You put the ingredients in the bowl, lock the top to which blades are attached, and fit it over base. Pushing the button activates the single-speed 500 watt motor. Bowl is dishwasher safe. **Manufacturers** of compact processors include 41, 84, 166, 299, 334, 381, 422. Cost is about $25 and up.

A full-sized food processor has a single plastic bowl that easily inserts and locks in place (Figure 20-30). The controls switch to chute operation for continuous processing of large amounts. The pusher keeps hands away from blade. Clear container is dishwasher safe. **Manufacturers:** 41, 45, 156, 166, 299, 329, 334, 381.

A small juice extractor is a single-purpose processor (Figure 20-31). Pressure on the center squeezer activates the 50 watt motor. Juice is collected in a seven-ounce serving carafe that detaches for easy serving. Convenient cord storage. UL listed. **Manufacturers:** 45, 89, 224, 299, 334, 416, 422. Cost is about $25 and up from housewares stores and mail-order firms.

A larger juice extractor works for fruits and vegetables. The single control turns easily. Tray holds food being fed into machine with pusher. High-speed blades pulverize and strain juice into a container for serving. Pulp and seeds go into a second holder for easy disposal. **Manufacturers:** 45, 166, 279, 299, 303. Cost is about $40 and up from housewares stores.

MISCELLANEOUS APPLIANCES

There are other special appliances you may want to consider: An automatic coffeemaker may be an important part of your wake-up routine. Before purchasing, check the following features:

- Handle design. Make sure you can safely pick up the container. A baffle will help keep your hand from touching a hot surface.
- Procedure for measuring and pouring in water. If you have marked incoordination or weakness, this may be more difficult than using a standard percolator.
- Features. These include wake-up programming so coffee is ready when you are and electronically controlled brewing in sizes that make from one to 10 cups.

If you have weakness or incoordination in your arms and hands, a non-breakable coffeemaker should be considered. A lightweight plastic, microwave coffee brewer makes two to five cups and is dishwasher safe. **Manufacturer:** 131. Cost is about $18 from housewares stores and mail-order firms. **Source:** 364.

A non-breakable, stainless-steel carafe that fits all machines is about $19 and up. Dishwasher safe. **Source:** 410. Small microwave coffee makers for single-cup servings cost about $10 from housewares and mail-order firms. **Source:** 378. The Cup-at-a-Time electric coffeemaker brews a single cup of coffee directly

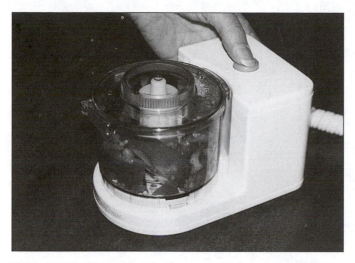

Figure 20-29. This compact food processor minces, chops, dices, and blends food like full-sized units. (Unit by Black & Decker® [U.S.] Co., Shelton CT. Photo by J.K.)

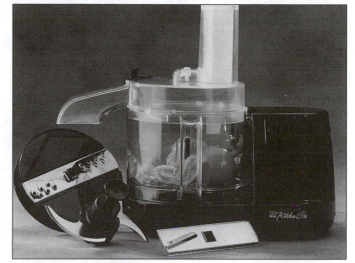

Figure 20-30. This full-sized food processor has a single plastic bowl that easily inserts and locks in place. (Photo courtesy of Regal® Ware, Inc., Kewaskum, WI.)

into a mug. **Manufacturer:** 41. Cost is about $20 and up from housewares stores.

If you love baking your own bread, adding whole grains, herbs, and other ingredients, a bread machine might be a luxurious addition to your repertoire. It mixes, kneads, lets dough rise, bakes, and cools automatically. On some units, a programmable clock/timer lets you set unit up to 13 hours ahead of time. Before purchasing, check out the features, including the types of breads and amounts that a particular appliance will handle. **Manufacturers:** 41, 159, 299, 303, 329, 346, 349, 381, 421. Cost is about $80 and up from housewares stores and gourmet mail-order firms. **Sources:** 65, 87, 176, 359, 381, 427.

GOING FURTHER

Addresses are given in the Appendices.

PUBLICATIONS

Anderson, J., & Hanna, E. (1997). *Microways: Every Cook's Guide to Successful Microwaving*. New York: Berkley. **Source:** 39B.

Best Recipes for Low Calorie Microwaving. (1990). Red Spoon Collection. New York: Prentice-Hall. **Source:** 316B.

Campbell Soup Microwave Institute. Write for current publications.

Castle, C. (1988). *The Complete Book of Steam Cookery*. Los Angeles: Jeremy P. Tarcher. **Source:** 206.

Claessons, S. (1992). *LoFat Microwave Cooking* .Emmaus, PA: Rodale Press. **Source:** 335B.

Crocker, B. (1990). *Betty Crocker's Microwave Cookbook*.

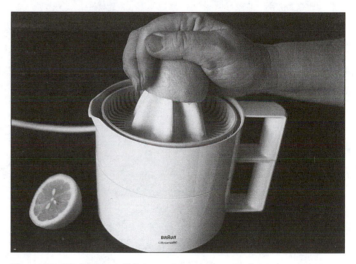

Figure 20-31. This small juice extractor is a single-purpose processor. (Unit by Braun, Inc., Lynnefield, MA. Photo by J.K.)

New York: Prentice-Hall. **Source:** 316B.

Hoffman, M. (1995). *Crockery Cookery* (rev. ed.). New York: Berkley-Putnam. **Source:** 39B.

Kenneally, J. (Ed.). (1990). *The Good Housekeeping Illustrated Microwave Cookbook*. New York: Hearst Books, Random House. **Source:** 326.

Reingold, C. B., & Chaback, E. (1990). *The Microwave Convection Oven Cookbook*. Mt. Vernon, NY: Consumers Union. **Source:** 75B.

21

Selecting and Caring for Kitchen Tools

Choosing proper cooking utensils will help compensate for difficulties caused by your physical disability or limited mobility. Certain principles apply to every item you use.

- Is it versatile? Can the utensil fill more than one need? A multipurpose tool takes less storage space than several single-purpose utensils. A good knife, for example, with a sharp, 8" to 10" blade and a comfortable handle can be used for many cutting tasks.
- Is it durable? The tool should be well made. Make sure the handle is securely attached to the utensil. Mechanical aids should work without frequent adjustments or repairs. Purchase reliable, high-quality brands.
- Is it easy to clean? Avoid decorative grooves that trap food and therefore require extra scrubbing. Non-stick finishes are easier to clean.
- Is it reasonably priced? Money does not always guarantee quality, but sometimes it is better to pay more for a superior product. Check advertisements to compare prices and look for sales. The costs listed in this book are suggested retail prices, but you may find items at a lower or discount price if you shop around.

KNIVES

Knives are the most frequently used food preparation tools. Three or four basic knives can serve most of your needs: a utility knife or a smaller paring knife, a larger serrated or straight blade for chopping, and a slicing or carving knife. If you have hand limitations, you may discover that one specially designed knife, like the Swedish knife in Figure 21-1, does most of your work.

When buying a knife, test to see how it feels in your hand. Is it balanced and comfortable to hold? Larger, shaped handles are more comfortable to grip. You don't want a knife that is too heavy, but you do need one that has the handle firmly attached to the tang of the blade. A full tang is an extension of the blade that extends to the end of the handle; a half tang extends to the middle. The tang should be fixed to the handle with two or more rivets. Other means of attachment may loosen with use and become annoying as well as dangerous.

Sharp knives are safer than dull ones. A sharp knife slices smoothly; a dull one requires more pressure and may slip while you're cutting. A serrated blade gives you additional control. When selecting a knife, consider your own needs and cooking style:

- If your grasp is weak, you will want a large, lightweight or open handle.
- If your hands are affected by arthritis, an angled knife gives more joint protection and greater power. Avoid extending your index finger while cutting, because it puts too much stress on joints.
- If you have poor coordination, you may prefer a heavier knife or an angled one that keeps your fingers out of the way.
- If you have hand limitations, you may prefer a larger knife for major cutting tasks plus a food processor for finer cutting.

A Swedish angled knife makes cutting more comfortable if you have limited motion, weakness in your arms, or poor coordination in your hands (see Figure 21-1). The grip-shaped, dishwasher safe handle keeps your hands away from the board. The force needed for cutting is reduced by up to 80%, because the power is transferred from your wrist to your shoulder. The molded handle keeps you from extending your index finger while cutting. The stainless-steel blade is serrated to increase control. **Manufacturer:** 122. Cost is about $20 and up from self-help firms. **Sources:** 5, 13, 122, 252, 264, 282, 290, 408.

An all-purpose E-Z Grip knife lets you chop, slice, and dice more comfortably (Figure 21-2). The cut-out handle with a blunt blade end requires a lighter grasp than a standard knife. It is set right above the blade, so you don't need as much pressure to cut. The stainless-steel blade is riveted to a hardwood handle. In various sizes from 7½" to 11" long, it costs about $6 and up from mail-order and self-help firms. **Sources:** 108, 252, 264, 378.

A pizza knife is not limited to slicing pizza but may be used for kitchen and at-the-table cutting (Figure 21-3). The one shown has a right-angle hand grip that increases power and protects your

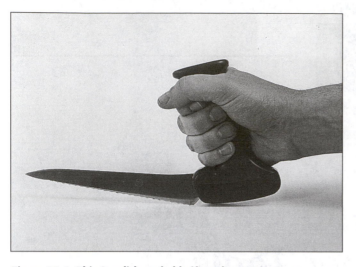

Figure 21-1. This Swedish angled knife makes cutting more comfortable if you have limited motion, weakness in your arms, or poor coordination in your hands. (Photo by J.K.)

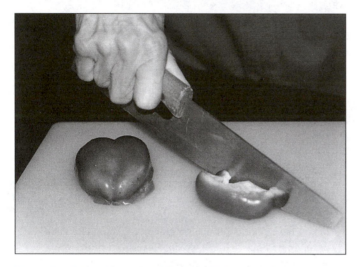

Figure 21-2. An all-purpose E-Z grip knife lets you chop, slice, and dice more comfortably. (Photo by J.K.)

wrist. **Manufacturer:** 122. Cost is about $18 from self-help firms. **Sources:** 5, 13, 120, 122, 252, 264, 290, 370, 408.

If grasp is weak or uncertain, a molded cuff may be riveted to a knife for more secure handling (Figures 21-4A and 21-4B).

CARING FOR KNIVES

A good knife should last for a lifetime, if you choose one of top quality and care for it correctly. Tips for caring for your knives:

- Never abuse a knife. Always use a cutting board to protect the blade as well as other surfaces.
- Clean the blade immediately after use with a damp cloth or soapy sponge, dry, and put away.
- If your knife is dishwasher safe, always place it so that it does not hit against other tools and become dulled and nicked.
- Store the knife so that the blade is not jostled and blunted in a drawer.
- Position your knives so they are convenient and safe to pick up, especially if you have poor coordination, weak hands, or limited vision.

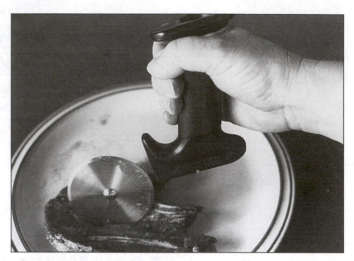

Figure 21-3. A pizza knife is not limited to slicing pizza but may be used for kitchen and at-the-table cutting. (Photo by J.K.)

A slanted knife block shields the blades yet keeps knives ready for grasping. You may purchase a block with or without knives. **Manufacturers:** 66, 111, 162, 201, 230, 321, 432. Cost of block without knives is about $12 and up; price with knives varies from about $19 to more than $200 from housewares stores and gourmet and mail-order firms. **Sources:** 65, 71, 82, 283, 373, 427.

A wall-hung knife rack also protects your hands from accidental contact with blades and keeps knives out of the reach of children. Handles are in a vertical position for efficient grasping. A sheet of plastic should cover the base so you can see exactly which knife you are pulling out. Racks are carried by housewares and gourmet stores. **Source:** 242. In-drawer knife racks hold blades at an angle so they do not hit each other. Cost is about $7 and up from housewares stores and kitchen/gourmet mail-order firms. **Sources:** 152, 283.

Knife sharpeners come in many designs. Electric can openers often have accessory sharpeners. If you are working with one hand, make sure that the unit automatically turns on when you apply pressure or that it has an on/off switch.

A Wilkinson® knife stays sharp because it is stored in a case that automatically hones the blade as it is put in and taken out (Figure 21-5). Stainless-steel blade knives are lightweight with comfort-grip handles and are dishwasher safe. The case may be kept on a counter or mounted on a wall. Cost is about $13 and up for a single knife and $20 and up for a set from housewares stores and mail-order firms. **Sources:** 49, 71, 359. A similar stainless-steel, self-sharpening utility knife is **manufactured** by 391. Cost is about $8 from housewares stores.

An all-metal, non-electric sharpener automatically places your knife at the correct angle for sharpening (Figure 21-6). **Manufacturer:** 63. Cost is about $38 from kitchen/gourmet firms. **Sources:** 65, 427.

Some electric knife sharpeners have a slot for pre-sharpening your knife and another for sharpening the entire length of the blade with revolving diamonds (Figure 21-7). You control the pressure on the knife. The four-pound sharpener is secured to the counter by suction cups. **Manufacturer:** 111. Cost is about $50 and up from housewares stores and mail-order firms. UL listed.

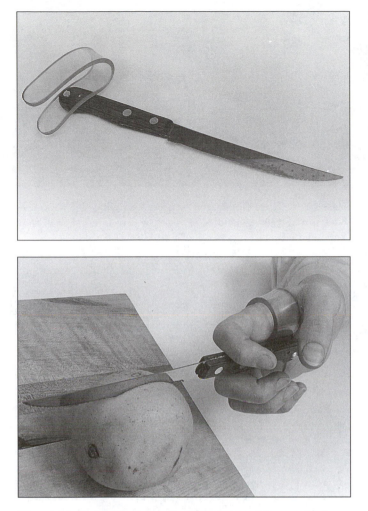

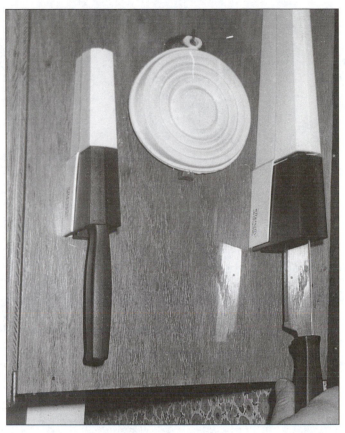

Figure 21-5. A Wilkinson® knife stays sharp because it is stored in a case that automatically hones the blade as it is put in and taken out. (Knife by Wilkinson Sword U.S.A., Atlanta, GA. Photo by J.K.)

Figures 21-4A, 21-4B. If grasp is weak or uncertain, a molded cuff may be riveted to a knife for more secure handling. (Photo courtesy of the O.T. Dept., Howard A. Rusk Institute of Rehabilitation Medicine.)

Sources: 167, 245, 283. Note: An electric knife sharpener requires even control to prevent burning the metal. If you have poor coordination, a non-electric sharpener is safer.

Additional aids for cutting in *Mealtime Manual* include the following:

- Adjustable slicing knife: See Chapter 9.
- Roller, rocker, and T-handle knives: See Chapter 22.
- Electric knives: See Chapter 20.
- Holders for meats and vegetables while cutting: See Chapter 1 and Chapter 28.
- A cake server: See Chapter 30.

KITCHEN SHEARS AND SCISSORS

Kitchen shears or scissors snip open plastic pouches, cut and trim meat, remove skin from poultry, divide dough, and chop fresh parsley, green onions, or other herbs. One or both blades may be serrated for greater control. Some kitchen shears come apart for cleaning. Decide what type of shears or scissors you need, then look for top quality. Keep them in prime condition and use them

correctly: wash then dry to prevent rusting and store so blades are protected.

Scissors are easier to handle if you have good use of one hand. Some styles, however, have self-opening springs that reduce the power required to use them. Scissors can be used with two hands if you have weak grasp. To use, stabilize the meat, other food, or plastic pouch on a non-slip surface, such as a textured cutting board or sponge cloth, then use both hands to operate the scissor blades. Do not use scissors if you have arthritis in your hands. Instead, use a compact or regular food processor for chopping.

Good Grips® scissors for right or left hand use have spring-opening handles (Figure 21-8). The wide handle distributes pressure over the whole hand. Precision ground, stainless-steel blades cut through meat and open packages and are dishwasher safe. **Manufacturer:** 301. Cost is about $15 from housewares stores and mail-order firms. **Sources:** 13, 16, 65, 71, 108, 238, 252, 261, 408, 427.

Adapted loop or Swedish scissors have a spring opening, cutting the amount of energy required in half (Figure 21-9). They work well for opening packages and cutting herbs. **Manufacturer:** 122. Cost is about $17 per pair from self-help firms. **Sources:** 1, 5, 13, 122, 252, 264, 290, 370, 408.

See additional scissors in Chapter 27 as well as grating and chopping aids in Chapter 28.

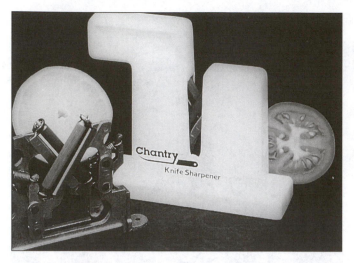

Figure 21-6. This all-metal, non-electric sharpener automatically places your knife at the correct angle for sharpening. (Photo courtesy of Chantry®, Clearwater, FL.)

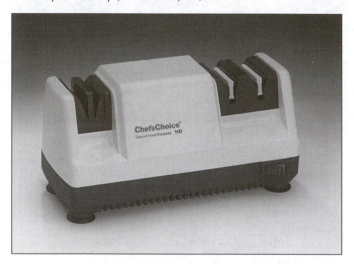

Figure 21-7. This electric knife sharpener has a slot for pre-sharpening your knife and another for sharpening the entire length of the blade with revolving diamonds. (Photo courtesy of Edgecraft® Corporation, Avondale, PA.)

POTS AND PANS

Pots and pans come in a wide variety of easy-to-care-for materials. If using a microwave oven, see Chapter 20 for specialized food containers and utensils.

If you have weak arms, lightweight aluminum pans conserve energy. Aluminum heats quickly and evenly. Since thinner-gauge pans tend to warp, cool any aluminum pot completely before washing. If the aluminum interior discolors from contact with minerals in food and water or from washing in an automatic dishwasher, remove stains by boiling 2 tablespoons cream of tartar for each quart of water in pan for 5 to 10 minutes. Cool, then scrub lightly with a soap-filled steel wool pad. Or cook an acidic food, such as tomatoes, rhubarb, or applesauce, in the pot.

Stainless steel, combined with copper or aluminum on the bottom and sides for better heat conduction, is durable, difficult to

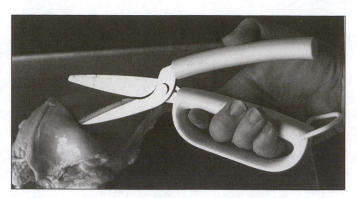

Figure 21-8. These Good Grips® scissors for right or left hand use have spring-opening handles. (Scissors by Oxo International, New York. Photo by J.K.)

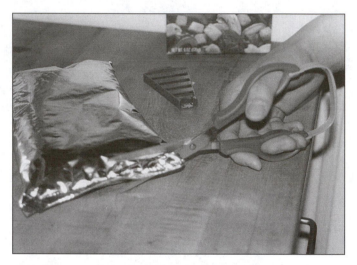

Figure 21-9. Adapted loop or Swedish scissors have a spring opening, cutting the amount of energy required in half. (Scissors from Etac USA, Waukesha, WI. Photo by J.K.)

dent, will not corrode, and is scratch-resistant. The slightly heavier weight may be preferred if you have poor coordination but no loss of strength.

When selecting a new pot or pan, judge it by your needs as well as its construction:

- Handles and lid knobs should be of non-heat-conducting materials so they remain cool, and extend out so they are easy for you to grip.
- The bottom should be flat and the sides straight for range-top use.
- Covers must fit securely to cut moisture loss.
- Non-stick finishes, both interior and exterior, reduce the use of fats and oils and also clean more easily.
- Manufacturer's instructions will tell whether the pan is dishwasher safe.

The Pro-Glide™ eight-piece set has a DuPont® non-stick surface inside and out (Figure 21-10). The handles are heatproof, and the knobs are open for easy grasp or lifting off with a utensil. The handles on the Dutch oven extend out far enough that you can pick it up without touching the metal, although pot holders are always recommended. **Manufacturer:** 329.

For other pans see the following:

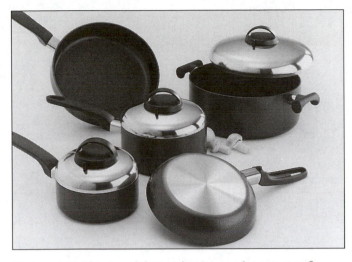

Figure 21-10. This Pro Glide™ eight-piece set has a DuPont® non-stick surface inside and out. (Photo courtesy of Regal® Ware, Inc., Kewaskum, WI.)

- Gripper pan and utensils, sauté or gourmet skillet: see Chapter 29.
- Two-handled pan and pan with assist handle: see Chapter 2.

Utensils of wood or coated with Teflon and plastic help protect non-stick finishes. **Manufacturers** include 112, 142, 273, 289. Cost is about $1 each and up from housewares stores and mail-order firms.

APRONS

Protect yourself against spills and splatters while you work in the kitchen. Make sure the material is not flammable: Do not use plastic or synthetics like nylon near the stove. Choose cloth or rubber.

A hoop apron eliminates the need to tie if you have use of one hand or limited range of motion (Figure 21-11). Plastic hoops cost about $1.50 and up from sewing stores and firms. **Sources** for hoops: 178, 187.

Also see cobbler's smock in Chapter 16.

HANDLING RECIPES

Keeping recipes handy and organized so you can vary meals is a task for any enthusiastic cook. Being able to read them easily while preparing meals is important. Suggestions to improve vision are given in Chapter 9.

A book stand keeps your cookbook at the proper angle and protects the pages from splatters (Figure 21-12). Select a stand that will hold various sizes of books. Stands for cookbooks often come with clear plastic shields that protect the open pages. **Manufacturers** include 63. Cost is about $8 and up from housewares stores and mail-order firms. Regular book holders cost about $3 and up from stationery stores and mail-order and self-help firms. A holder called the Book Butler has spring-held posts to keep pages flat and costs about $16 and up. **Sources:** 120, 196, 252, 264, 290, 370, 408.

A rotary file keeps favorite recipes within fingertip reach

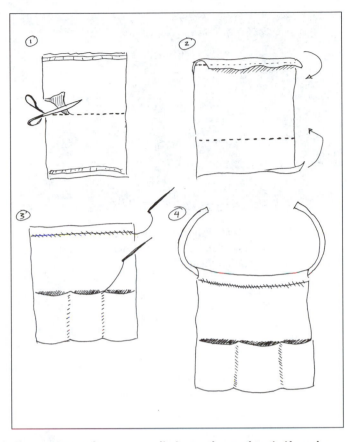

Figure 21-11. A hoop apron eliminates the need to tie if you have use of one hand or limited range of motion. (Illustration by G.K.)

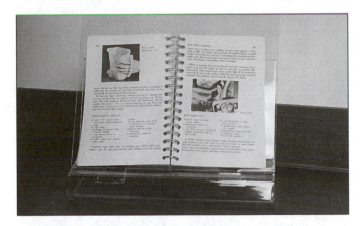

Figure 21-12. A book stand keeps your cookbook at the proper angle and protects the pages from splatters. (Photo by J.K.)

(Figure 21-13). The 3½" x 5" plastic envelopes file up to 500 recipes. Cost is about $16 and up for unit with 160 envelopes from stationery stores or mail-order firms. **Source:** 377.

A custom cookbook lets you keep favorite recipes as well as new ones you want to try right at hand. You insert recipes in a three-ring binder, equipped with clear vinyl, slip-in pocket pages for 3" x 5" cards or 5" x 8" cards. It costs about $20 from photographic supplies firms. **Source:** 405.

If reading is difficult, you may record recipes on a cassette tape. You can stop the machine while you complete the given task. See Chapter 9.

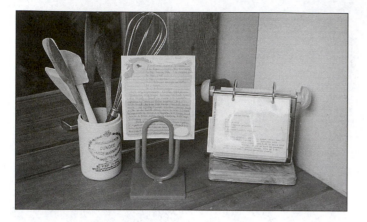

Figure 21-13. A rotary file keeps favorite recipes within fingertip reach. (Photo courtesy of the O.T. Dept., Howard A. Rusk Institute of Rehabilitation Medicine.)

CHAPTER 22

Selecting
Eating Aids

Mealtime is more enjoyable if you are able to eat with ease. If you have weakness, arthritis, or incoordination in your hands and arms, a change in the style of dishes and utensils you use may help. The items shown here are commercially available or easily devised at home.

A pleasant place to eat should be part of your meal. Make sure that you have a comfortable chair and the right level surface. When sitting in a wheelchair, you may want to use a lapboard. See Chapter 7. If transporting food is difficult, use a wheeled table. See Chapter 16.

Many eating aids come in designs that the whole family will like using. When choosing dishes and utensils, here are a few tips:

- Plates with straight rims give you an edge to push food against while picking it up. These plates are available in plastic or acrylic designs from stores selling informal housewares.
- Mugs are easier to hold than glasses and come in a variety of designs. Look for lightweight plastic mugs with large handles to accommodate your whole hand.
- Flatware is available with built-up handles that are easier to grip than metal utensils. Look for informal flatware.
- A non-slip placemat, HandyAid®, Dycem® non-slip products, or another small rubber pad keeps dishes from sliding. See Chapter 1. If the surface is waterproof, use a damp sponge cloth or paper towel.

A plate with a right-angle rim lets you push food being picked up with a fork or spoon against it (Figure 22-1). The large handled mug is easy to pick up. Rimmed plates are often found among informal settings for use at picnics or events where handling a plate is difficult for anyone.

Lightweight forks and spoons with extra large handles make holding easier if you have weak grasp or stiff fingers (Figure 22-2). **Manufacturers:** 128, 193, 331, 394. Twenty-piece, stainless-steel flatware sets with ribbed plastic, bamboo, wood, or "bistro" handles cost about $15 and up per set from department stores and mail-order firms. Before purchasing, make sure that they are dishwasher safe. **Sources:** 71, 82, 98, 242, 359, 373.

If you have tremors or incoordination, a weighted spoon may

be helpful. **Manufacturers:** 103, 393. Cost is about $4 each from self-help firms. **Sources:** 5, 16, 120, 130, 252, 264, 290, 370, 393, 408.

You can build up the handle of a standard eating utensil with a foam curler or cylindrical closed-cell foam padding. The rough surface increases friction on the handle for a more secure grip. Foam curlers in various diameters cost about $1.50 per set from variety and department stores. Strips of cylindrical foam padding that you can cut to size for various utensils are available from hospital supply and self-help firms. **Distributor:** 103. **Sources:** 1, 5, 13, 16, 108, 120, 130, 138, 252, 264, 265, 290, 368, 370, 393, 408.

Commercially available eating utensils with built-up handles include teaspoons, tablespoons, forks, and knives (Figure 22-3). Handles may be ribbed, molded for easier approach to mouth, attached to angled utensils, extended in length, or shaped to fit hand. **Manufacturers/Distributors:** 103, 122, 393. Cost is about $4 each and up from self-help firms.

The Arthwriter, originally designed for holding a pen or pencil, also holds an eating utensil when grasp is weak or affected by arthritis (Figure 22-4). Cost is about $10 from self-help firms. **Sources:** 15, 120, 290, 306.

Some scoop plates have non-slip bases to keep them from sliding and a curved inner rim to guide food onto the spoon or fork (Figure 22-5). **Manufacturers** include 122. Plates cost about $5 each and up from self-help firms. **Sources:** 1, 5, 8, 15, 16, 108, 120, 130, 138, 155, 238, 247, 252, 264, 265, 290, 370, 393, 408.

A vertical handle on an eating aid may be easier to manage than a horizontal one if you have marked loss of grasp and motion in your arm. **Manufacturer:** 393. Cost is about $7 each and up from self-help firms. **Sources:** 5, 8, 120, 252, 264, 290, 370, 408.

If reaching your mouth is difficult because of limited range due to arthritis or other reasons, a lengthened eating utensil may solve the problem (Figure 22-6). These lightweight utensils come with straight, bent, or adjustable handles for easier approach to your mouth. **Manufacturer:** 122. Cost is about $7 each and up from self-help firms. **Sources:** 5, 108, 120, 122, 290, 408.

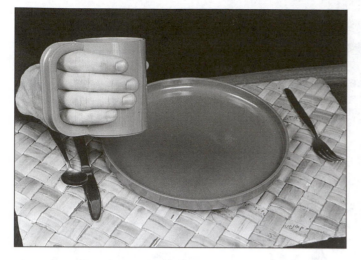

Figure 22-1. This plate with a right-angle rim lets you push food being picked up with a fork or spoon against it. (Photo courtesy of the O.T. Dept., Howard A. Rusk Institute of Rehabilitation Medicine.)

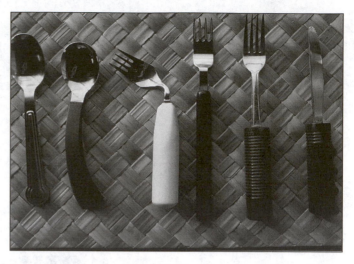

Figure 22-3. Commercially available eating utensils with built-up handles include teaspoons, tablespoons, forks, and knives. (Photo by J.K.)

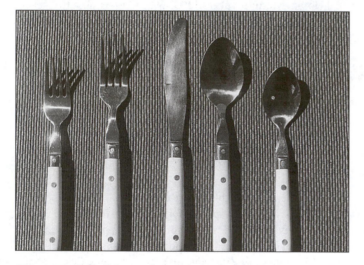

Figure 22-2. The flatware here is by Excel. (Cutlery, Inc., Garden City, NY. Photo by J.K.)

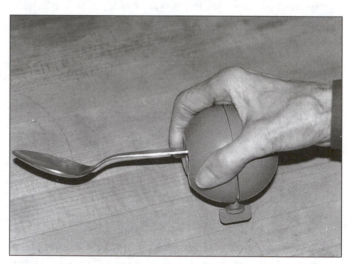

Figure 22-4. The Arthwriter, originally designed for holding a pen or pencil, also holds an eating utensil when grasp is weak or affected by arthritis. (Photo courtesy of the O.T. Dept., Howard A. Rusk Institute of Rehabilitation Medicine.)

A snap-on plate guard provides a rim to push the food against and onto the utensil (Figure 22-7). Plastic and metal guards come in several sizes to fit plates. **Manufacturers** include 122. Cost is about $5 each from self-help firms. **Sources:** 5, 13, 108, 120, 122, 138, 238, 247, 252, 264, 290, 368, 370, 394, 408.

If you have difficulty rotating your forearm or have poor coordination, an angled spoon or fork may be more comfortable (Figure 22-8). **Manufacturer:** 122. Cost is about $30 per set or $11 each for right- or left-handed use from self-help firms. **Sources:** 5, 108, 120, 122, 252, 264, 290, 368, 408.

An angled knife reduces pressure on your hand and transfers it to your upper arm. See Chapter 2.

A swivel spoon rotates to keep the bowl of the utensil level as you lift it to your mouth if you cannot rotate your forearm or have marked incoordination (Figure 22-9). **Manufacturers** include 122. Cost is about $3 each and up from self-help firms. **Sources:** 1, 5, 16, 108, 120, 122, 130, 238, 252, 264, 290, 368, 370, 408.

If you have loss of grasp, a universal cuff with a palmar pocket will hold an eating utensil or other tool (Figure 22-10). Velcro® fasteners make putting on the cuff easier. **Sources:** 5, 16, 108, 120, 238, 252, 264, 265, 290, 370, 408.

If you have marked weakness in your wrists as well as loss of grasp, a cock-up splint with a palmar pocket will hold an eating utensil. See Chapter 2. For more information about the type of splint best for you, contact a local rehabilitation center, occupational therapist, or visiting nurse service.

Cutting food with one hand is easier with a rocker knife (Figure 22-11). The curved blade cuts as you rock the handle. **Manufacturers** include 122, 226. Cost is about $9 and up from self-help firms. **Sources:** 1, 5, 108, 120, 130, 155, 238, 252, 264, 290, 368, 370, 382, 408.

A T-handled knife also cuts in a rocking motion. Rest your full

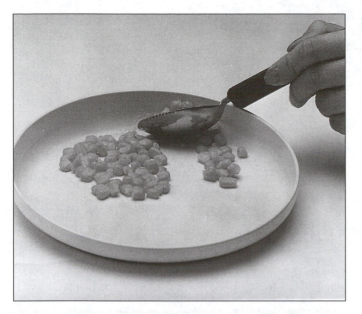

Figure 22-5. This scoop plate has a non-slip base to keep it from sliding and a curved inner rim to guide food onto the spoon or fork. (Photo courtesy of Enrichments®, a Bissell Healthcare Company, Bolingbrook, IL.)

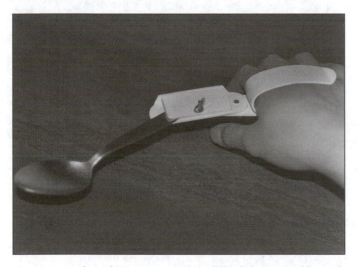

Figure 22-6. If reaching your mouth is difficult because of limited range due to arthritis or other reasons, a lengthened eating utensil may solve the problem. (Photo by J.K.)

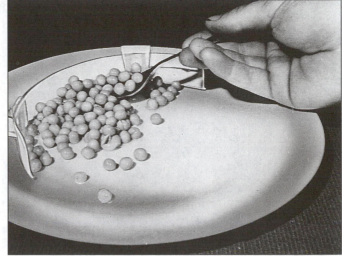

Figure 22-7. A snap-on plate guard provides a rim to push the food against and on to the utensil. (Photo courtesy of Maddak®, Inc., Pequannock, NJ.)

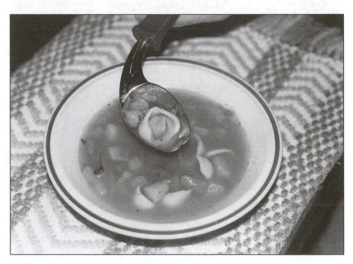

Figure 22-8. If you have difficulty rotating your forearm or have poor coordination, an angled spoon or fork may be more comfortable. (Photo by J.K.)

hand on the top, applying pressure when cutting. **Manufacturer:** 219. Cost is about $17 from self-help firms. **Sources:** 5, 120, 155, 252, 264, 290, 370, 408. Also see Chapter 2 for folding knife and Chapter 21 for angled knife and pizza cutter.

A sandwich holder inserted into the palmar pocket of a wrist support makes reaching your mouth easier when grasp is lacking (Figure 22-12). Cost is about $7 from self-help firms. **Sources:** 5, 16, 108, 120, 238, 252, 264, 290, 370, 408.

DRINKING

Long straws eliminate the need to pick up a glass or mug if your arms are weak or you have poor coordination. Eighteen-inch-long polyethylene reusable straws cost about $3 for 10 and up from hospital supply and self-help firms. **Sources:** 5, 16, 108, 120, 155, 252, 264, 265, 290, 368, 393, 408. Straws may also be cut from surgical tubing and bent to the angle you desire.

A straw holder keeps the straw upright (Figure 22-13). You may use a small bulldog clip, a pencil clip, or a commercially available holder. The one shown has several holes, so you select the most comfortable angle. Cost is about $4 from self-help firms. **Sources:** 5, 16, 120, 238, 368, 408. If you are able to lift a cup or glass but still need a straw to drink, look for flex-neck straws, which have a spiral corrugation so you can bend them to stay in any position. Cost is about $1 per box from grocery stores and hospital supply houses.

A T-handled mug is easier to pick up when fingers are stiff (Figure 22-14). Cost is about $3 and up from self-help firms. **Sources:** 5, 108, 120, 290, 368, 408. Large-handled mugs of var-

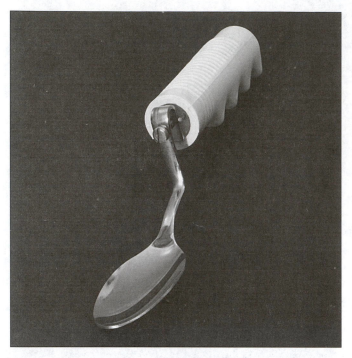

Figure 22-9. A swivel spoon rotates to keep the bowl of the utensil level as you lift it to your mouth if you cannot rotate your forearm or have marked incoordination.

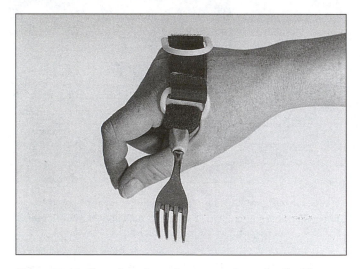

Figure 22-10. If you have loss of grasp, a universal cuff with a palmar pocket will hold an eating utensil or other tool. (Photo courtesy of AliMed®, Inc., Dedham, MA.)

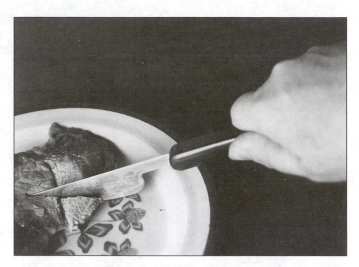

Figure 22-11. Cutting food with one hand is easier with a rocker knife. (Knife by Etac USA, Waukesha, WI. Photo by J.K.)

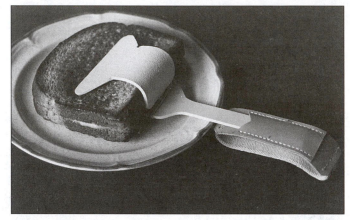

Figure 22-12. A sandwich holder inserted into the palmar pocket of a wrist support makes reaching your mouth easier when grasp is lacking. (Photo by J.K.)

ious designs cost about $3 and up from housewares stores.

A two-handled mug gives better control and divides the weight if you have arthritis or weakness in your hands (Figure 22-15). The plastic glass is in an insulated holder that lets you slip one hand through the handle and steady the cup with the other hand under a lip on the opposite side. It can be used for hot or cold drinks and has an optional lid with a spout. **Manufacturer:** 122. Cost is about $17 from self-help firms. **Sources:** 5, 8, 108, 120, 122, 130, 138, 155, 252, 264, 290, 368, 370, 394, 408.

A similar two-handled poly mug with thumb rests has been designed for the person with arthritis. Dishwasher and microwave

safe. Cost is about $5 from mail-order and self-help firms. **Sources:** 5, 138, 171, 173, 290.

A goblet of lightweight plastic is designed with a thick stem for easier grip (Figure 22-16A). The bowl of the glass rests on your hand to distribute weight. The height makes it easier to bring to your mouth. **Manufacturer:** 122. Cost is about $10 each from self-help firms. **Sources:** 5, 108, 120, 252, 264, 290, 368, 370, 408. A similar plastic goblet shown in Figure 22-16B also is supported by the hand and costs about $2 in the seasonal sections of variety stores.

If you have limited neck motion or dysphagia, this nose cup may be helpful (Figure 22-17). The cutout area lets you tip the cup up without bending your head back. You can make a similar cup by cutting a notch in a regular plastic glass. Cost is about $6 from self-help firms. **Sources:** 5, 8, 16, 108, 120, 138, 252, 264, 290, 368, 408.

A covered mug prevents spilling if you have incoordination or want to carry your cup (Figure 22-18). Commuter's cups, which hold up to 14 ounces are often available from fast food chains or through mail-order firms. Some microwave cups also come with

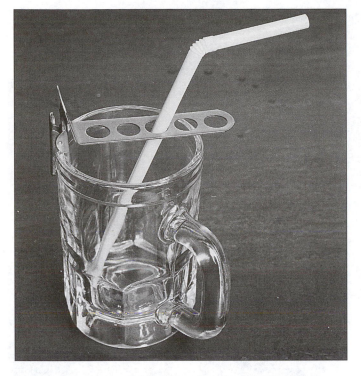

Figure 22-13. A straw holder keeps the straw upright. (Photo courtesy of the O.T. Dept., Howard A. Rusk Institute of Rehabilitation Medicine.)

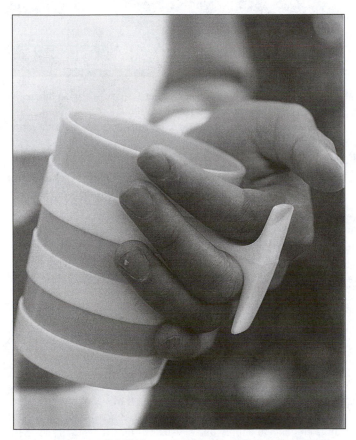

Figure 22-14. A T-handled mug is easier to pick up when fingers are stiff. (Phoyo by J.K.)

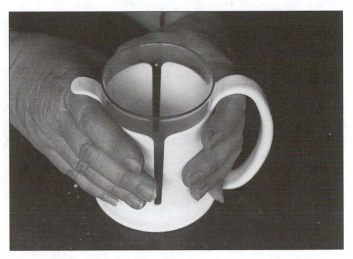

Figure 22-15. A two-handled mug gives better control and divides the weight if you have arthritis or weakness in your hands. (Photo by J.K.)

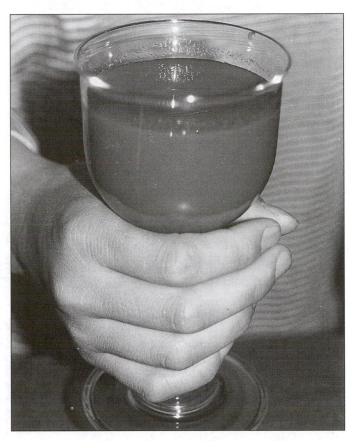

Figure 22-16A. This goblet of lightweight plastic is designed with a thick stem for easier grip. (Goblet from Etac USA, Inc., Waukesha, WI. Photo by J.K.)

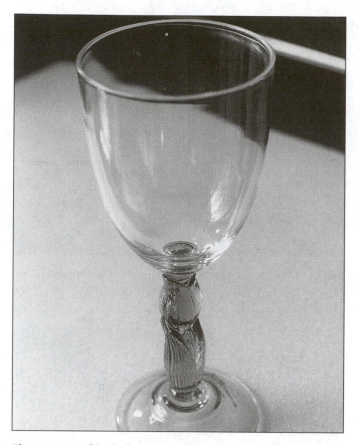

Figure 22-16. This similar plastic goblet also is supported by the hand and costs about $2 in the seasonal sections of variety stores. (Photo by J.K.)

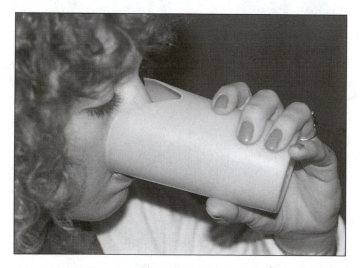

Figure 22-17. If you have limited neck motion or dysphagia, this nose cup may be helpful. (Photo by J.K.)

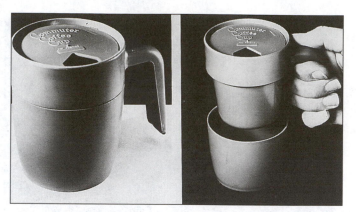

Figure 22-18. A covered mug prevents spilling if you have incoordination or want to carry your cup. (Photo by J.K.)

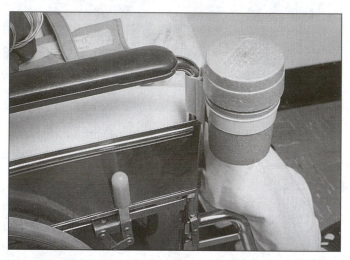

Figure 22-19. This clip-on drink holder fastens to a wheelchair arm or other tubular furniture to keep a drink near at hand. (Photo courtesy of the O.T. Dept., Howard A. Rusk Institute of Rehabilitation Medicine.)

lids. **Sources:** 5, 16, 120, 252, 264, 270, 290, 368, 370, 408.

This clip-on drink holder fastens to a wheelchair arm or other tubular furniture to keep a drink near at hand (Figure 22-19). You can also use it on a walker to carry a covered drink to another place. Cost is about $1 and up from department stores and self-help firms. **Sources:** 5, 120, 265, 290, 370, 404, 408.

Terrycloth covers aid grasp by providing extra friction and also

protect your hands from cold (Figure 22-20). Cost is about $7 for a set of six to eight from housewares stores and mail-order firms. **Sources:** 270, 410.

If sensation in your hands is impaired, a thermal mug is an excellent safety precaution. The double-wall construction protects your hands from heat or cold. Make sure that the mug is dishwasher safe. **Manufacturers** include 157, 343, 404. Cost is about $2.50 each or $8 and up per set from department stores and mail-order and self-help firms. **Sources:** 5, 16, 82, 120, 290, 368, 370, 408.

If you cannot lift a cup or glass, a glass holder tilts toward you (Figure 22-21). The glass is held by a well in the holder. Cost is about $10 from self-help firms. **Sources:** 1, 5, 108, 155, 252, 264, 290, 408.

A sipping cup is for drinking while lying down (Figure 22-22). When you stop drawing liquid, it stops flowing. White nylon lid and cup can be sterilized. **Distributor:** 103. Cost is about $3 and up from hospital supply and self-help firms. **Sources:** 1, 5, 8, 16, 108, 120, 138, 155, 252, 264, 267, 370, 408.

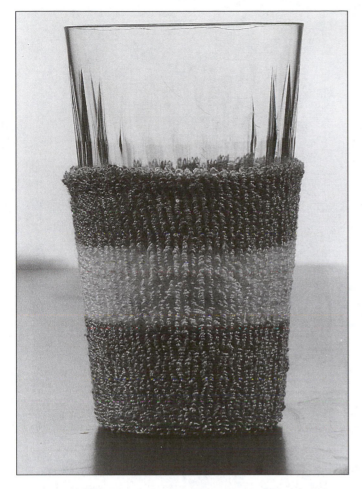

Figure 22-20. Terrycloth covers aid grasp by providing extra friction and also protect your hands from cold. (Photo courtesy of the O.T. Dept., Howard A. Rusk Institute of Rehabilitation Medicine.)

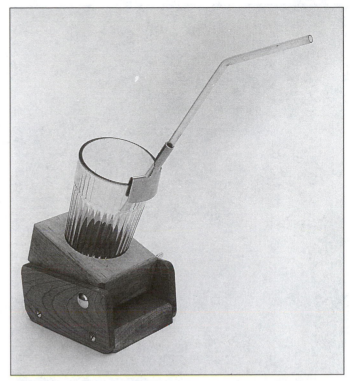

Figure 22-21. If you cannot lift a cup or glass, this glass holder tilts toward you from 0° to 24°. (Photo courtesy of the O.T. Dept., Howard A. Rusk Institute of Rehabilitation Medicine.)

MISCELLANEOUS

Staying neat while eating may be difficult if you have poor vision or incoordination. A comfortable eating arrangement as well as the proper eating utensils help. An adult bib is one answer. A bib with a Velcro® closure allows more independence. Cost is about $6 each and up from hospital supply and self-help firms. **Sources:** 1, 50, 100, 120, 132, 138, 175, 265, 290, 370, 408, 410.

Keeping children's clothes clean while they are eating reduces your laundry basket (Figure 22-23). This plastic molded bib has a slot fastener and rinses clean easily. **Source:** 1. Also see Chapter 26.

A table tray with a slide-under frame allows you to pull it closer to a chair while eating or doing other activities. Look for one with height adjustments and a surface that folds flat when not in use. Cost is about $25 and up from mail-order firms. **Sources:** 50, 100, 270, 364, 387. Also see Chapter 16.

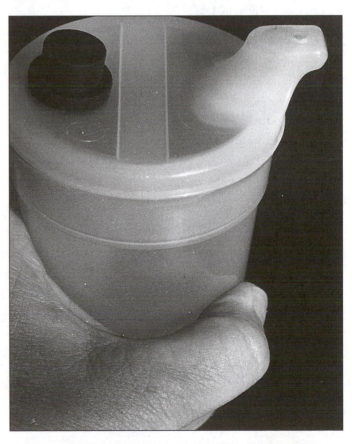

Figure 22-22. This sipping cup is for drinking while lying down.

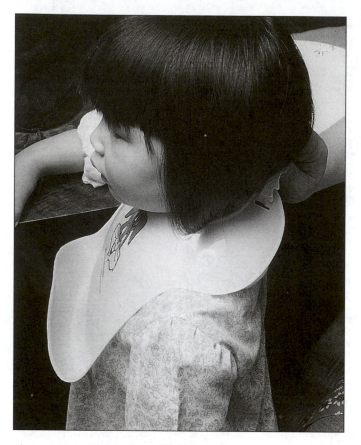

Figure 22-23. This plastic molded bib has a slot fastener and rinses clean easily. (Photo by J.K.)

Section Four

MEAL PLANNING

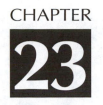

Cooking for One or Two

More than 19 million Americans cook only for themselves. Their biggest challenge is to plan interesting, healthy meals. Often physical and even mental problems of advancing age can be traced to inadequate nutrition and poor eating habits. If you find yourself skimping on meals and nutrition, talk to a home economist or registered dietitian about ideas for delicious, balanced meals and ways to add fresh fruits, vegetables, and grains to your diet.

Researchers have some good news for those watching their weight about eating alone. A study at a Georgia State University indicates that solo meals, on the average, were about 45% lower in calories and fat than meals eaten with others. Furthermore, as more people joined the table, more food was eaten per person.

With a little planning, good nutrition for one person can be easy to prepare and exciting. These tips will help keep meals interesting:

- Plan your meals for the whole week. Shop with a checklist to make sure your food purchases include a variety of all the food groups: green, leafy, and yellow vegetables; fruits; low-fat dairy products; fish; lean meat and poultry; enriched breads; and whole-grain products. Select fresh foods as your first choice and processed frozen or canned foods as alternatives.
- Try at least one new recipe each week. See sample recipes and cookbooks listed at the end of this chapter.
- Scan magazines and newspapers for suggestions on cooking for one or two. The articles often show how to scale down family-sized recipes, split mixes for two meals, or stretch a roast into three or more meals. Seniors' columns frequently give two-serving recipes.
- To save money, purchase meats on sale. Then divide meat into smaller portions and freeze for upcoming meals. Form ground meat into patties for future use in sauces, casseroles, or by themselves.
- Cook extra quantities of fruits and vegetables, or even entire meals, to store in your freezer. Date each package before you freeze it.
- Use custard cups or small plastic containers to freeze individual portions of soups, vegetables, or casseroles. The single servings will defrost faster than an entire casserole and can be transferred to a proper heating container.
- Purchase loose-pack frozen vegetables and fruits in plastic bags that allow you to use them one serving at a time.
- Look for food products sold in single-size servings. Soups, stews, vegetables, fruits, yogurts, and puddings are a few foods marketed in small packages. Since these products tend to be expensive, watch supermarket ads for sales.
- When you use only half an onion or green pepper, chop the whole vegetable, then freeze the remainder in a small plastic bag or airtight container.
- Ask your supermarket butcher to repackage meat in smaller portions. Many stores offer senior citizens the lower bulk price as well as a discount for shopping on a certain day, usually the middle of the week.
- Take time to eat. Do not eat while standing. When you are ready to eat, set the table with attractive dishes; add a flower, music, soft lights, and enjoy.
- Share cooking talents with a friend or neighbor. Cook up a batch of chicken soup, stew, oatmeal cookies, or apple crisp while a friend cooks a complimentary dish. Then divide into equal portions, give out, and receive a bonus in taste and time.
- Encourage children and grandchildren to bring individually portioned food gifts of homemade stew, even meals. They will find this doubly rewarding, because often it is hard to think of something you might like or need and they get a chance to receive your fellowship and thanks.
- Plan a "share-a-meal" night at least once a week with a neighbor or friend. The food feeds your body and the companionship your spirit.

A microwave oven is an indispensable tool when cooking for one (Figure 23-1). Individual portions cook or reheat in just minutes. Lightweight containers, available in all sizes, can go from refrigerator or freezer into the microwave oven. **Manufacturers:** 28, 343. Cost is about $2 each and up from housewares stores.

Use a two-egg poacher to make breakfast for one or two. Cost

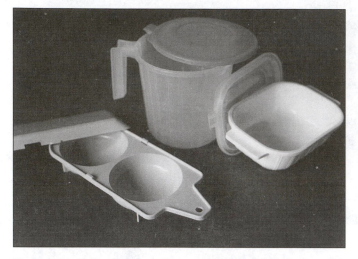

Figure 23-1. Lightweight containers, available in all sizes, can go from refrigerator or freezer into the microwave oven. (Photo by J.K.)

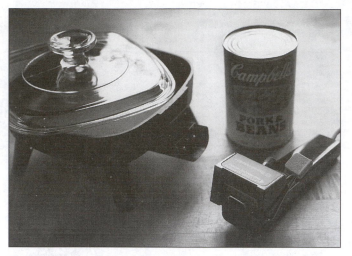

Figure 23-2. This lightweight, 7" square electric Handi-Pan® has all the features of its bigger skillet relatives. (Photo courtesy of Toastmaster®, Columbia, MO.)

is about $3 from housewares stores and mail-order firms. See Chapter 28.

Single-serving or small appliances include coffee makers, food processors, woks, electric slow cookers and skillets, countertop ovens, and water heaters. These are described in Chapter 20.

Small saucepans, roast/lasagna pans, and whistling teakettles are available through housewares stores and mail-order firms. **Sources:** 65, 270.

The lightweight, 7" square electric Handi-Pan® shown in Figure 23-2 has all the features of its bigger skillet relatives. The handle has an adjustable heat control, which removes for cleaning. The interior has a non-stick coating, and the pan has a tempered glass lid. It is UL approved. **Manufacturer**: 399. Cost is about $35 from housewares stores and mail-order firms. **Sources:** 71, 283, 410.

Here are a few recipes to whet your appetite.

CREAM OF CORN SOUP

2 servings

A versatile, calcium- and fiber-rich lunch or light supper. Serve with green salad and whole-wheat bread or rolls.

1 10-ounce can creamed corn
1 10½-ounce can cream soup (mushroom, chicken, celery)
½ cup plain low-fat yogurt
1 teaspoon chopped fresh dill or parsley or ½ teaspoon dried

Blend ingredients in small saucepan or a quart-size microwave-safe bowl. Heat to simmering point, stirring occasionally. Serve immediately.

MEATLOAF FOR TWO (WITH VARIATIONS)

2 to 3 servings

½ pound lean ground beef or ground turkey

½ cup dried bread crumbs or oatmeal
½ cup (1 small) finely diced onion
1 egg , slightly beaten, or equivalent egg substitute
$^1/_3$ cup ketchup
Dash pepper
Variations—add one or two or the following:
½ cup sliced fresh mushrooms
½ cup shredded low-fat cheese
½ chopped green or sweet red pepper
1 grated carrot
1 teaspoon chopped fresh parley
1 chopped tomato and generous dash dried basil

Mix all ingredients thoroughly together. Shape into loaf or two patties; place in shallow baking pan. Bake at 350°F for 35 minutes.

ZIPPY HONEY-MUSTARD CHICKEN BREASTS

2 servings

2 skinless boneless chicken breast halves
2 tablespoons liquid honey
2 tablespoons Dijon or other mustard
$^1/_3$ cup dried seasoned bread crumbs

Preheat oven to 350°F. Grease or non-stick spray a small baking pan.

In flat bowl, mix honey and mustard.

On waxed paper or in a second flat bowl or pie pan, sprinkle bread crumbs.

Spread honey mixture on both sides of one chicken breast, then press both sides into bread crumbs. Place on greased baking pan. Repeat with second breast half.

Bake in 350°F oven for 15 to 20 minutes, or until chicken is no longer pink.

Serve with baked potato (put in oven ½ hour before chicken) or rice, and green salad or vegetable. Elegant enough for company!

BANANA CRISP DESSERT

2 to 3 servings

2 ripe bananas
Topping:
2 tablespoons cold margarine or butter
2 tablespoons all-purpose flour
2 tablespoons brown sugar
½ cup rolled oats
½ teaspoon ground cinnamon
Dash nutmeg

Preheat oven to 375°F. Grease or non-stick spray small baking dish.

Peel bananas; slice in half lengthwise, then crosswise, to fit in one layer in dish.

Mix flour, sugar, oats, and spices together. With hand, mix margarine into dry ingredients until crumbly.

Bake in 375°F oven 15 minutes or until bananas are soft. Cool slightly. If desired, serve with vanilla or frozen low-fat yogurt.

Variations: use peaches, nectarines, or apples, but double topping ingredients, and increase cooking time to 25 minutes at 350°F.

GOING FURTHER

PUBLICATIONS

Cooking for One or Two. Program Aid #1043. $1.25 Washington, DC: Superintendent of Documents.

Crocker, B. (1990). *Betty Crocker's New Microwaving for 1 or 2*. New York: Prentice-Hall. **Source:** 316B.

Margo Oliver's Cookbook for Seniors: Nutritious Recipes for One, Two, or More. (1990). Bellingham, WA and Vancouver, BC: Self-Counsel Press. **Source:** 357A.

Microwave Cooking for One or Two. (1994). Better Homes and Gardens. Des Moines, IA: Meredith. **Source:** 267B.

24

Meal Planning and Nutritious Eating

Good nutrition is essential to your health. Eating the proper amounts and kinds of foods helps your body function at its best. You can choose from a variety of foods including fresh, frozen, canned, and dried in supermarkets and grocery stores. Taking time to plan ahead and prepare meals lets you eat well, even on a budget.

All through life you need the same nutrients. As you grow older, however, caloric needs decrease, especially if you are less active. It is particularly important at this time to keep variety in your meals. Often, there is a tendency to select foods that do not supply enough proteins, vitamins, and minerals in relation to the requirement for less calories. In some cases, a special diet may be necessary. This should always be recommended by your doctor, a registered dietitian, or other qualified professional trained in nutrition.

A variety of foods usually provide the proper amount and balance of nutrients. You will enjoy your meals more and find them satisfying if you eat in a leisurely fashion and in pleasant surroundings.

PLANNING AHEAD

As you read through this section, think about setting up your shopping list for the week so that all the foods you need for good health are included. Make out a schedule of meals for the week; fill in ideas as you read the weekly circulars from local stores. Start keeping extras on hand not only for emergencies but to round out your daily nutrition quota.

TECHNIQUES TO REDUCE WORK

Making meal preparation easier is the goal of this manual. Many techniques help speed individual tasks:
- Learn to work when you are at your energy peak.
- Use blocks of time to cook ahead.
- Combine convenience foods with fresh produce.

- Select quality tools and appliances to increase efficiency and reduce preparation time.

Trying new foods and recipes helps turn meal preparation into fun rather than a chore. A few recipes that will help you try out new techniques are given in Chapter 23. Since we all have our own personal, family, and ethnic preferences, use these as a guide, then adapt your dishes to the new techniques.

COOKING ON A BUDGET

When planning meals, you are probably conscious of your budget. You may even be saying "I can't afford good nutrition on my budget." Good nutrition is not necessarily more expensive. Planning cuts costs. Using meat as a condiment rather than a main course and adding low-cost beans, pasta, and grains to main dishes are beginning steps. Read the circulars, and have chicken when it is on sale—not next week when the price doubles. All foods go in cycle by supply and demand. "To every food there is a season" means you can be the reaper if you follow the trends of the food market. The seasons for fresh vegetables and fruits are not just in the summer, but when the Florida green beans are ripe and strawberries fly in from southern and western fields in mid-winter.

GUIDELINES TO PLANNING A DAY'S MEALS

Foods supply the nutrients required for proper functioning of your body. Although there are more than 50 specific nutrients, they may be divided into six types: proteins, carbohydrates, fats, vitamins, minerals, and water. Each performs a different role.

Proteins are made up of building blocks called amino acids. They build, maintain, and repair body tissues.

Carbohydrates are the sources of energy for work and maintenance of body temperature. Starches like cereals, breads, flours, as well as sugars, fall into this group.

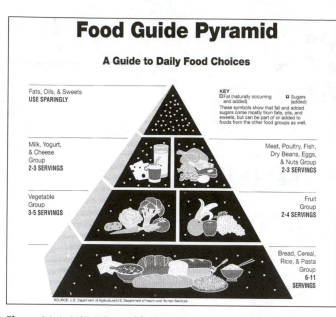

Figure 24-1. USDA Pyramid. (U.S. Department of Agriculture/U.S. Department of Health and Human Services, Washington, DC.)

Fats are also primary sources of energy but for the health of your heart should be limited to 30% or less of the calories you eat each day.

To figure out what percentage of your calories are fat, multiply the number of grams of fat in what you eat by seven calories each. If a slice of bread has 100 calories and two grams of fat, it means that the percentage of fat is two times seven or 14 calories, which in this case is 14%. A Fat Finder® can help you understand and reduce calories. **Source:** 133.

Vitamins have many different roles for proper utilization of foods and healthy functioning of your body.

Minerals are needed for the formation of teeth, bone, and red blood cells, and for many vital body functions. Women need more calcium than men to prevent osteoporosis, the disease where bones begin to become soft and deteriorate. Three glasses of milk a day, or the equivalent in yogurt and low-fat cheese, provide the daily suggested requirement.

If you eat a well-balanced diet, you should not need food supplements. The vitamins and minerals our bodies usually require are found in adequate supply in a carefully planned diet.

Water is required for all the chemical reactions that occur in your body. It transports the nutrients, is needed for blood, regulation of body temperature, and elimination. You should drink six to eight glasses of water every day to keep your body at its best. This is in addition to coffee, tea, and other beverages.

The jobs of all the nutrients are interrelated. One cannot do its job without all the others being present. For example, the proteins in cereal are more nutritious if they are consumed with milk. No one food contains all the essential ingredients in proper balance except mother's milk for newborn infants. Thus, you need an assortment of foods at every meal.

Fiber is a part of food that cannot be digested. Though not a nutrient, it is important in your diet to provide bulk, keep your arteries clear, and your system functioning regularly.

GUIDELINES FOR PLANNING A FULL WEEK'S MEALS

When planning your menus for the week, it is important to start with an understanding of the food pyramid (Figure 24-1). It serves as your guide for the daily selection of the foods that supply adequate amounts of nutrients needed by your body. Foods should be selected from each of the following groups every day in the proportions shown by the pyramid.

The basis of your diet should be six to 11 servings of the bread and cereal group per day; a minimum of three to five servings of the vegetable group and two to four of the fruit group. The dairy group requires two to three servings as does the meat group. And at the top, fats and sweets should only be used sparingly. There are, however, differences dependent on age and gender.

BREAD-CEREAL GROUP

These foods supply many of the vitamins in the B group, iron, and carbohydrates as well as fiber. You need six to 11 servings of enriched or whole-grain breads and cereals. Included are enriched flour, macaroni, spaghetti, noodles, rice, and rolled oats.

One bread-cereal serving is one slice of bread, one ounce or ½ to ¾ cup of ready-to-eat cereal, ½ to ¾ cup cooked cereal, cornmeal, pasta, grits, or noodles.

VEGETABLE-FRUIT GROUP

The foods in this group supply most of your ascorbic acid (vitamin C) as well as much of the vitamin A, some iron, and other minerals. Four or more servings are needed daily, including one serving of citrus fruit or juice, or tomato (for vitamin C); a serving of a dark green or deep yellow vegetable (for vitamin A); and two or more servings of other vegetables and fruits, including potatoes.

One vegetable serving is one cup of raw leafy vegetables, ½ cup of other vegetables, cooked or raw, or ¾ cup of vegetable juice. A fruit serving is a portion as ordinarily served, such as one medium banana or apple, ½ cup sliced fruit, or ¾ cup of fruit juice. This group also provides fiber that helps keep your circulatory and elimination systems healthy.

DAIRY GROUP

Items in this group are a primary source of calcium. They also provide protein, riboflavin, and usually vitamins A and D. Men and children under nine need two or more cups of milk a day; children nine to 12 and women need three or more cups. Teenagers need four or more cups. This can be milk (skim or 1% preferred), evaporated skim or dry milk, or buttermilk. Cheese, low-fat ice cream, yogurt, and soups or sauces prepared with skim or 1% milk contribute to this group.

A dairy serving is one cup of milk or low-fat yogurt or 1½ ounces of natural cheese.

If you have a lactose intolerance and do not digest milk well, don't give up the calcium from milk. Talk with your doctor about lactose-free milk that you can buy in local grocery stores or tablets that allow you to drink regular milk and eat dairy products.

MEAT GROUP

Foods in this group supply protein, iron, riboflavin, and niacin.

You need two to three servings daily. One meat group serving is only 2 to 3 ounces of lean cooked meat, poultry, or fish, all without bone; one egg or two tablespoons of peanut butter; ½ cup cooked dry beans. The food value of beans is increased when served with a small amount of animal protein, such as a glass of milk or serving of yogurt.

The food pyramid serves as a guide for meal planning. Plan your meals around it, and if you have difficulty, talk with your physician, nurse, or a registered dietitian. See going further at the end of this chapter for free or very low-cost meal planning and nutrition resources.

CHOOSING AND USING FOODS

Nutrition is what we eat and how our body uses it. You must consider all of the food you consume in a day, from the time you get up until you retire at night.

The amount of food you need depends on your age, sex, and amount of activity. Each person has slightly different nutritional needs; these are constantly changing. Children's needs are dictated by their growth patterns. Adult needs change with age. One set of rules does not apply to everyone.

All food is helpful if you are in need of the nutrients it contains, but this should not be your only guide. Some foods are more helpful than others because they contain substances that are vital to growth, repair, and regulation of body machinery.

A good rule to follow is to eat a sufficient quantity to achieve proper weight. If you are slightly overweight and must lose a few pounds, continue to eat a variety of foods, but reduce the size of servings. Of course, if you need to gain a little weight, have slightly larger portions. Your doctor should advise you as to the necessity of changing your weight.

The following principles will result in a balanced diet:
- Always eat breakfast, which leads to regular eating habits.
- Eat foods that have nutritious rather than empty calories.
- Eat meals that have variety.
- Eat foods properly prepared. Some vitamins and minerals dissolve in water, so cook these foods with as little water as possible. Some vitamins are destroyed by heating, so food should not be overcooked. Rather than boiling, microwaving or steaming vegetables helps conserve vitamins.
- Learn and follow what is an average portion size for various foods. See earlier in this chapter. Measuring portions for weight control may be easier to do with a scale for some foods (Figure 24-2). An electronic or digital scale is more accurate. Look for a model with a dish to hold the portion and a dial large enough to read easily. Make sure that you can re-set the dial to use with other plates or containers. **Manufacturers** of electronic scales: 84, 308, 381. **Sources:** 65, 194, 283.

Carefully trim serving sizes to suggested portions, like 3 ounces of meat. This way you'll be able to judge accurately and learn to cut down for life-long weight control.

HEALTHY SNACKING

If you like to snack, choose foods that add to your daily nutri-

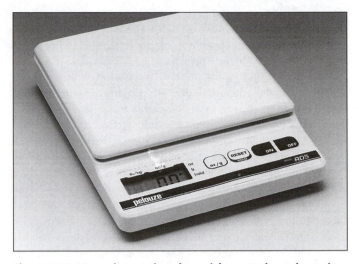

Figure 24-2. Measuring portions for weight control may be easier to do for some foods with a scale. (Photo courtesy of Pelouze Scale Co., Evanston, IL.)

tion needs. This is especially true if you only eat small meals and must add to your nutritional quota or if you eat small meals because you cannot tolerate heavier ones, as with COPD. See Chapter 8.

Foods that are low in calories include vegetable and fruit juices, celery and carrot sticks, unsugared cereals, one or two whole-grain crackers, non-fat milk, low-fat yogurt with fresh or canned fruit, and unsweetened applesauce or gelatin with fruit. It is the foods (like soda and chips) that fall outside the food groups, those high in appeal, fat and calories that usually make one put on extra pounds. If watching your weight, get a calorie table, and circle low-calorie treats that you enjoy. Make sure you have those rather than the no-no's on your shelves.

DIABETES

If you have diabetes, it is important to follow food plans and medication schedules carefully. Staying in contact with your physician or Visiting Nurse Association is important. They can teach you to check your own glucose level and give suggestions on controlling it. Several publications provide helpful information for the person with diabetes. See Going Further at the end of this chapter.

SPECIAL DIETS

Although the techniques in this manual are designed to help you manage more easily in your kitchen, they are not planned for the person on a special diet or with food allergies. There are, however, several places where you can get information and help. See Going Further at the end of this chapter.

If your doctor recommends a special diet to you and gives you a general plan, ask for specifics. You'll want to know which foods you can eat and which you cannot and the daily amounts of each. Ask for printed materials including recipes for your diet. If your physician is connected with a hospital, an interview with the hospital dietitian should be arranged to help you with menu planning.

Or you could be referred to a dietetic consulting service in your area. A few cities now have a Dial-A-Dietitian telephone service run by the American Dietetic Association. See helpful organizations and agencies in the Appendix.

If you are given a diet during a hospital stay, then you, the dietitian, and the person who does the cooking at home should sit down before you leave so you completely understand the diet.

County extension services are usually staffed with home economists who can answer questions on special diets or recommend available services. Look under Home Economics Extension Service or Extension Service in your phone book. The local Department of Health or Visiting Nurses Association may have a dietitian who can help. In some towns, there is a Meals-on-Wheels program that will bring food to your home when you cannot get out. They will adjust your meals for low-salt or diabetic needs if requested. The home economics teacher in your local school can often assist. Utility companies often have home economists on their staff who are glad to help.

Local booksellers have suitable books on diet planning or will order them for you. Check with your library before purchasing. Your doctor, dietitian, or health agency personnel can suggest specific recommended titles. Many of these books are available in paperback. The federal government also publishes books to help with special meal planning. See Going Further at the end of this chapter.

Organizations concerned with health problems publish materials. These include the American Diabetes Association, the American Dietetic Association, the Allergy Foundation of America, the American Heart Association, and The Arthritis Foundation. Addresses are given in Appendix B. Before writing the national office, check your phone book for a local chapter near you.

Major food companies often have booklets and information about their products in relation to special diets. Write to the Consumer Services Department. The address of the company is on the product label.

Shopping has become easier and more exciting for the person on a special diet. Many large supermarkets carry an extensive variety of dietetic foods. If you have any doubts about the product being right for your diet, ask your doctor. (Dietetic foods are not necessarily low-calorie.)

CONVENIENCE FOODS

The changes we have seen in cooking methods (i.e., the microwave) and in food processing, frozen, packaged, and canned, allow you to fix exciting meals in less time than it took grandmother to heat the range. Foods, from appetizers to desserts, are available with built-in convenience.

With more American families having two workers outside the home, the market for prepared foods has multiplied. Produce sections and salad bars in grocery stores offer cut-up vegetables and fruits for at-home stir-fry meals or salads. Meats are packaged for quicker preparation, i.e., boneless chicken breasts and ground turkey. On the shelves, canned, low-salt vegetables, condensed soups, and cooked beans may be mixed with meat or fish for quick main courses. Some convenience foods are low-fat and choles-

terol-free, i.e., meatless chili and burger mixes, such as those from Dixie USA, Inc. **Source:** 97.

Plan how you can adapt favorite recipes for easier preparation by substituting convenience foods for items that normally require chopping, slicing, or shredding, and long cooking items, such as sauces and dry beans.

Read the labels, which have been redesigned to offer clearer information, including serving sizes and the percentage of total fat and cholesterol for the day.

SUBSTITUTIONS

These substitutions will help decrease preparation time, and may be used when your pantry or refrigerator does not have the original item.

1 cup fresh milk—½ cup evaporated milk plus ½ cup water or 1 cup reconstituted non-fat dry milk

1 cup sour milk or buttermilk—1 tablespoon lemon juice or vinegar plus enough milk to make 1 cup

1 tablespoon fresh herbs—1 teaspoon crumbled dry herbs

1 medium garlic clove—⅛ teaspoon garlic powder or instant minced garlic

¼ cup chopped fresh or frozen onion—1 tablespoon instant minced onion or onion flakes; or 1 teaspoon onion powder

¼ chopped fresh or frozen green pepper—1 tablespoon dried sweet pepper flakes

½ medium stalk celery—1 tablespoon dried celery flakes

Juice and rind of one lemon—3 tablespoons bottled juice and 1 tablespoon fresh rind, or 1½ teaspoons dried rind

Juice and rind of one orange—⅓ to 1½ cup juice and 2 tablespoons of fresh rind, or 1 tablespoon dried rind

1 strip cooked bacon—1 tablespoon real bacon bits or bacon-flavored bits

1 cup diced cooked chicken—1 can (5 ounces) boned chicken

If using dried onion, pepper, or celery flakes in a recipe that requires less than 10 minutes cooking time, reconstitute them first, according to package directions, then add.

LOW-FAT, LOW-CHOLESTEROL FOODS

One of the problems in selecting foods is choosing those low in cholesterol and fat. The American Heart Association has recommended that no more than 30% of the calories in your diet come from fat. Even better, some physicians and scientists feel, would be 20%.

Reducing fat in the diet takes perseverance and new ways of eating and cooking.

DAIRY FOODS

Use polyunsaturated margarine or oil, and monosaturated oil instead of butter, lard, and animal fats.

Use skim or 1% milk instead of whole or 2% milk.

Use evaporated skim instead of evaporated whole milk.

Use low-fat cheeses instead of whole milk cheeses.

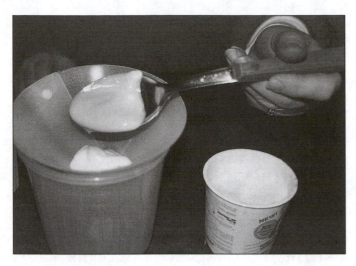

Figure 24-3. This micromesh drainer with stand holds one pint of yogurt. (Drainer by Chantry®. Photo by J.K.)

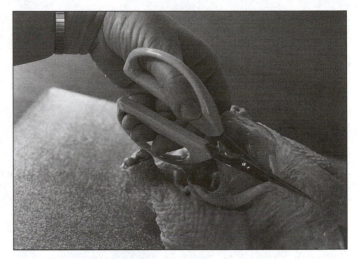

Figure 24-4. These small Scissors Unlimited snip out corners and pockets of fat. (Scissors Unlimited by Joyce Chen Products, Billerica, MA. Photo by J.K.)

Use low-fat yogurt instead of sour cream.

Use egg whites or egg substitutes including tofu instead of whole eggs.

Use olive oil instead of butter, margarine, or lard.

Use fruit purees in place of oils when baking.

Yogurt cheese is low in fat, cholesterol, and lactose, but high in calcium and protein. It is easy to make with a micro-mesh drainer, funnel, or a cheesecloth in a drainer that strains the liquid out of low-fat yogurt in 8 to 14 hours. You are left with a thick creamy cheese to spread on bagels and bread, top fruits and desserts, even baked potatoes instead of sour cream. It can be mixed with herbs for a spread or dip, or made into cheesecake, ice cream, and pies. See Going Further.

A micromesh drainer with stand holds 1 pint of yogurt (Figure 24-3). **Manufacturer:** 63. Cost is about $12 and up from housewares stores and mail-order firms. A similar mesh funnel for making yogurt cheese folds flat when not in use and is dishwasher safe. **Distributor:** 402. Cost is about $11 from gourmet and mail-order firms. **Sources:** 65, 402.

A good pair of scissors is a great investment in really cutting down your fat intake (Figure 24-4). These small Scissors Unlimited snip out corners and pockets of fat. The flexible handles are designed for cutting chicken bones and other heavier foods as well as fine dicing and slicing or opening packages. The no-stain, no-rust, stainless-steel blades are attached with a heavy-duty rivet. Dishwasher safe. **Manufacturer:** 213. Cost is about $17 from self-help and gourmet firms. See other shears and scissors in Chapter 21.

MEATS

- Start trimming the amount—3 ounces is a normal portion.
- Start trimming the fat—even on lean meat.
- Cut away any visible fat.
- Cook on a rack to drain away fat when roasting, broiling, or baking. See Chapter 29.
- Broil rather than pan-fry.
- Select non-stick pans that require no added fat for browning.

- Make stews the day ahead, refrigerate, and then remove fat that has hardened on top.
- Omit gravies; baste with fruit and vegetable juices, wine, oil-based marinades.

For draining fat while cooking, see the low-fat meatloaf pan, Chapter 28.

LOW-SODIUM COOKING

If you must cut down your intake of salt because of medical reasons, such as high blood pressure, kidney problems, congestive heart failure, or to cut the risk of heart disease, there are many ways to keep foods exciting. Labeling of the sodium content in foods is easier to find on the new labels. The availability of no-salt and lowered-salt convenience foods have increased.

- Begin by never adding salt to your food in the kitchen or at the table. Remove the salt shaker from the table and the salt box from the cupboard.
- Read labels; avoid sodium in its many forms. Ask your doctor, visiting nurse, home economist, or a dietitian for a list. Some of the types include sodium phosphate, monosodium glutamate, sodium alginite, sodium bisulfite, sodium benzoate, sodium caseinate.
- Look for reduced-sodium foods including low-sodium soups, cheeses, tuna fish, soy sauce, vegetable and tomato juices, no-salt ketchup, low-salt cereals, frozen dinners, herb mixtures, and other condiments.
- Omit salt from the cooking water for vegetables, rice, or pasta. Get the flavor from foods you serve with it.
- Substitute herbs, spices, lemon and lime juice and zest, garlic, and vinegar for salt in main dishes and salads.
- Avoid salt substitutes. Too much potassium can lead to other problems, i.e., nausea, diarrhea, muscle weakness.
- Buy no-salt processed foods when possible. When not, rinse vegetables, fruits, meats, and poultry to remove some of the excess salt.
- Watch for salt-free seasonings recipes, often given in family

service magazines. Try your own, blending garlic powder, oregano, dill weed, paprika, marjoram, pepper, and dry mustard. For cooked vegetables, combine celery seed, marjoram, thyme, and basil. Try the same mixture for stews with some rosemary added. Salads perk up with thyme, rubbed sage, savory, basil, and marjoram. Put your favorite mixture in a shaker and enjoy.

- Avoid recipes that combine high-sodium foods, such as cheese and soup, in the same recipe.
- The final thought is that after 8 to 12 weeks on a low-sodium diet, your taste preferences will shift, and you automatically want less salt.

FOOD AND DRUG INTERACTIONS

Some foods and drugs may react with each other. To avoid an undesirable reaction, some medications must be taken with food, some must never be taken with food, and some react only with certain foods. Talk with your physician and pharmacist about food-related side effects whenever you are given a new medication. Alcohol consumed with certain medicines can be very dangerous. Caffeine can also affect the action of some drugs. Aspirin and ibuprofen both tend to affect some people's stomachs and should be taken with food, but not with fruit juice. Sodium (salt) is often restricted with vasodilators and anti-hypertensive drugs.

GOING FURTHER

Addresses are listed in the Appendices.

PUBLICATIONS

Atwater-McClay, S., & Miech, M. *4-Ingredient Cookbook*, and *Trim & Thin 4-Ingredient Cookbook*. $9 each through Laurel Designs. **Source:** 229.

Cooking for People with Food Allergies. Washington, DC: U.S. Government Printing Office. $1.50. Forty pages of information on preparing foods that do not contain milk, corn, wheat, eggs. Tips to help recognize these ingredients in prepared foods. Recipes.

Diabetes Self-Management. See Periodicals.

Dustan, H. (1988). *Cookbook for Diabetics and Their Families*. Birmingham, AL: University of Alabama at Birmingham, Oxmoor House. **Source:** 300.

Eating for a Healthy Heart: Dietary Treatment of Hyperlipidemia, and Recipes for Low-Fat Low-Cholesterol Meals. Both free from the American Heart Association.

Food & Drug Interactions. Free from the Food & Drug Administration.

Goulder, L., & Lutwak, L. (1988). *The Strong Bones Diet: the High Calcium Low Calorie Way to Prevent Osteoporosis*. Gainesville, FL: Triad. **Source:** 402.

Grundy, S. M. (Ed.). (1989). *American Heart Association Low Fat Low Cholesterol Cookbook*. New York: Times Books, Random House. **Source:** 326.

Healthy Heart Cookbook. (1990). Washington, DC: U.S. Government Printing Office. $3. Recipes, advice on shopping wisely, substituting ingredients, lowering cholesterol levels, cooking.

Hooper, L. H. (Ed.). (1992). *The Healthy Heart Cookbook*. Birmingham, AL: Oxmoor. Excellent recipes, easy- to-read print. **Source:** 300.

Jacobson, M. F., & Fritschner, S. (1991). *The Completely Revised and Updated Fast-Food Guide*. New York: Center for Science in the Public Interest, Workman. **Source:** 431B.

Jones, J. (1992). Eating Smart: ABCs of the New Food Literacy. New York: Macmillan Publishing. **Source:** 251B.

MacDonald, H. B., & Howard, M. (1990). *Eat Well, Live Well: The Canadian Dietetic Association Guide to Healthy Living*. Toronto, ON: MacMillan of Canada.

Margen, S., & the editors of the University of California at Berkeley Wellness Letter. (1992). *The Wellness Encyclopedia of Food and Nutrition: How to Buy, Store, and Prepare Every Variety of Fresh Food*. New York: Health Letter Associates. Distributed by Random House. **Source:** 326.

Schlesinger, S. (1994). *500 Fat-Free Recipes: A Complete Guide to Reducing the Fat in Your Diet*. New York: Villard Books, Random House. **Source:** 326.

Starke, R. D., & Winston, M. (1991). *American Heart Association Cookbook* (rev, 5th ed.). New York: Times Books, Random House. **Source:** 326.

Stern, B. (1995). *Simply Heart Smart Cooking*. Toronto: Heart and Stroke Foundation of Canada. Random House. **Source:** 326B.

Stone, M., Melvin, S., & Crawford, C. (1988). *Not Just Cheesecake: The Low-Fat, Low-Cholesterol, Low-Calorie Great Dessert Cookbook*. Gainesville, FL: Triad. **Source:** 402.

Wilson, J. W. (1988). *Eating Well Cookbook: When You Just Can't Eat the Way You Used To*. New York: Workman. **Source:** 431B.

A Word About Low-Sodium Diets, #FDA 87-2179. U.S. Department of Health and Human Services, Public Health Service, Food and Drug Administration. Free.

For additional suggestions on meal planning see Chapter 11 , Chapter 23, and Chapter 25.

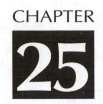

Shopping

PLANNING

Good organization of your kitchen and food storage areas makes it easier to plan for grocery shopping. Here are some helpful tips:

- Store foods of the same category together so you can tell at a glance what is needed.
- Use storage aids that let you see what is in the cabinets and refrigerator without lifting and reaching. See Chapter 14.
- Keep a list of needed items attached to a stick-on or magnetic pad on the refrigerator door where you can immediately add to it.
- To reduce walking in the store, organize your list by the order in which items are shelved in your favorite store.
- Teach family members to write down foods that they know need to be replaced.
- Let family contribute menu ideas on a memo pad next to the shopping list. They'll be motivated to help prepare these meals.
- Keep a file handy of favorite and new recipes, then include the ingredients for one or two new dishes each week on your grocery list.
- Make out a weekly menu plan. It saves energy as well as money. See Chapter 24.
- Saving money when shopping is important, whether purchasing for your family on a limited budget or cooking for one on a fixed income. Work out your week's list with the newspaper specials right at hand.
- Choose the best shopping time for you when the stores are not crowded. Quiet hours with the shortest lines are usually in the middle of the week, in the morning or early afternoon.
- If you cannot shop alone, ask your family, a friend, or community volunteer to take you shopping. Check with your church or Visiting Nurse Association for a group that provides volunteer drivers.
- Although weekly shopping is suggested, you may want to make another arrangement. If a family member or friend is only available once every 2 or 3 weeks, rethink your shopping schedule. Follow the tips but work out the full time span of menus so you only have small pick-ups to do in between.
- If you cannot go out and shop, be very specific on your list as to brand, size of package, and price range you desire.
- If writing or remembering is difficult, you may purchase preprinted lists from a mail-order firm. Or ask someone to type out a personalized master list, then duplicate it. You just have to check off what you need.

A permanent shopping list attaches to your refrigerator with magnetic tape (Figure 25-1). When you need any of the 181 items, slide over the product's colored indicator tab. List folds neatly to go with you and even carries coupons. Cost is about $9 from mail-order firms. **Sources:** 152, 364.

A magnetic or stick-on memo pad lets you jot down items as you remember. Cost is about $2 and up from variety and stationery stores or mail-order firms. You might even consider an electronic memo-minder that records your list as you speak into it. Cost is about $25 and up from business and stationery firms. **Sources:** 167, 176, 177, 325.

"Let your fingers do the walking." Use your telephone to cut down on shopping trips. See the flexible gooseneck arm, which holds the phone handset at a comfortable angle and leaves your hands free to take notes, in Chapter 11. If your fingers are weak or affected by arthritis, try a phone handle that fastens over the receiver with Velcro®. The frame bends to fit your palm size and rests on your hand leaving fingers free. Cost is about $6 from self-help firms. **Sources:** 120, 393. A giant push-button phone or attachment for your phone helps with dialing if you have incoordination or limited vision. Keep your telephone area comfortably set up with a chair and writing surface.

If you have difficulty writing due to weak and stiff hands or incoordination, a felt-tip pen or soft pencil with a foam curler handle reduces grasp and pressure (Figure 25-2).

A special writing device can make a difference when doing shopping lists and other correspondence (Figure 25-3). The Steady Write® lets your hand rest on the smooth base, rather than gripping

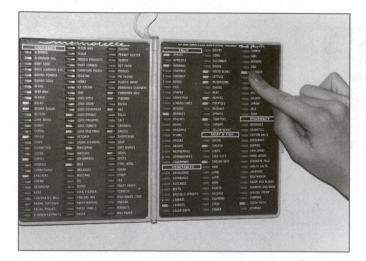

Figure 25-1. This permanent shopping list attaches to your refrigerator with magnetic tape. (Photo by J.K.)

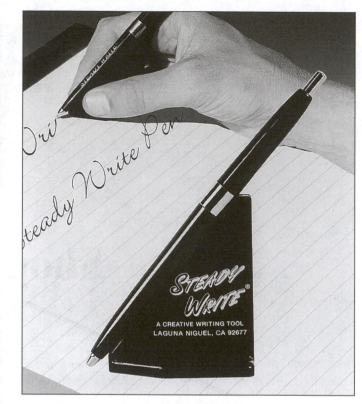

Figure 25-3. This Steady Write® lets your hand rest on the smooth base, rather than gripping a pen. (Photo courtesy of Steady Write®, Laguna Niguel, CA.)

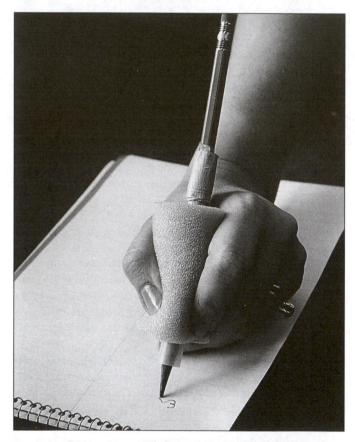

Figure 25-2. If you have difficulty writing due to weak and stiff hands or incoordination, a felt-tip pen or soft pencil with a foam curler handle reduces grasp and pressure. (Photo courtesy of the O.T. Dept., Howard A. Rusk Institute of Rehabilitation Medicine.)

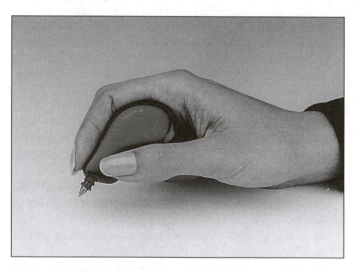

Figure 25-4. The Evo-Pen™, originally designed for people with arthritis, fits right in your palm, allowing your hand to rest as you write. (Manufactured by Evo-Pen™, New York. Photo by J.K.)

a pen. The permanently mounted, ball-point pen or pencil slides over the paper as you form the letters. For right- or left-handed writers. **Manufacturer:** 379. Cost is about $7 or $13 for a set with pen, pencil, and refills, from mail-order and self-help firms or directly from the manufacturer. **Sources:** 1, 50, 108, 238, 270, 379.

The Evo-Pen™, originally designed for people with arthritis, fits right in your palm, allowing your hand to rest as you write

(Figure 25-4). Cost is about $4 from self-help firms or directly from the **manufacturer:** 127. Contact an occupational therapist for other writing solutions.

A clipboard with a storage base organizes not only your shopping but your whole day or week for a balance of work and leisure (Figure 25-5). It holds the paper steady while writing and can be set on your lap as a small writing desk. Cost is about $6 and up from department and stationery stores.

A small calculator helps you stay within limits of your budget

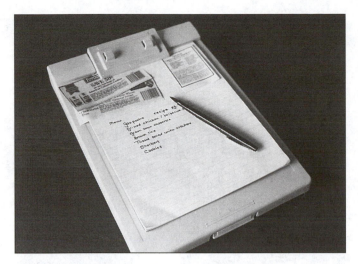

Figure 25-5. A clipboard with a storage base organizes not only your shopping but your whole day or week for a balance of work and leisure. (Photo by J.K.)

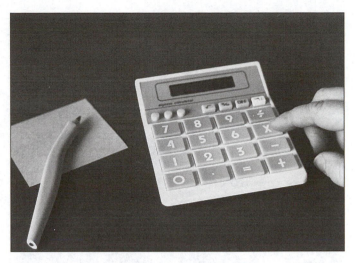

Figure 25-6. Look for a calculator with big keys that are easy to see and operate if you have poor vision or incoordination. The Bio-Curve pen is designed to reduce pressure on the wrist and fingers while writing. (Photo by J.K.)

(Figure 25-6). Look for a unit with big keys that are easy to see and operate if you have poor vision or incoordination. The calculator shown and those that run on solar or ambient light are about $15 and up from department stores and mail-order firms. **Sources:** 50, 242, 270, 415.

The Bio-Curve pen is designed for people with arthritis. The non-slip outer surface is sueded for extra friction, which means less grasp is needed, and angled to reduce pressure on the wrist and fingers while writing. Cost is about $3 and up from self-help firms. **Sources:** 15, 108, 382.

Other writing aids include small triangular or shaped grips that slip onto the shaft of a pen or pencil. **Manufacturer:** 190. Cost is about $.50 each and up from stationery stores and self-help firms. **Sources:** 1, 5, 15, 394.

CARRYING

- Limit carrying as much as possible to conserve your energy.
- If you use a cane or walker, you may be able to switch to a large grocery cart while shopping. Try this out initially, however, with supervision by someone in your family, a visiting nurse, or therapist.
- Roll, don't carry, heavy loads. A variety of carts are available for use both within the store and for transport to your car and home. Some large stores even have wheelchairs for shoppers' use.
- If you are eligible, apply for a special permit to park near the stores to reduce walking with packages and to allow you more room to maneuver in and out of your car. This is usually done through your Town Hall.
- Paper bags permit better body mechanics than plastic. If you have arthritis, they let you use your whole arms and trunk to carry.
- If carrying puts a strain on you, request help in loading the car and plan to shop so that your family or a neighbor can unload on return home.
- Try to use a shopping cart or bag on wheels that meets your needs. If you are walking and doing a small amount of shop-

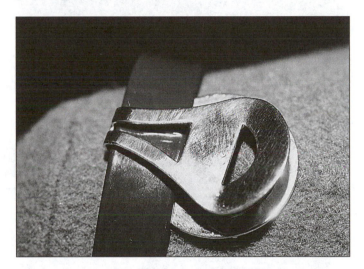

Figure 25-7. A shoulder bag pin keeps the bag from slipping off your shoulder. (Photo by J.K.)

ping, models that roll on four rather than two wheels are more stable. A liner helps keep items from slipping out. Carts cost about $23 and up from department stores and mail-order firms. **Sources:** 100, 270, 387.

- If you are shopping with a young child, train him or her from the start to stay seated in the basket. Some stores provide seat belts or devise your own with a stretch webbed belt that threads through the carriage spokes.

A shoulder bag transfers the weight of carrying from your hands to your trunk (Figure 25-7). This is especially important if you use one hand to manage a cane or have arthritis, which makes it imperative to avoid static holding with your hands. A shoulder bag pin keeps the bag from slipping off your shoulder. Pins are about $16 and up from department stores and mail-order firms. **Source:** 270.

Eliminate the hassle of a handbag with a fanny pack or small knapsack (Figure 25-8). Either keeps necessities safe and handy, distributes weight over your trunk, and leaves both hands free to

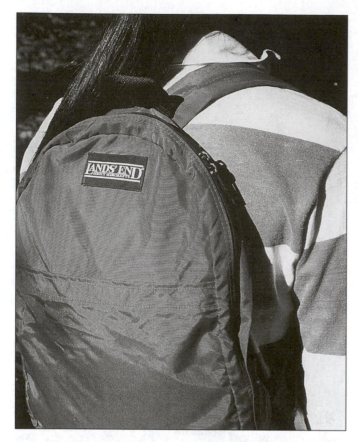

Figure 25-8. Eliminate the hassle of a handbag with a fanny pack or small knapsack. (Photo by J.K.)

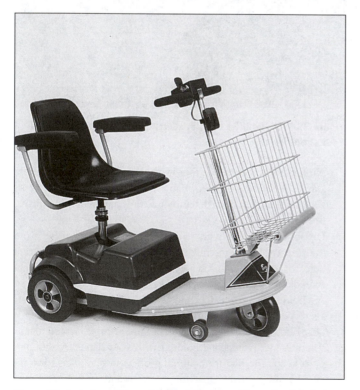

Figure 25-9. A shopping cart basket for use with a wheelchair is frequently provided by the store. (Photo courtesy of Amigo® Mobility International, Inc., Bridgeport, MI.)

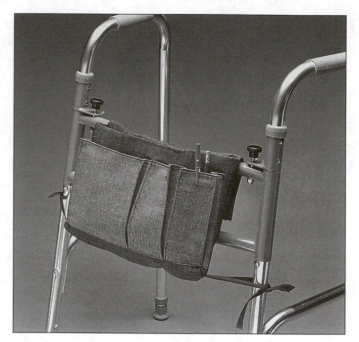

Figure 25-10. When shopping from a wheelchair or with a walker, a basket or carry-all that attaches to the walker bar or arm may be helpful. (Photo courtesy of North Coast Medical, Inc., San Jose, CA.)

manage a walking aid or packages. **Manufacturers:** 106, 110, 227, 245. Belt bags and day packs of nylon and canvas cost about $8 and up from department stores and sporting goods and mail-order firms. **Sources:** 53, 106, 110, 152, 196, 245, 270, 298, 364, 378.

A shopping cart basket for use with a wheelchair is frequently provided by the store. If one is not available where you shop, ask if the management might consider one. In larger stores and malls, the Smart Shopper by Amigo® is a popular energy saver (Figure 25-9).

A reacher is a helpful aid for groceries stacked on high shelves. See Chapter 14. For heavy items, ask a passing shopper for assistance, rather than risk broken goods.

When shopping from a wheelchair or with a walker, a basket or carry-all that attaches to the walker bar or arm may be helpful (Figure 25-10). The basket can be fitted with a transparent acrylic liner to keep small items from slipping through and may be removed for cleaning. **Manufacturer:** 163. Cost is $21 and up from self-help firms. **Sources:** 13, 120, 240, 252, 261, 264, 368, 290, 370, 408. The bag shown has a deep pockets and a zipper closure. **Manufacturer:** 163. Gardening stores often carry a metal-framed, mesh lawn mower bag that has Velcro® so you can attach it to a baby carriage or walker. Cost is about $6. **Source:** 270. Also see Chapter 4.

A fabric shopping bag on wheels rolls on two rubber casters to save you the stress of carrying (Figure 25-11). It starts the trip as a tote bag and unfolds into a 21" x 12" x 7" size with a top zippered compartment, front pocket, and stand-up bracket. It works for laundry as well as groceries. If you are tall, make sure the handles adjust, or add an extra loop so you do not have to bend while using. **Distributor:** 61. Cost is about $20 and up from department stores

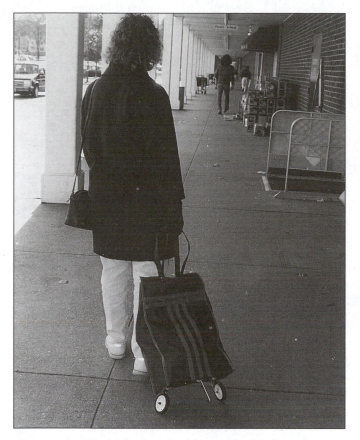

Figure 25-11. This fabric shopping bag on wheels rolls on two rubber casters to save you the stress of carrying. (Photo by J.K.)

and mail-order firms. **Sources:** 152, 270, 378, 387, 407, 415.

An accordion tote expands in size to accommodate shopping, for use at home, or for use on wider travels (Figures 25-12A and 25-12B). It starts as a 14" x 14" shoulder bag, then unzips by sections to reach a height of 23". The water-resistant, nylon taffeta bag has a zippered top, four ball-bearing casters, large stitched handles, an outer zippered pocket, and a removable shoulder strap for use when empty or as a tote. **Manufacturer:** 160.Cost is about $18 and up from department stores and mail-order firms. **Sources:** 169, 364, 407.

If you prefer a solid shopping cart, one with four wheels will roll more smoothly. Cost is about $25 from department stores and mail-order firms. **Source:** 100.

Even if you are carrying only a few items in a plastic bag, a bag handle is in order, especially if you have any arthritis in your hands (Figure 25-13). The wide padded handle distributes the weight, eliminating painful hands and pinched fingers, while the plastic-coated hook grasps the loops of the bag. Cost is about $5 from self-help firms. **Sources:** 15, 59, 252.

If you live within walking distance of your stores, but have weak lower extremities, respiratory problems, poor balance, or back pain, ask your physician, nurse, or therapist about carrying groceries with a rolling walker (Figure 25-14). Walkers designed for outdoor use must have large wheels to accommodate bumpy terrain. **Manufacturers:** 25, 122 (illustrated), 414. Also see Chapter 4.

If getting things into and out of a car trunk is difficult, ask for

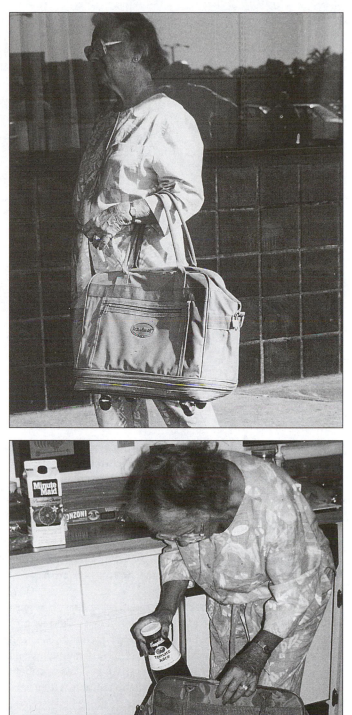

Figures 25-12A, 25-12B. This accordion tote expands in size to accommodate shopping at home or for use on wider travels. (Manufactured by Goodhope Bags Industries, Inc., La Puenta, CA. Photo by J.K.)

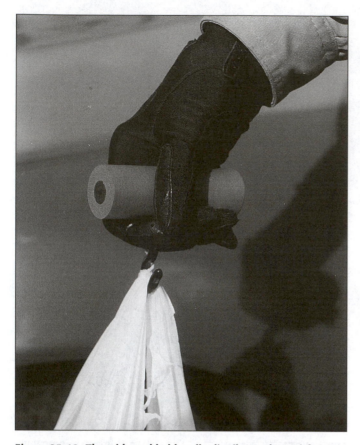

Figure 25-13. The wide padded handle distributes the weight over your arm, eliminating painful hands and pinched fingers, while the plastic-coated hook grasps the loops of the bag. (Photo by J.K.)

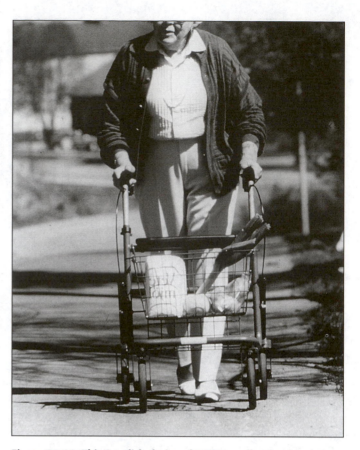

Figure 25-14. This Swedish-designed NOVA walker has hand brakes and carries a large basket. (Photo courtesy of Etac USA Inc., Waukesha, WI.)

help. Leave heavier items until someone is available. A trunk rack or bag holder for any automobile keeps food bags from spilling while you drive (Figure 25-15). Cost is about $15 from department stores and mail-order firms. **Sources** for grocery bag holders: 49, 194.

If you are a slower shopper, have a distance to travel, or need help unloading your car later, refrigerated items should be protected from heating and spoiling. A large picnic cooler will accommodate bags if you ask the packer to separate items and not fill the bags too full. **Manufacturers:** 70, 397. Cost is about $20 and up. Help prolong the cold by taking reusable frozen containers with you.

Insulated food carriers keep foods like meat and milk cold for hours or take-out foods hot until you get home and are ready to eat. A 15" x 18" bag holds up to 26 pounds. **Manufacturer:** 27. Cost for a soft-sided cooler, constructed of Dacron or polyethylene with Dacron® or Thinsulate® insulation, is about $15 each and up from department stores and mail-order firms. **Sources:** 270, 387.

If walking or wheeling a chair is fatiguing so that you need a little more power for shopping and other activities, see Chapter 7 for information on powered scooters and other units.

HANDLING MONEY AND KEYS

A key holder eliminates the frustration of trying to handle a

small key or keys if your hands are weak, incoordinated, or affected by arthritis (Figure 25-16). Built-up key holders provide leverage in turning one or more keys. A dual-purpose key holder/car door opener shown solves two problems with one aid. The padded handle has an adjustable gripper at one end for depressing door buttons and a removable fob on the other for keys. Cost is about $25 from self-help firms. **Sources** for this and other similar units cost about $5 and up from self-help firms: 13, 15, 108, 120, 238, 252, 264, 290, 370, 393, 408.

A raised rim on a horseshoe purse keeps coins from spilling, so that you can pick them up with more control. Cost is about $8 and up from department stores and mail-order firms. **Source:** 270.

A sectioned coin purse to separate coins is helpful if you have loss of vision or incoordination (Figure 25-17). Cost is about $2 and up from department and variety stores.

GETTING AROUND

Getting in and out of your house does not have to be a barrier to going shopping. The entrance ways to your home can be remodeled to allow greater independence. A ramp to replace steps lets a wheelchair or walker come and go more easily. For entrances with higher grades, a lift may be required. Stair lifts and elevators also make the interior of your house completely accessible. Contact your local Vocational Rehabilitation Office for planning and possi-

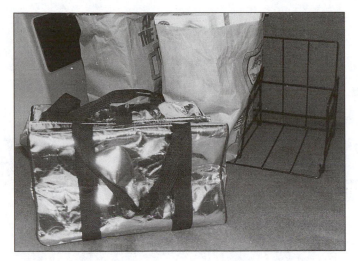

Figure 25-15. A trunk rack or bag holder for any automobile keeps food bags from spilling while you drive. (Photo by J.K.)

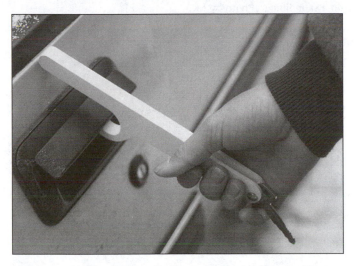

Figure 25-16. A key holder eliminates the frustration of trying to handle a small key or keys if your hands are weak, incoordinated, or affected by arthritis. (Key holder by North Coast Medical, Inc., San Jose, CA. Photo by J.K.)

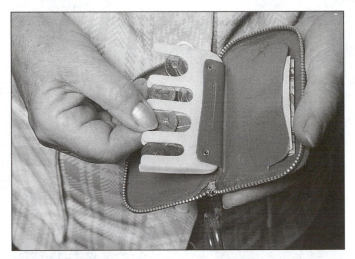

Figure 25-17. A sectioned coin purse to separate coins is helpful if you have loss of vision or incoordination. (Photo courtesy of the O.T. Dept., Howard A. Rusk Institute of Rehabilitation Medicine.)

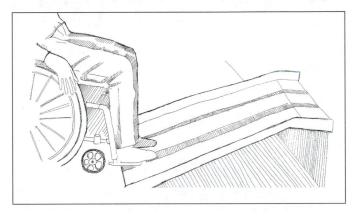

Figure 25-18. A ramp may be designed to fit your home. (Illustration by G.K.)

ble financial assistance. See Appendix B.

A ramp may be designed to fit your home (Figure 25-18). For apartment use or outside travel, a portable ramp may be an adequate answer. Lightweight ramps of aluminum attach to the back of a wheelchair. Solid ramps, rather than two channel ramps, are easier to use if someone is going to help push you up the ramp, because they give the person a place to walk. Cost is about $125 and up. **Sources:** 5, 19, 168, 252, 264, 313.

A porch lift raises you to a level where you can wheel or walk directly into your house (Figure 25-19). For information, contact the following: 195, 286, 418, and local hospital supply firms.

Getting into and out of a car may be difficult if you have limited use of your lower extremities, or hip or back problems. A portable swivel cushion of closed-cell foam with a removable velour cover turns 360°, eliminating the weight of your body (Figure 25-20). A padded cushion rests on a plywood base, rotating on steel ball-bearings, much like a lazy susan, as you turn to enter or leave your car. Always wear your seat belt to maintain a

stable balance while driving or riding. Cost is about $19 and up from mail-order and self-help firms. **Sources:** 50, 59, 175, 238, 364, 382, 387, 415.

If you have little natural bottom padding, you may prefer a softer swivel seat, designed with two cushions that slide on a satin lining (Figure 25-21). Bottom cushion stays stationary while the top cushion turns so you do not have to lift your buttocks or legs and are in best position for sitting or rising. **Manufacturers:** 103, 243. Cost is about $25. **Sources:** 15, 243, 382.

If you sit in a wheelchair to drive or as a passenger, a wheelchair lift may simplify your coming and going (Figure 25-22). Ask your therapist for assistance in locating the best unit to meet your needs. Visit local rehabilitation suppliers, and try before you buy. **Manufacturer:** 45.

If driving is a problem, talk with your therapist or visiting nurse, or contact your local Vocational Rehabilitation Office or nearest rehabilitation center. You may need some small changes within your car, such as wide-angle mirrors, a riser cushion, or adaptations in the controls. They can help solve the problems or refer you to a specialized drivers' training program. The major automobile manufacturers, i.e., Chrysler, Ford/Lincoln-Mercury, and General Motors, have automobile mobility programs for

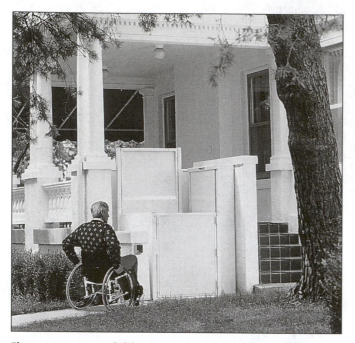

Figure 25-19. A porch lift raises you to a level where you can wheel or walk directly into your house. (Photo courtesy of Access Industries, Inc., Grandview, MO.)

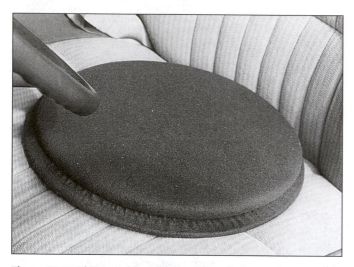

Figure 25-20. This portable swivel cushion eliminates the weight of your body as you rotate into the car. (Photo by J.K.)

adapting cars to an individual's needs. The American Automobile Association publishes a book of suggestions for drivers with physical limitations and gives courses for older drivers. The American Association for Retired Persons gives a defensive driving course, called 55-Plus. Contact your Senior Center. See Going Further at end of this chapter.

Moving groceries from the car to the house is eased when you use wheels. Hand trucks or carts designed for carrying garden supplies or loading pleasure boats may be used to transfer groceries. Small folding or pop-carts cost about $35 and up from department stores and mail-order firms. **Sources: 49, 50.** Larger units are about $50 and up from gardening stores and boating suppliers. **Sources: 49, 50, 87, 374.**

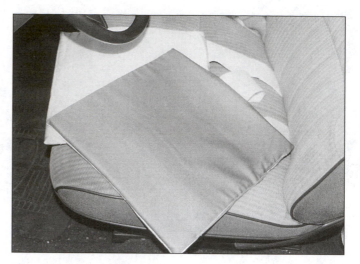

Figure 25-21. If you have little natural bottom padding, you may prefer a softer swivel seat, designed with two cushions that slide on a satin lining. (Photo by J.K.)

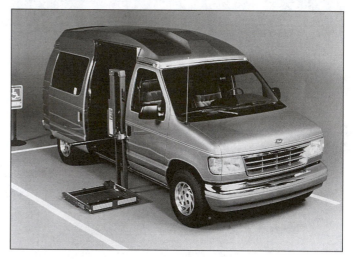

Figure 25-22. If you sit in a wheelchair to drive or as a passenger, a wheelchair lift may simplify your coming and going. (Photo courtesy of the Braun Corporation®, Winimac, IN.)

Although we have a long way to go, public transportation has improved in some communities, often with buses that have lift access for wheelchairs and alternate bus services for senior citizens and people with disabilities. Contact your local Social Services or Senior Services department for up-to-date information. Special cab services are available in many towns and cities. Since these may be expensive, first find out about volunteer services.

DIFFERENT WAYS OF SHOPPING

No longer do you have to trudge to the store for many of your purchases. The world of mail order comes to you, often in overwhelming amounts. Television shopping reaches your armchair. Computer programs for in-home banking and grocery shopping exist in many parts of the country. All of this means, however, that you have to be a more wary consumer.

Basic rules to be a wiser, safer consumer include the following:
• Read all ads carefully and completely. If it seems too good to

be true, it usually is.

- When ordering from a post office box, make sure the company's name and full address is listed for follow-up.
- Check the company's return policy before ordering. If there is no guarantee, call and ask about their method of handling returns.
- Remember, if you telephone your order, you may forfeit legal protection. Federal law requires that a company fill your written mail order within 30 days. If the wait is longer, notice must be sent to you with an estimated time of delivery. You may choose to wait or cancel your order and receive a full refund. Only if you live in a state that protects telephone orders can you be certain of these rights. To have it in writing, follow up a phone order with a written note confirming your order. Keep a copy for yourself.
- Never send cash: Always send a check or money order. If you want to pay by credit card, you have extra protection. Should you have a complaint, write to the credit card company. The company may tell you that your payment is late, but the credit company must, by law, investigate and cannot bill you until the dispute is resolved. But put it in writing. You lose this legal right if you call in your complaint.
- Note the date you placed your order, whether in writing or by telephone. Keep this with a copy of the advertisement or catalog and completed catalog form. Most catalogs have duplicate forms. If paying by check, write the company's address on the check so you can follow up if the item should not arrive, but the check is cashed. Keep the canceled check or charge-account record with your order information until you receive the merchandise.
- You may want to set up a single form if you do a lot of mail-order shopping.

  The following headings will help keep track of purchases:
  - Order Date.
  - Company or Catalog Name and Address.
  - Merchandise Description.
  - Special Instructions.
  - Discounts or Coupons.
  - Total Cost.
  - Method of Payment.
  - Expected Date of Arrival.
  - Date of Receipt.

  If you often return items, add two extra columns for Return of Item and Receipt of New Product or Refund.
- Check the company's policy on delivery time. If the item is not delivered within 30 days, the company should have contacted you. You are not required to accept a substitute.
- If you receive an item that does not meet your expectations, follow the company's directions exactly for return. Do it promptly, and fill in the reason. If there are no instructions, call the company. This saves aggravation, even when there is no toll-free number.
- If you receive a package damaged in delivery, notify the post office immediately. If the outer wrapping is broken, request that the delivery person wait until you have opened it, or get a receipt stating that the package was damaged. Keep all invoices and packing slips to accompany request for replacement. If the company has a toll-free number, call and ask how to handle the return. Sometimes they do not require return of the item, just a note. Other companies want the item returned, but will first send a postage-paid label.
- If you receive something you did not order, you may consider it a gift. The sender cannot ask you to return or pay for it. If you believe you are a victim of mail fraud, call the Postal Inspection Service.

Consumer publications listed at the end of this chapter provide additional information to protect yourself as a consumer and mail-order shopper.

GOING FURTHER

Addresses in the Appendices.

PUBLICATIONS

Consumer's Resource Handbook, #582T. Published annually. Free from Department 46, Consumer Information Center. Tips and information plus more than 700 addresses for corporate consumer offices, Better Business Bureaus, trade associations, federal, state and local government consumer offices. Suggestions on writing a complaint letter and what to do if you do not get desired results.

The Handicapped Driver's Mobility Guide. Directory lists services for handicapped drivers. Free from the American Automobile Association.

How to Write a Wrong, #447T. Free from the Consumer Information Center. How to complain and get results, door-to-door sales, and "the Cooling Off Rule" for contracts.

Twenty Ways Not to Be Swindled, #08029. Illustrated booklet. South Deerfield, MA: Channing L. Bete Co., Inc. Twenty common consumer rip-offs. $1.25. **Source:** 62.

What Senior Citizens Should Know About Crime Prevention. South Deerfield, MA: Channing L. Bete Co., Inc. Tips for at home, going out, in the car, and as a consumer. $1.25. **Source:** 62.

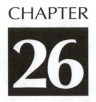

Involving Your Family and Handling Children

If you teach your children to enjoy food preparation activities, before long you will have assistant chefs at your side wanting to measure, mix, and cook. Encourage their culinary talents by getting a cookbook geared to their age level or by writing out recipes so that they can follow them. The ultimate reward is when a son or daughter fixes the whole meal for you, and cleans up afterward!

Establish a routine for chores, such as carrying in the groceries, taking out the trash, and helping you shop. You may have to adjust your own standards of housekeeping and let your family help clean the house in their own manner. The joy of family participation is more important than sweeping away every cobweb.

Set up a communication center with a large calendar on the refrigerator door. Cost is about $15 from stationery stores and mail-order firms. **Source:** 364.

From about the age of four, children can help set and clear the table, scrub vegetables, and sweep the floor (Figure 26-1). A six-year-old can use his energy and muscles to help bring in groceries (Figure 26-2).

HANDLING CHILDREN

Children younger than four years of age must be taught about safety, including the dangers of heat, electricity, and cleaning materials. If you have difficulty moving quickly or keeping a constant eye on your children, take safety precautions.

A gate at the kitchen door keeps your child in sight and provides a play area while you work (Figure 26-3). If you have limited use of your hands, make sure that you can easily operate the gate's latch. **Manufacturers** include 136 (gate opens with one hand). Cost is about $33 and up from department stores and mail-order firms. **Source:** 345.

A baby carriage may be used indoors as an alternative place to keep an infant near you or to move the infant around the house. The safety belt secures the child within the stroller, and brakes keep the stroller stationary. An infant beginning to climb is too old and mobile for a baby carriage.

A motorized scooter speeds carrying of an infant and other items around the house (Figure 26-4). It might be indicated if you find propelling a wheelchair or walking difficult or fatiguing. See Chapter 7 for a discussion of scooters.

Your safety belt can be extended to hold an infant in your wheelchair. For a very young infant, a baby sling or carrier secures your infant while maneuvering your wheelchair or scooter. Try various styles of slings in the store before you buy, and talk with other mothers about their preferences. **Manufacturers** include 136, 400B.

If your balance is good, you might carry your infant or young child in a backpack child carrier (Figure 26-5). This leaves your hands free for shopping and other tasks. Share the carrying with other family members on longer outings, and encourage your child to walk as soon as possible. Look for a carrier with easy-to-adjust control straps, padded shoulder straps, and a hip belt to distribute the weight. A frame stand that provides a solid base allows you to put it on more easily. **Manufacturers** include 400B.

An intercom reduces steps and helps you keep an "ear" on a child or children while sleeping. Wireless intercoms require no wiring changes in the home. **Manufacturers:** 136, 325, 344. Cost is about $30 per pair and up from department and electronic stores and mail-order firms. **Sources:** 87, 175, 176, 177, 194, 325, 345, 369. If you want to keep an eye on your child, you can install a Baby View Monitor by the crib. **Manufacturer:** 344. Cost is about $200 from department stores.

A stove shield or guard rail at the front of your range top keeps tiny hands away from hot pans. A plastic unit attaches to the stove with adhesive-backed clips and slides out for easy cleaning. Cost is about $20. **Source:** 345. Suction cups may also be used to hold a home-devised guard in place. A disadvantage of a guard rail is that you must lift pans over the bar. You may, however, slide them back and forth at the sides.

Electrical outlets conveniently located for you may be dangerous for an inquisitive toddler (Figure 26-6). A safety outlet cover keeps small fingers out of electrical sockets. Look for covers in the children's section of department stores or through mail-order firms. **Manufacturers:** 157, 344. A set of two is about $8. **Source:** 345.

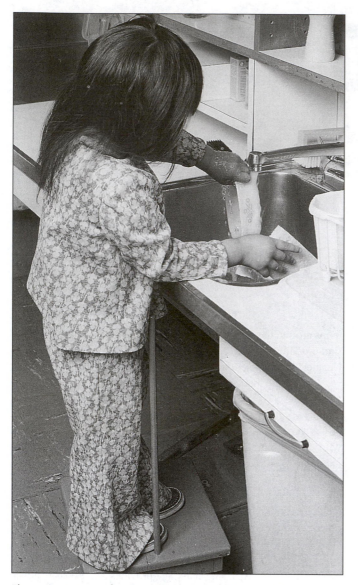

Figure 26-1. From about age four years, children can help set and clear the table, scrub vegetables, and sweep the floor.

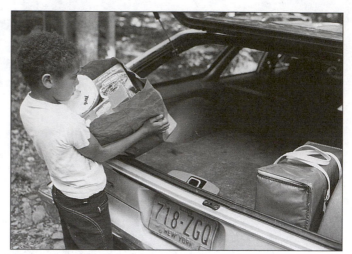

Figure 26-2. This six-year-old uses his energy and muscles to help bring in groceries.

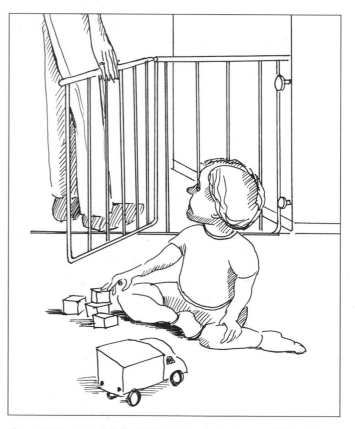

Figure 26-3. A gate at the kitchen door keeps your child in sight and provides a play area while you work. (Illustration by G.K.)

Latches installed on cabinet doors keep out curious tots. **Manufacturers** include 157, 311. Cost is about $6 and up per set of two. A variety of latches are carried by **source** 345. As an added precaution, store dangerous cleansers and chemicals out of reach, rather than under the sink. Mark the bottles with a red "X," a skull and crossbones, or another symbol that your child can be taught to identify and understand means "danger.".

Other areas and safety aids to consider include corner protectors on tables and raised hearths, cord shorteners on blinds, door knob covers to prevent opening by inquisitive searchers, toilet cover locks, and window or railing bars. **Manufacturer** of several types of locks: 157. **Source** for all these items: 345.

Feeding a small child is easier if you can avoid or minimize lifting. Choose a low chair for the child that is level with your chair. **Manufacturers** include 80, 311. The legs on an older-style, wooden high chair can sometimes be shortened to lower the seat. Make sure you can easily remove the chair's tray to slide the child into your lap. Attach toys or utensils to the tray with a plastic coated

spring coil or suction cups so that you do not have to retrieve them. Keep a plastic sheet under the chair to reduce cleanup. **Manufacturer:** 344. Cost is about $7 from department stores and mail-order firms. **Source:** 242.

If you have weak hands or arthritis, use a jar opener for baby foods and bottles (Figure 26-7). See details in Chapter 1.

Reduce cleanup with an easy-to-clean bib (Figure 26-8). Check for large plastic or vinyl-coated styles in local department stores and through mail-order firms. The bib shown has a Velcro® closure. **Source:** 1, original design by 170, who makes only infant-

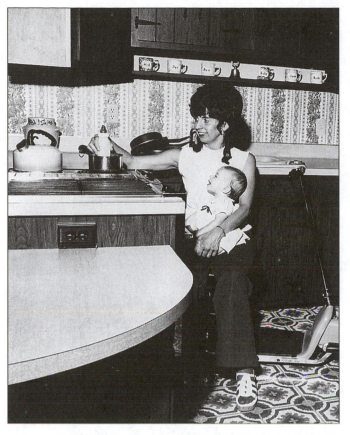

Figure 26-4. A motorized scooter speeds carrying of an infant and other items around the house. (Photo courtesy of Amigo® Mobility International, Inc., Bridgeport, MI.)

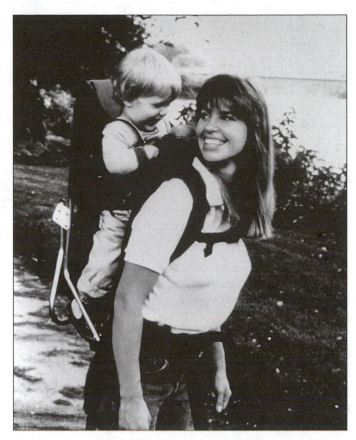

Figure 26-5. If your balance is good, you might carry your infant or young child in a back pack child carrier. (Photo courtesy of Touch Traveler®, Schenectady, NY.)

sized bibs but carries a wide range of easy-care, easy-to-don clothing for children.

A non-spillable training cup also lessens cleanup and encourages your child to be self-feeding. **Manufacturer:** 157. Cost is $1.50 and up from housewares stores and mail-order firms.

If you have incoordination or partial loss of vision, a plastic- or rubber-coated spoon will help protect your child's mouth during feeding (Figure 26-9). The easy-hold bowl shown here has a finger grip to help you hold the bowl securely while feeding your infant with the other hand. Microwave and dishwasher safe. **Manufacturers:** 157, 350. Bowl and spoon set is about $4 from children's departments. Additional **source** for spoons: 393.

Other feeding aids include easy-grip feeding utensils, suction-based feeding bowls, and cups with specialized grips and spouts. **Manufacturers**: 157, 350.

Here are some more tips for organizing your work with young children:

- Share baby-sitting duty with your friends.
- Plan an activity that engages your child's attention while you cook.
- A baby walker is not a safe place to leave your child. He or she will quickly learn to propel himself or herself. In 1993, there were injuries to 25,000 children in the United States due to falls with baby walkers. Use a chair swing or chair.
- Hire a reliable neighborhood adult or teenager to play with or care for your children two or three times a week. Use this time

to accomplish chores, such as meal preparation or home money management, that require you to work uninterrupted. Or use the time to take a rest and pamper yourself with some relaxing reading.

- Secure your child with a safety belt in the grocery cart while you are shopping. Most supermarkets now provide safety belts. Bring along a sitting activity or treat for your child to enjoy as you shop. Even a three-year-old likes to "write" or check off lists as Mom or Dad shops.
- Use a harness or leash to keep your child beside you while you shop or travel.
- Always use the proper car seat, designed for the age and weight of your child. Before buying, be certain that you can operate the latches and belts. Also, make sure that your vehicle's seat belt system is suitable for the car seat requirements.
- Teach your child to pick up toys and clothing.
- Join a mother's group for sharing ideas.

GOING FURTHER

Addresses are listed in the Appendices.

PUBLICATIONS

Beebe, B. M. (1982). Best Bets for Babies. New York: Bantam Doubleday Dell.

Beebe, B. M. (1983). *Tips for Toddlers*. New York: Bantam Doubleday Dell.Berman, E. (1977). *The Cooperating Family:*

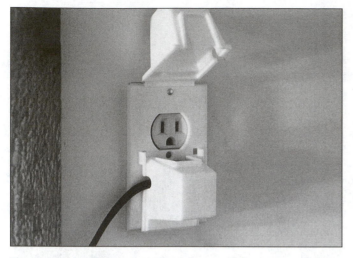

Figure 26-6. A safety outlet cover keeps small fingers out of electrical sockets. (Photo courtesy of the O.T. Dept., Howard A. Rusk Institute of Rehabilitation Medicine.)

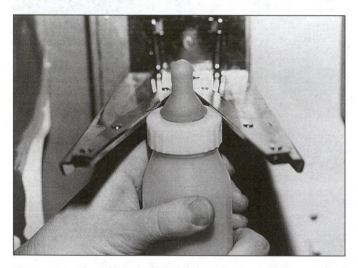

Figure 26-7. If you have weak hands or arthritis, use a jar opener for baby foods and bottles. (Opener by Zim Manufacturing Co., Chicago, IL. Photo courtesy of the O.T. Dept., Howard A. Rusk Institute of Rehabilitation Medicine.)

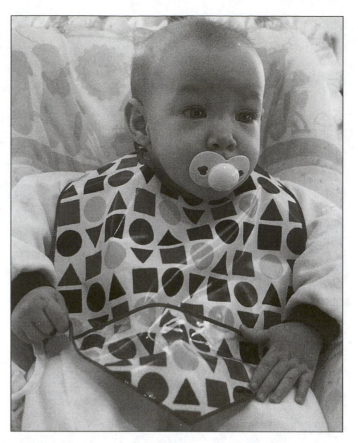

Figure 26-8. Reduce cleanup with an easy-to-clean bib. This bib has a Velcro® closure. (Bib by Hanna Andersson®, Portland, OR. Photo by L.K.)

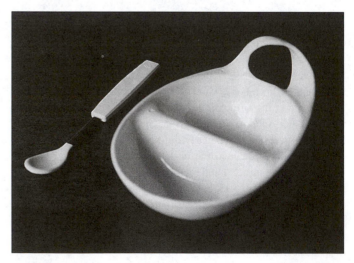

Figure 26-9. The Easy-Hold bowl shown here has a finger grip to help you hold the bowl securely while feeding your infant with the other hand. (Bowl and spoon by Sassy, Inc., Grand Rapids, MI. Photo by J.K.)

How Your Children Can Help Manage the Household—For Their Good As Well As Yours. New York: Prentice-Hall, Simon and Schuster.

Cunningham, M. (1995). *Cooking with Children: 15 Lessons for Children Age 7 and Up*. New York: Alfred Knopf, Random House.

Demoss, A., Rogers, J., Tuleja, C., & Kirshbaum, M., with support from the National Institute of Disability and Rehabilitation Research. (1995). *Adaptive Parenting Equipment: Idea Book*, and the *Parenting with a Disability Newsletter*. Berkeley, CA: Through the Looking Glass. Book illustrates equipment available and modified from cribs, chairs, and carrying aids, to bathing units, modified splints for feeding a child, and play. $10 individual, $25 professional. Subscription to the three-times-a-year newsletter is free. See Periodicals.

Faber, A., & Mazlish, E. (1975). *Liberated Parents—Liberated Children*. New York: Avon Books.

Kelly, M., & Parsons, E. (1992). *Mothers Almanac*. New York: Bantam Doubleday Dell. **Source:** 34C.

Parent News. Center for Persons with Disabilities, Utah State University. See Periodicals.

Section Five

PREPARING AND SERVING, AND APPENDICES

CHAPTER 27

Opening Containers

Convenience and prepared foods are packaged in containers designed to keep flavor in, preserve freshness, and prevent contamination by bacteria. If, however, you have weak hands, use of only one hand, incoordination, arthritis, or poor vision, these same packages may present barriers to you. Simple techniques and aids can overcome these problems.

CANS

If you are using one hand, have arthritis, or weakness in both hands, an electric can opener is an essential appliance. See Chapter 20.

A manual can opener with gears reduces pressure on your hands and works well if you have moderate strength in both hands (Figure 27-1). This Swiss opener locks onto the can so that no pressure is required while turning the key. It may be even be used with one hand after a little practice. Dishwasher safe. **Manufacturer:** 435. Cost is about $15 and up from department stores and mail-order firms. **Source:** 427.

The large key on this gear-driven manual opener distributes pressure on your hand, protecting your fingers while turning (Figure 27-2). **Manufacturers:** 193, 201, 384. Cost is about $10 and up from housewares stores and mail-order firms. **Source:** 410.

The strip-top opening on some cans may be removed with one hand by putting your hand on top of the can while pulling the tape up with your fingers (Figure 27-3A). If you cannot release the cover with a slight push upward, a bottle-cap opener makes the job easier. If you have weak pinch in your fingers, try catching the tab between two fingers and release it enough to wrap around one finger for better leverage. Two other answers: use a pair of pliers or if the can has a rimmed bottom, turn it upside down and open with an electric can opener.

Needle-nose pliers quickly release the foil tab or safety seal on single serving-size cans of juices, half-gallon juice containers, medicines, and other foods. Try the stainless-steel, self-opening Swedish loop pliers. See matching scissors in Figure 27-15B. The spring-loaded pliers have ribbed polypropylene handles to make gripping easier. Try pliers for tubes, very small jar tops, and flip-top cans. If you are using one hand, put the container on a damp sponge cloth, then lever the pliers against the top of the can as you pull the tab free. **Manufacturer:** 122. Cost of loop pliers is about $18 from self-help firms. **Sources:** 5, 13, 252, 264, 290, 368, 408.

A tab grabber lifts and removes the metal key tab on pop-top cans (Figure 27-3B). The opposite end has a circular gripper for twist-off bottle caps. Some come with a magnetized case to hang on refrigerator. Set of two is about $6 from housewares stores and mail-order and self-help firms. **Manufacturers:** 107, 142, 181, 289. **Sources:** 5, 6, 13, 71, 120, 252, 264, 290, 408.

If your hands are weak or affected by arthritis, a ring-topped can may be opened by applying simple leverage against the side of the can (Figure 27-4). Use a table knife or fork.

Pressing down the button of an aerosol container, such as used for cooking sprays, is easier with an aerosol dispenser handle (Figure 27-5). Light pressure on the wide handle releases the contents. Cost for this and similar units is about $7 each and up from self-help firms. **Sources:** 5, 252, 264, 290, 368.

JARS

Getting the lid off a jar is difficult for anyone, but almost impossible if your hands are weak or if you are working with one hand, and is actually damaging to joints if you have arthritis in your hands. Jar opening and openers are described in Chapters 1 through 3 as well as here. The wall-mounted Zim wedge jar opener is best if you have severe loss of strength, incoordination, or arthritis in your hands (see Figure 27-5). The Swedish Rehab Fixer-board holds the jar in a vise while you turn with one or both hands (see Chapter 28). The Capscrew works well when you have weak hands, poor vision, or incoordination.

Opening even a new jar with one hand is easy with a wedge-type opener (Figure 27-6). Steel teeth grasp the cover as you turn the jar. Installing the opener above a counter or small shelf gives you a place to set the can immediately after opening. The Zim jar

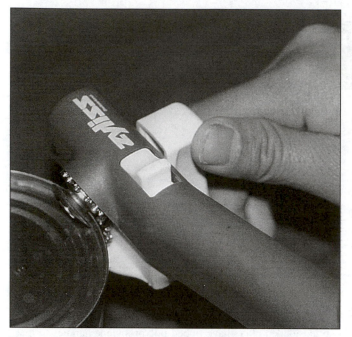

Figure 27-1. This Swiss opener locks onto the can so that no pressure is required while turning the key. (Opener by Zyliss Wabe Co., Lyss, Switzerland. Photo by J.K.)

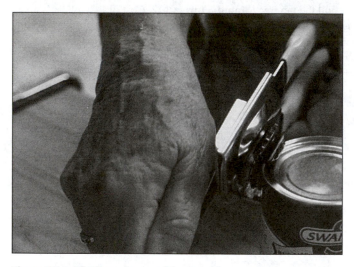

Figure 27-2. The large key on this gear-driven manual opener distributes pressure on your hand, protecting your fingers while turning. (Opener by Swing-A-Way Manufacturing Co., St. Louis, MO. Photo by J.K.)

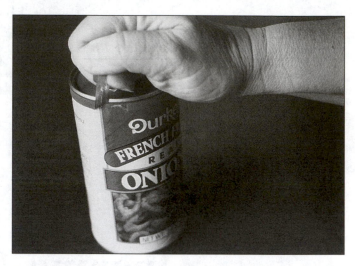

Figure 27-3A. The strip-top opening on some cans may be removed with one hand by putting your hand on top of the can while pulling the tape up with your fingers. (Photo courtesy of the O.T. Dept., Howard A. Rusk Institute of Rehabilitation Medicine.)

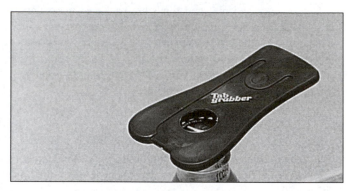

Figure 27-3B. A tab grabber lifts and removes the metal key tab on pop-top cans. The opposite end has a circular gripper for twist-off bottle caps. (Photo courtesy of North Coast Medical, Inc., San Jose, CA.)

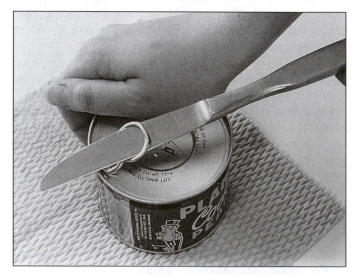

Figure 27-4. If your hands are weak or affected by arthritis, a ring-topped can may be opened by applying simple leverage against the side of the can. (Photo courtesy of the O.T. Dept., Howard A. Rusk Institute of Rehabilitation Medicine.)

opener comes in two models: one that folds down against the wall when not in use, and another that installs under a cabinet. **Manufacturer:** 434. Cost is about $9 from self-help and mail-order firms. **Sources:** 5, 6, 13, 15, 16, 120, 252, 264, 290, 408.

Good Grips® also makes a wedge-shaped jar opener with a built-up handle for use with both hands, and you do not need the device attached to a wall. **Manufacturer:** 301. Cost is about $8 from housewares stores and mail-order firms. **Sources:** 5, 13, 15, 16, 65, 252. See other jar openers in Chapters 1, 2, and 28.

Small, portable jar openers help when you are occasionally faced with a stubborn jar or are camping or traveling. A Plumber's

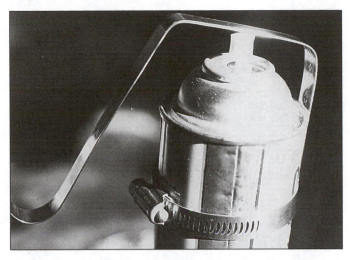

Figure 27-5. Pressing down the button of an aerosol container, such as used for cooking sprays, is easier with an aerosol dispenser handle. (Photo by J.K.)

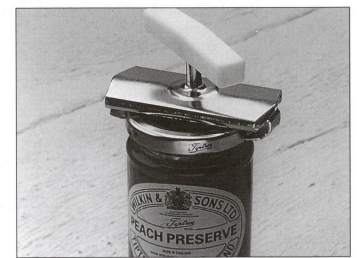

Figure 27-7A. This rachet type jar opener releases the top with one or two hands. Base may be stabilized to reduce holding. (Photo courtesy of Rowoco, Wilton Industries, Woodridge, IL.)

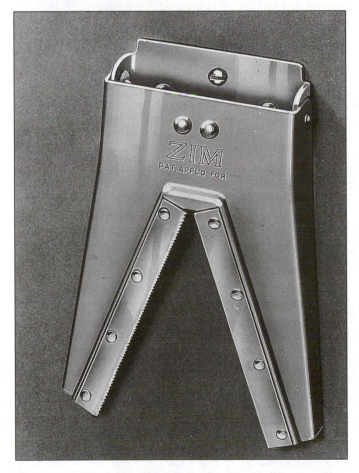

Figure 27-6. Opening even a new jar with one hand is easy with a wedge-type opener. Steel teeth grasp the cover as you turn the jar. (Photo courtesy of North Coast Medical Inc., San Jose, CA.)

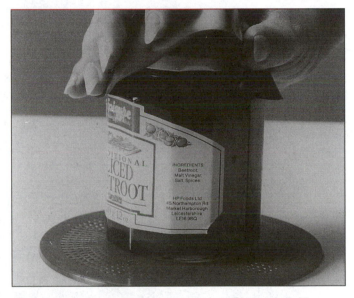

Figure 27-7B. The flexible, rubber HandyAid® gripper pad has hundreds of tiny suction cups that grasp the jar cover while you turn it. (Photo courtesy of AliMed®, Inc., Dedham, MA.)

Wrench jar opener has a closed loop with a wooden handle that lets you loosen as well as tighten jar tops from ½" to 3½" in diameter. You slip the friction belt around the cover. As you press against the wood lever, the belt adjusts to cap size to loosen the top in one push. Cost is about $3 and up from hardware stores and mail-order firms. **Sources:** 5, 49, 290. A rachet-type jar opener (Figure 27-7A) will allow you to open a jar with one hand if the base is stabilized on a rubber mat or wedged in a drawer. **Manufacturer:** 339. Cost is about $3 from housewares stores and mail-order firms.

The flexible, rubber HandyAid® gripper pad has hundreds of tiny suction cups that grasp the jar cover while you turn it (Figure 27-7B). Pad may also be used under the jar or under a bowl or pan to hold it steady while you are stirring. Cost is about $3 each from mail-order firms. **Sources:** 252, 410.

The Capscrew (Figure 27-8) helps open tops with diameters from 1½" to 4¾" if your hands are weak or affected by arthritis. It is designed with interior folds that fit over objects, including knobs, while you twist the handle. Cost is about $11 and up from self-help firms. **Sources**: 5, 120, 252, 368.

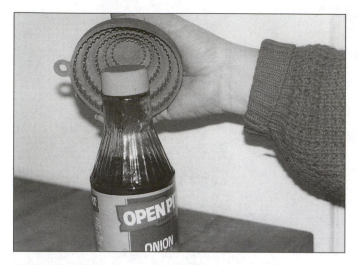

Figure 27-8. This Capscrew helps open tops with diameters from 1½″ to 4¾″ if your hands are weak or affected by arthritis. (Photo courtesy of the O.T. Dept., Howard A. Rusk Institute of Rehabilitation Medicine.)

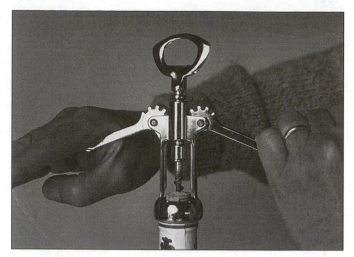

Figure 27-10. This winged cork screw is a good stand-by for use with two hands. After unit is screwed into cork, push down on both wings to raise cork. (Photo courtesy of the O.T. Dept., Howard A. Rusk Institute of Rehabilitation Medicine.)

Pump tops for condiments like mustard, ketchup, and smooth, pourable salad dressings eliminate the need to remove a cap before serving or to shake out contents (Figure 27-9). Pumps are removable and dishwasher safe. **Manufacturers** include 154. Cost is about $1.25 each and up from housewares stores.

If you don't have someone else around to do the honors of opening wine, a winged corkscrew is a good stand-by for use with two hands (Figure 27-10). After unit is screwed into cork, push down on both wings to raise cork. **Manufacturers:** 181, 201, 289. Cost is about $5 and up from department stores and mail-order firms.

A second kind of corkscrew has a shield that slips over the top of the bottle to align it with the opener. You may stabilize the bottle in a drawer or between your knees, if necessary, and turn the large handle with one hand. Cost is about $25 from wine stores and mail-order firms. **Source:** 369.

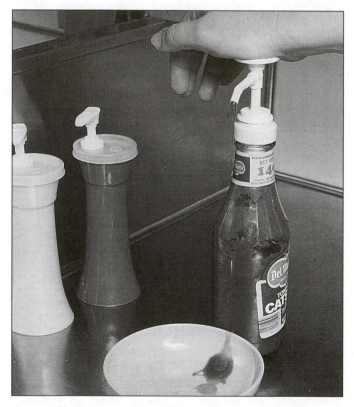

Figure 27-9. Pump tops for condiments like mustard, ketchup, and smooth, pourable salad dressings eliminate the need to remove a cap before serving or to shake out contents. (Photo courtesy of the O.T. Dept., Howard A. Rusk Institute of Rehabilitation Medicine.)

Some spice and food containers open more easily with a pill cap opener. The device is placed on top of the bottle, and upward pressure is exerted to release the cap. The opposite end works as a lever on twist-top bottles, while a wedge slips between the cap and lip for lift-tops. Cost is about $1 and up from pharmacies and mail-order firms. **Sources:** 5, 15, 120, 252, 264, 290, 408.

BOXES AND PAPER CONTAINERS

If you have weakness in your fingers or must avoid stress on finger joints because of arthritis, use a knife with a serrated blade to open boxes (Figure 27-11). Place the box on its side, stabilized by a damp sponge cloth if necessary. Cut around three sides. If you have loss of grasp in both hands, choose a knife with a small handle that slips into the pocket of an elastic cuff (see Chapter 2).

A lightweight, plastic box opener has a sharp protected blade. Some models come with a ribbed or built-up rubber-coated handle for more secure grasp (Figure 27-12). Cost is about $2.50 and up from self-help firms. **Sources:** 5, 15, 120, 252, 264, 290, 408.

Designed for cutting linoleum, a knife with a curved blade also works well for opening boxes. The sharp hooked blade of carbon steel cuts through cardboard while the large handle has a built-up grip. **Manufacturer** of both the knife and the box opener: 376. Cost is about $4 and up from hardware stores.

Some paper cartons for juice now come with screw-type spouts that open with one hand (Figure 27-13). Use pliers to open the safety seal underneath the cap.

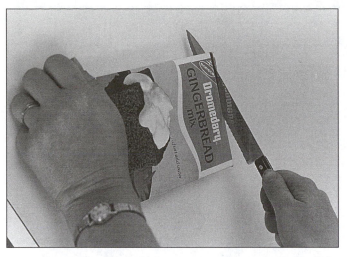

Figure 27-11. If you have weakness in your fingers or must avoid stress on finger joints because of arthritis, use a knife with a serrated blade to open boxes. (Photo courtesy of the O.T. Dept., Howard A. Rusk Institute of Rehabilitation Medicine.)

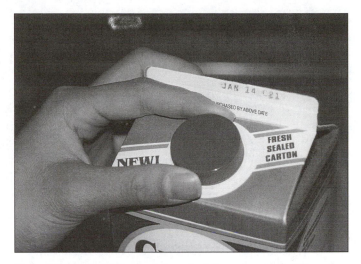

Figure 27-13. Some paper cartons for juice now come with screw-type spouts that open with one hand. (Photo by J.K.)

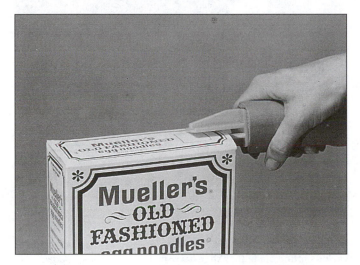

Figure 27-12. A lightweight, plastic box opener has a sharp protected blade. (Photo courtesy of AliMed®, Inc., Dedham, MA.)

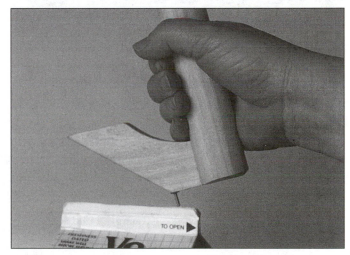

Figure 27-14. This milk/juice carton opener is designed for use if your hands are weak or affected by arthritis. (Photo by J.K.)

A milk/juice carton opener is designed for use if your hands are weak or affected by arthritis (Figure 27-14). The metal device breaks the "V" seal, then opens the top seal with a stainless-steel prong. The built-up wooden handle may be used with one or two hands. Cost is about $14 from self-help firms. **Sources:** 5, 252, 264, 368.

Refrigerated dough provides quick toppings or bases for casseroles, pizzas, and fruit desserts. To make opening the container easier if you are working with one hand or have weak grasp, stabilize the package in a corner or wedge it between two heavier objects to prevent rolling. Then pull off the outer wrapping with your fingers or a pair of pliers. Light pressure with a spoon will release the seal so the package partially opens. Then bend back the container to expose all the dough. A damp sponge cloth helps keep the can from rolling.

PLASTIC BAGS AND POUCHES

If weak grasp makes it difficult to hold a knife with one hand, try both hands for greater stability. Choose a utility knife with a sharp point and a scalloped or serrated blade to pierce and cut open a plastic pouch. A damp sponge cloth keeps the plastic bag from sliding.

Scissors with contoured handles or the Swedish loop-handled scissors make opening cellophane or plastic bagged foods easier (Figures 27-15A and 27-15B). **Manufacturers** of contoured scissors include 137 (illustrated), 182. Spring-loop scissors are **manufactured** by 122. Cost is about $10 and up from housewares stores, self-help firms, and sewing suppliers. **Sources:** 122, 187, 252, 264. Also see scissors in Chapter 21.

Try out shears before purchasing them. The sharpness of the blade reduces the effort required to cut (Figure 27-16). A smaller handle may also fit your hand better. **Manufacturer:** 201. Cost is about $15 from housewares departments and mail-order firms. **Sources:** 65, 427.

A plastic bag opener mounts on the wall or under your counter (Figure 27-17). To open a paper or plastic bag, you slide it through a slot concealing a razor blade. Fingers do not touch the recessed blade. Cost is about $4 from self-help firms. **Sources:** 5, 120.

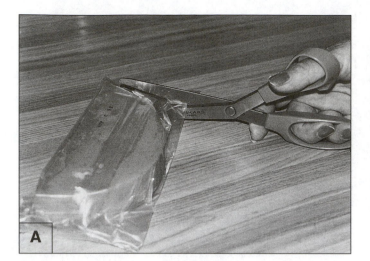

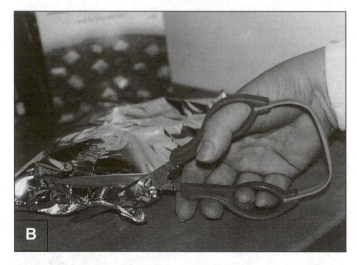

Figure 27-15A. Scissors by Fiskars, Inc. Figure 27-15B. Scissors by Etac USA, Waukesha, WI. (Photos by J.K.)

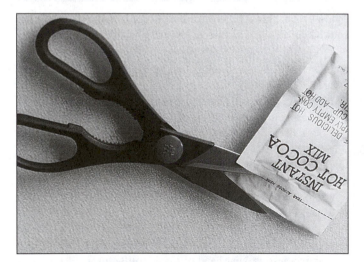

Figure 27-16. The sharpness of the blade, as on these kitchen shears, reduces the effort required to cut. (Shears from J.A. Henckels Zwilling, Inc., Hawthorne, NY. Photo by J.K.)

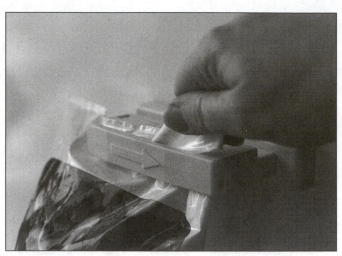

Figure 27-17. To open a paper or plastic bag, you slide it through a slot concealing a razor blade. (Photo by J.K.)

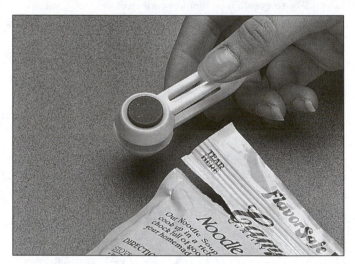

Figure 27-18. This portable, plastic or foil bag opener has a concealed cutting blade that slices across the top of the package. (Photo courtesy of North Coast Medical, Inc., San Jose, CA.)

A portable plastic or foil bag opener also has a concealed cutting blade that slices across the top of the package (Figure 27-18). Cost is about $3 each from housewares stores and self-help firms. **Source:** 290.

If you have difficulty handling plastic tags on bread, try a Twix-It® (see Chapter 15), a spring-type clothespin, or bread clip. A set of two bread clips is about $1 from housewares stores.

To open a heated, immersible pouch of food with one or two hands, place the pouch in a shallow serving dish and cut across the top with a pair of kitchen shears, regular scissors, or a knife. If you have loss of grasp in both hands, put a thumb or fingers from each hand in both of the scissors handle holes to control the blades.

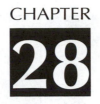

Handling Ingredients

MEASURING

There are two kinds of cooks in this world: those who carefully measure everything and those who make approximations. The latter use the palm of one hand to figure out how much seasoning is needed or judge an onion to be ½ cup size. But when trying a new recipe, even the most experienced cook uses measuring aids. For more information on measuring, see also Chapter 9.

Long-handled measuring cups are easiest to manage with weak hands or incoordination (Figure 28-1). If you are lacking grasp, the long handle may be manipulated with both hands. **Manufacturers:** 33, 112, 142, 181, 273, 289, 321. Cost is about $8 and up for a set of metal cups, and $3 for a set of plastic cups, from housewares stores and mail-order firms. **Sources:** 65, 71, 196, 231, 256, 364, 410.

When measuring and pouring liquids from one container to another, keep the containers as close to each other as possible (Figure 28-2).

If you use only one hand or have poor coordination, it helps to place the measuring spoon or cup flat on the counter while you fill it. Long handled, flat-bottomed measuring spoons are more stable and easier to pick up than rounded ones. See Chapter 9.

If you have incoordination or use of just one hand, try bent measuring spoons (Figure 28-3). Gently bend the handles of aluminum measuring spoons until the bowls are at right angles to the handles. The spoons will still nest for storage. **Manufacturers:** 112, 142, 289, 321. Cost is about $1.50 per set from housewares stores and mail-order firms. **Sources:** 196, 231.

Dispensers for sugar, instant coffee, or iced tea release one teaspoon at a time. **Manufacturer:** 154. Cost is about $2 each and up from housewares stores and self-help and mail-order firms. **Sources:** 196, 231.

The lid of a plastic pasta dispenser may be adjusted to measure long pasta goods (like spaghetti) for one, two, or three portions (Figure 28-4). **Manufacturer:** 343. Cost is about $4 from housewares stores and mail-order firms. Another pasta measurer is a disk with different sized circumference holes designating the amount of pasta needed for that number of servings. **Manufacturer:** 107. Cost is about $2 from housewares stores.

CUTTING AND SLICING

TIPS FOR CUTTING

- Select a knife and work surface that make cutting foods easier, especially if you have weakness or incoordination in your hands and upper extremities.
- Place your cutting board at a comfortable height to increase efficiency and permit greater control.
- Use an angled knife to keep your wrist straight for greater power while cutting and slicing.
- Select a textured cutting surface to prevent slipping of food.

Care and choosing of knives and scissors or shears is discussed in Chapter 21. Adapted cutting boards are shown in Chapter 1.

CUTTING BOARDS

An adapted cutting board can be designed for use if you have poor grasp, incoordination, or the use of only one hand (Figure 28-5). Suction-cup feet on the 10½" x 12" Swedish cutting board provide stability. The polyethylene surface is easy to clean; stainless-steel nails anchor food to be cut. A sliding clamping device adjusts to securely hold jars, cans, or boxes to be opened, secures food (like a loaf of bread) to be sliced, and braces bowls while food is mixed or stirred. The board is dishwasher safe. **Manufacturer:** 122. Cost is about $55 and up from self-help firms. **Sources:** 120, 122, 252, 264, 290, 370, 408.

Note: Plastic and wood boards should be scrubbed after each use, between cutting vegetables or fruits and meat, and washed frequently with bleach and water to kill bacteria. One company now manufactures a board with an antibacterial finish. **Manufacturer:** 213.

You may make an adapted board at home. Use a standard cutting board and two stainless-steel or aluminum nails. Drill two holes, slightly smaller than the diameter of the nails to be insert-

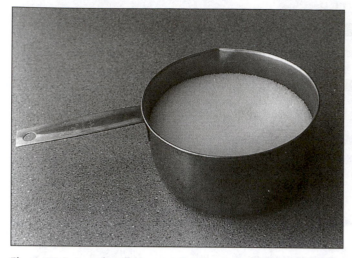

Figure 28-1. Long-handled measuring cups are easiest to manage with weak hands or incoordination. (Measuring cups by Mirro®/Foley, Manitowoc, WI. Photo by J.K.)

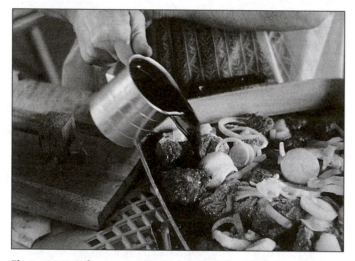

Figure 28-2. When measuring and pouring liquids from one container to another, keep the containers as close to each other as possible. (Photo by J.K.)

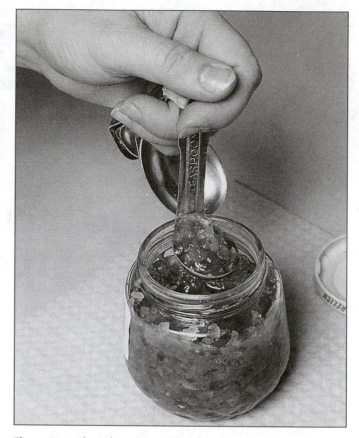

Figure 28-3. If you have incoordination or use of just one hand, try bent measuring spoons. (Photo courtesy of the O.T. Dept., Howard A. Rusk Institute of Rehabilitation Medicine.)

ed, about 1¼" apart. Support the board upside-down so the nail points will not be dulled; hammer them gently into place. **Manufacturers/distributors** of wood and polyethylene boards include 9, 33, 126, 142, 162, 181, 207, 289, 321. These include paddle boards, which are easier to pick up with one hand.

Four rubber tips or suction cups under a board keep it from sliding. For safety when not using the board, cover the nails with a cork or foam block. A raised plastic guard holds bread or a sandwich in place for spreading; a corner slit in the guard lets you cut the sandwich in half. Kits of hardware for making an adapted board cost about $10. **Source:** 393.

If picking up cut foods is difficult, try an elevated cutting board (Figure 28-6). With the extra clearance of 2" to 3", a bowl or plate easily slides underneath the board, so all you have to do is push the food off the board into the container. **Manufacturer:** 207. Cost is about $15 and up from gourmet specialty and mail-order firms.

An acrylic cutting board is easy to clean and does not retain food odors (Figure 28-7). Some boards have rounded edges to fit over your countertop edge, protecting the counter from scratches. Acrylic boards are available with textured or plain surfaces; some come with rubber feet in each corner to stabilize the board while in use. **Manufacturer:** 33. Cost is about $15 and up from housewares stores and mail-order firms. **Sources:** 71, 231, 242, 270, 364, 407, 415.

An over-the-sink board is another cutting surface option. Available in wood or polyethylene, it fits over the sink, creating a lowered working height, which reduces lifting when doing food preparation. Adjustable arms fit sinks up to 20" wide. Over-the-sink boards come with or without a built-in strainer so foods drain into sink. **Manufacturers:** 112, 207. Cost is about $13 and up from housewares stores, self-help, and mail-order firms. **Sources:** 71, 231, 242, 427.

If you have incoordination or limited vision, a funnel cutting board with a narrowed end can help you transfer cut food with greater ease (Figure 28-7). **Manufacturer:** 142. Cost is about $10 and up from self-help and mail-order firms. **Sources:** 196, 240. A similar solution is a flexible cutting board, which you pick up with all the cut-up food on it and bend to slide the foods into a pan or serving dish. **Manufacturers/Distributors:** 216, 289. Cost is about $3 from housewares stores and mail-order firms. **Sources:** 240, 270, 378.

SLICING AIDS

A molded plastic cutting center adjusts to make slices of vari-

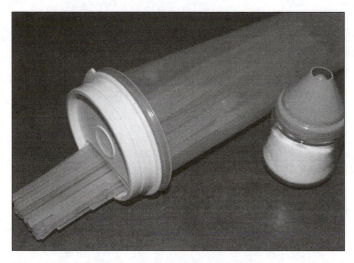

Figure 28-4. The lid of this plastic pasta dispenser may be adjusted to measure long pasta goods (like spaghetti). (Photo by J.K.)

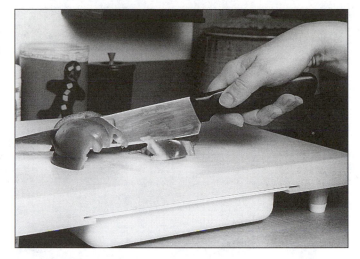

Figure 28-6. If picking up cut foods is difficult, try an elevated cutting board. (Photo courtesy of the O.T. Dept., Howard A. Rusk Institute of Rehabilitation Medicine.)

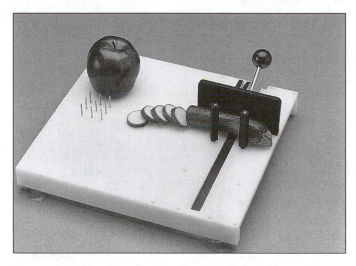

Figure 28-5. This adapted cutting board is designed for use if you have poor grasp, incoordination, or the use of only one hand. (Photo courtesy of North Coast Medical, Inc., San Jose, CA.)

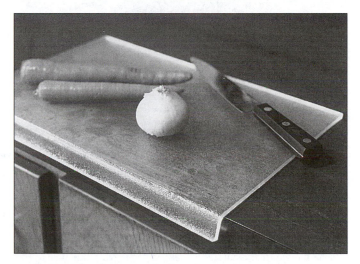

Figure 28-7. An acrylic cutting board is easy to clean and does not retain food odors. (Photo by J.K.)

ous thicknesses (Figure 28-8). If you have incoordination, weakness, or limited vision, the pair of vertical knife slots are positioned to direct the knife to make slices of even thickness. This one is shown with a 13½" polypropylene open-handled knife with a stainless-steel blade. The knife is designed to evenly distribute pressure on your hand, which is especially important if you have weak grasp. Both board and knife are dishwasher safe. **Manufacturer:** 122. Cost is about $20 and up for the cutting aid, $40 and up for the center and knife. **Sources:** 16, 120, 122, 247, 252, 264, 370, 408.

A foldable bread slicer allows you to slice a whole loaf in even thicknesses (Figure 28-9). Available in wood or polyethylene, it may be used with any bread knife. **Manufacturer:** 162. Cost is about $14 and up from housewares stores and mail-order firms. **Sources** for this and similar holders: 71, 173, 231, 270, 364, 387.

Serious cuts from slicing bagels have joined the list of most common kitchen accidents (Figure 28-10). Avoid this mishap with a bagel slicer. The device holds bagels or English muffins vertical

while you guide a serrated knife down through the slot. Some holders have three slots to cut thinner slices for making bagel chips; others are designed to cut rolls as well. **Manufacturers:** 10, 74, 142, 162. Cost in wood or acrylic is about $5 from housewares stores and mail-order firms. **Sources:** 59, 65, 71, 231, 245, 270, 364, 410, 427.

Slicing soft-skinned fruits and vegetables (like tomatoes) is easier with a tong holder if you have visual limitations or incoordination (Figure 28-11). Use the holder in a horizontal position on the cutting surface. The tong end cups the food to prevent it from being squashed. The tines of the holder are spaced to make slices of even thickness. To slice, insert the knife blade between the tines. **Manufacturers:** 142, 289. Cost is about $7 and up from housewares stores and mail-order firms. **Sources:** 59, 71, 171, 173, 270, 364, 407, 410.

A roast holder tong, larger than the vegetable one, stabilizes a cooked piece of meat for carving. It is used in a vertical position. Insert the knife point between the tines for uniform slices.

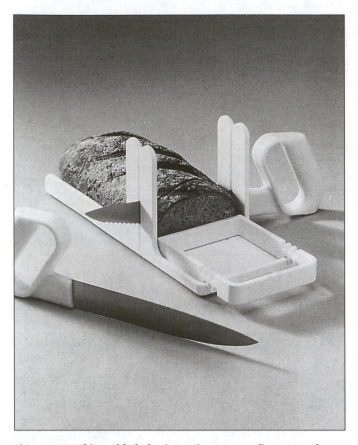

Figure 28-8. This molded plastic cutting center adjusts to make slices of various thicknesses. (Photo courtesy of North Coast Medical, San Jose, CA.)

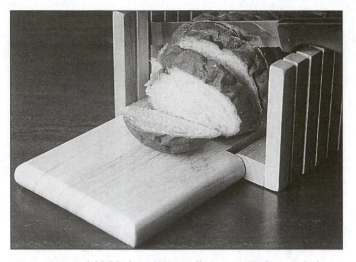

Figure 28-9. A foldable bread slicer allows you to slice a whole loaf in even thicknesses. (Slicer by Great Lakes Designs, Cleveland, OH. Photo by J.K.)

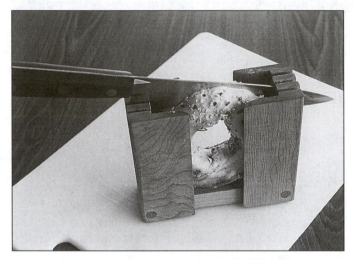

Figure 28-10. The device holds bagels or English muffins vertical while you guide a serrated knife down through the slot. (Bagel slicer by Concept Design, Inc., Saco, ME. Photo by J.K.)

Available in aluminum or stainless steel, the tongs accommodate roasts up to 12" in diameter and may also be used for bread. **Manufacturer:** 289. Cost is about $10 and up from gourmet stores and mail-order firms. **Sources:** 59, 196, 252, 264, 370, 408.

The handle of this angled cheese slicer is perpendicular to the cutting surface, so your wrist stays straight for stronger grip and better joint protection while slicing (Figure 28-12). Unit is dishwasher safe. **Manufacturer:** 122. Cost is about $13 and up from self-help firms. **Sources**: 120, 122, 252, 264, 370, 408.

Use versatile kitchen utensils to reduce or simplify work (Figure 28-13). An egg slicer may also be used to cut tofu, mushrooms, and bananas, or you may use a mushroom slicer. **Manufacturers/distributors:** 9, 142, 289. Cost is about $2 and up from housewares stores and mail-order firms. **Sources:** 270, 283.

CHOPPING AND GRATING

An electric food processor speeds food preparation, such as cutting, slicing, or grating, especially if you have weakness, limited vision, use of one hand, or incoordination. See Chapter 20. In recipes that call for minced or grated foods, you may substitute prepared products like instant minced onions or frozen, chopped onions and green peppers, freeze-dried citrus peel, or parsley flakes for the fresh ingredient.

When a food item is not available in a convenient prepared form (example: shredded carrots for salad), rely on your food processor to make quick work of shredding or dicing. Food processors are ideal for handling large quantities of food, but if you need to prepare small amounts (less than one cup), you may prefer a manual chopper. For more suggestions, refer to Chapter 21.

There are also times when an item is not available in a ready-to-use form or you want the additional flavor of freshly grated or minced food. Nothing rivals fresh lemon peel. Then you need an easy-to-use grater or grinder.

A hand grater with a plastic base has two stainless-steel or three plastic grating and slicing rasps that are graded from fine to coarse (Figure 28-14). The slanted surface is more energy efficient than a vertical surface. On some models, suction feet secure grater to the counter. With others, you may stabilize the grater by putting a damp sponge cloth underneath. **Manufacturer:** 122. Cost is about $15 and up from kitchen/gourmet specialty and housewares stores or self-help firms. **Sources:** 5, 13, 120, 122, 252, 264, 370, 408.

Some folding graters have different grades on each side and a container at the bottom to catch food (Figure 28-15). It folds for

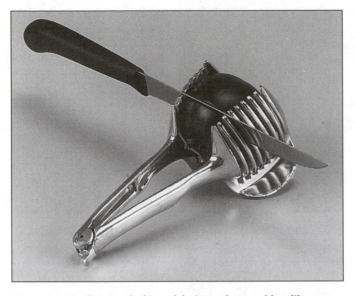

Figure 28-11. Slicing soft-skinned fruits and vegetables (like tomatoes) is easier with a tong holder if you have visual limitations or incoordination. (Photo courtesy of Norpro, Inc., Everett, WA.)

storage and is dishwasher safe. **Manufacturer:** 343. Cost is about $8 from housewares stores.

To operate a manual rotating chopper, you must have adequate hand strength (Figure 28-16). As you depress the handle, the spring-loaded, stainless-steel blades rotate. This implement is handy for small amounts of food, such as hard-cooked eggs, fresh herbs, nuts, and soft vegetables. Look for a chopper that opens completely for cleaning. If you have loss of vision or poor coordination, ask someone to clean the blades for you. Top rack dishwasher safe. **Manufacturers/distributors:** 67, 142, 154, 235, 278, 289. Cost is about $10 from housewares stores and mail-order firms. **Sources:** 71, 152, 283, 364.

MIXING

Mixing bowls with non-slip, rubber ring bases stay stationary while you combine ingredients. Some plastic or Melamine bowls have U.S. standard and metric measure marks. The molded handle is easy to grip; the pouring spout aids in transferring ingredients. Five-cup, seven-cup, and 10-cup bowls nest for storage. Top rack dishwasher safe. **Manufacturers:** 78, 142, 343. Cost is $10 and up per set from housewares stores and mail-order firms. Graduated bowls with rubber ring bases are also available without handles or measurements in 1½-, 2-, and 3-quart capacities. **Sources:** 231, 242, 283, 364, 410, 427. Check instructions before purchasing if you wish to use bowls in a microwave oven.

Use a wire whisk to beat light batters or eggs and to blend ingredients for gravies or soups. If your arms are weak or tire easily, the thin wires of a whisk require less exertion for stirring than a solid utensil, such as a spoon. If your grasp is weak, choose a large-handled whisk or adapt a small-handled whisk by inserting it into a foam curler or piece of foam tubing. If you have almost complete loss of grasp, consider using a Universal Cuff. The small, coiled handle of a whisk will slip into the palmar pocket of the cuff. See Chapter 2. **Manufacturers/distributors** of whisks: 112,

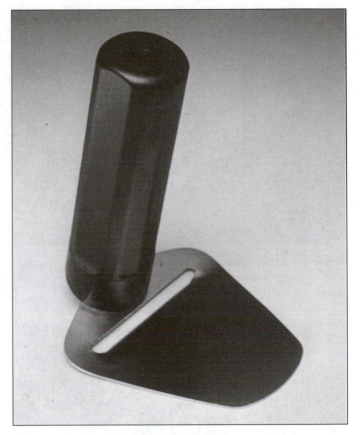

Figure 28-12. The handle of this angled cheese slicer is perpendicular to the cutting surface, so your wrist stays straight for stronger grip and better joint protection while slicing. (Photo courtesy of Etac, USA, Inc., Waukesha, WI.)

142, 289. Cost of whisk is $2 and up from housewares stores and culinary specialty and mail-order firms. **Sources:** 65, 231, 256, 283, 427.

A bowl or pan may be kept from sliding by putting an octopus pad, a Dycem® non-slip mat, or damp sponge cloth under it (Figure 28-17). **Manufacturer:** 104 (Dycem®), 112 (Octopus), 289. **Sources:** 13, 120, 231, 252, 264, 290, 408.

Some bowls have suction disks with levers to secure them to a non-porous surface. A bowl with a suction lever base is about $15 from self-help firms. Suction disk alone is $4 and up. **Sources:** 120, 290, 408.

If your arms are weak or you have poor coordination, it may be easier for you to stir ingredients in a bowl if you sit down and hold the bowl in your lap (Figure 28-18). Another alternative is to sit on a high kitchen chair with the edge of the bowl resting on the countertop edge. A damp sponge cloth between the bowl and counter keeps the bowl from rotating.

You may also try putting the bowl in the sink while mixing. Wedge the bowl in a corner, and stabilize it with a damp sponge cloth. Spatters are confined to the sink. Balance your forearms on the sink edge.

When you bake, consider making muffins or cupcakes. It is easier to remove muffins or cupcakes baked in paper liners from a muffin pan than it is to remove a baked cake from a cake pan. Measure the batter into the prepared muffin pan by using an ice

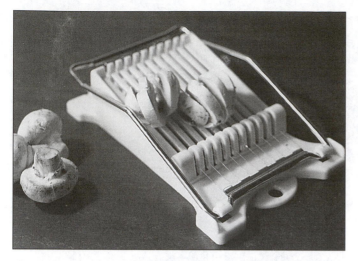

Figure 28-13. Use versatile kitchen utensils to reduce or simplify work. An egg slicer may also be used to cut tofu, mushrooms, and bananas. (Photo by J.K.)

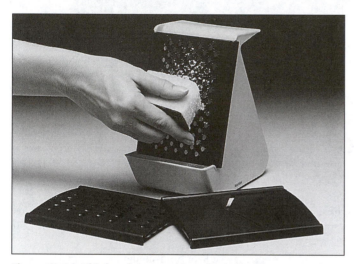

Figure 28-14. This hand grater with a plastic base has two stainless-steel or three plastic grating and slicing rasps that are graded from fine to coarse. (Photo courtesy of the O.T. Dept., Howard A. Rusk Institute of Rehabilitation Medicine.)

cream scoop or a dry measuring cup. To eliminate frosting, sprinkle cinnamon sugar or a streusel topping over batter before baking. If you are cooking for one or two, freeze muffins or cupcakes, then take out as needed. A rubber, spoon-shaped spatula helps scrape out batter more efficiently than a flat spatula. **Manufacturer:** 343. Cost is about $2 each or $6 for a set with one large and one small from housewares stores and kitchen specialty firms. **Sources:** 65, 71, 231, 283, 410, 427.

PREPARING VEGETABLES AND FRUITS

Scrubbing vegetables with one hand is easier to do using a suction-based brush. Two suction cups anchor the brush handle to the sink or countertop so the bristles are upright. You may want two brushes, because one can also be used to help clean flatware and dishes. Cost is about $5 each from self-help firms. **Sources:** 120,

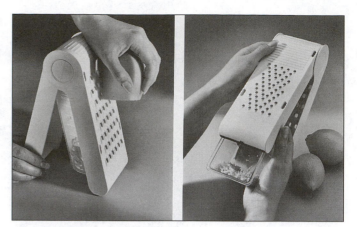

Figure 28-15. This folding grater has different grades on each side and a container at the bottom to catch food. (Photo courtesy of Rubbermaid®, Inc., Wooster, OH.)

290, 368, 408.

Serving vegetables and fruits in their skins is nutritious and saves time and energy. If you want to peel them, here are few tips:

- Always put a paper towel on the working surface before you begin peeling. When done, pick up the towel with the peels.
- If using a board with nails to hold the vegetable, put the towel over the nails.
- Select a peeling device that is comfortable for you to hold, especially if you have arthritis or weakness in your hands.

A loop-handle peeler lets you grasp with less force than is needed for a straight-handled tool (Figure 28-19). The swivel action blade follows the contour of the vegetable. Use it with the right or left hand. **Manufacturers:** 112, 142, 180, 181, 278, 435 (illustrated). Cost is about $1.25 and up from housewares stores and mail-order firms. **Sources:** 120, 231, 247, 283, 290, 427.

The rubber-ribbed handle of a Good Grips® cushioned-grip peeler is easier to hold; dishwasher safe (Figure 28-20). **Manufacturer:** 301. Cost is about $6 for the peeler alone or $10 in a set with a cushioned-grip paring knife, from housewares stores or self-help and mail-order firms. **Sources:** 65, 108, 120, 231, 238, 290, 408, 410.

Tip: When a recipe calls for small whole onions, you may use canned ones. If you like your onions fresh, here's a simple way to peel them. First, stabilize the onion on the cutting board nails, or hold it with one hand. Then carefully cut through the entire outer layer of onion, from top to bottom; peel off the outer layer. If a recipe calls for sliced or diced onion, cut the onion in half, then lay it on its flat side to prevent sliding while you're slicing.

SALAD GREENS

A variety of salad greens adds nutrition and interest to meals. Experiment with lettuce, raw spinach, escarole, arugula, raddichio, chicory, endive, Chinese cabbage, and sprouts. Rinse and drain salad greens using a large plastic colander in the sink. Let them drain until you are ready to use. **Manufacturers** of colanders include 112, 142, 278, 289, 343.

A salad spinner removes excess water from washed salad greens quickly and easily. Put the washed greens in the basket insert. Replace the lid. To operate, you pull a cord, turn a knob,

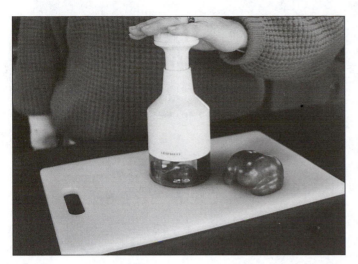

Figure 28-16. This implement is handy for small amounts of food, such as hard-cooked eggs, fresh herbs, nuts, and soft vegetables. (Photo by J.K.)

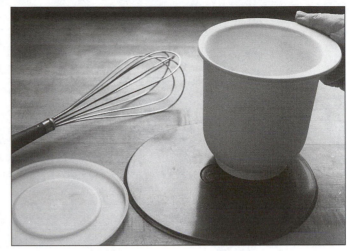

Figure 28-17. A bowl or pan may be kept from sliding by putting an octopus pad, a Dycem® non-slip mat, or damp sponge cloth under it. (Photo by J.K.)

or press a lever on the lid to activate the spinning mechanism. The force of the spin causes the excess water to drain out the bottom. **Manufacturers:** 142, 215, 278. Cost is about $6 and up from housewares stores and mail-order firms. **Sources:** 71, 378, 390, 427.

If dried thoroughly and stored properly, greens washed in advance store well. You may purchase a ready-made, or stitch your own, terrycloth drying/storage bag. **Manufacturer:** 142. Cost is about $4 and up from housewares stores and mail-order firms. **Sources:** 71, 242, 427. To sew your own salad crisper, fold a terrycloth kitchen towel in thirds. Stitch up both sides of two-thirds, leaving the other third as a flap. Shake off the washed greens, place them in cloth bag, and store in refrigerator. Lettuce keeps crisp for several days.

An airtight lettuce crisper keeps greens like cabbage, lettuce, and cauliflower fresh. Remove core from head, then stand on raised trivet for refrigerator storage. Check top before purchase to make sure you can remove it without too much effort.

MOLDED SALADS

Make a gelatin salad in an attractive serving dish so you will not have to transfer it. You might also try individual molds, which are easier to handle than a single large mold.

To make unmolding easier and reduce cleanup, lightly oil molds, and put them on a tray before filling. Pour liquid into molds right next to the refrigerator so you do not have to transport them. If after jelling, the gelatin is stuck in the mold, dip the bottom of the form into a bowl of warm water, and immediately invert it onto the serving plate. Molds in many designs and sizes are sold by housewares stores and mail-order firms. **Manufacturers/distributors:** 112, 142, 404.

PREPARING POULTRY AND MEAT

Removing the skin and fat from poultry is easier and safer when you use a pair of sharp kitchen or poultry shears, rather than a knife.

Stabilize the chicken on a textured cutting surface or between the nails on an adapted cutting board. Cut the skin of each piece from one end to the other, then pull off the skin. Use pliers if you cannot grasp the skin securely. See Chapters 21 and Chapter 24.

Coating meat and chicken with a dry mixture, such as flour or crumbs, is easier if you use a plastic bag. Measure the dry ingredients into the bag, gather the bag to close the opening, and shake it to mix. Add chicken or meat, a few pieces at a time, and shake again to coat. If you work with one hand, use a thicker plastic bag, like those designed for freezer storage, so you can more easily grasp the top without the bottom giving way.

To crush stuffing, crackers, dry bread, or chips, use a rolling pin and two plastic food storage bags or one heavy-duty freezer bag. Place the food to be crushed in the bag; close the opening. Press and roll the rolling pin over the bag until the contents are crushed. A blender or food processor will also produce crumbs for coating mixtures.

PREPARING GROUND MEAT

Ground meat can be made into patties and frozen until you need to prepare a quick meal.

A patty press shapes the meat into patties of a uniform thickness and diameter (Figure 28-21). It is especially helpful if you work with one hand, have severe arthritis, or loss of vision. **Manufacturers/distributors:** 142, 289. Cost is $4 and up from housewares stores and mail-order firms. **Sources:** 173, 270. Put dry waxed paper or "hamburger separators" between patties for easier dividing after freezing. **Manufacturers/distributors:** 142, 289. Cost is about $8 per package of 350 separators from housewares stores and mail-order firms. **Source:** 270.

A multiple patty press features a plastic press and shallow, ring-shaped containers that stack to form and store hamburgers or ground turkey for freezing (Figure 28-22). **Manufacturer/distributor:** 404. Cost is about $9.

For meatloaf, whether you choose to use ground beef, ground

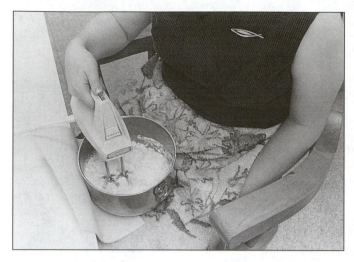

Figure 28-18. If your arms are weak or you have poor coordination, it may be easier for you to stir ingredients in a bowl if you sit down and hold the bowl in your lap.

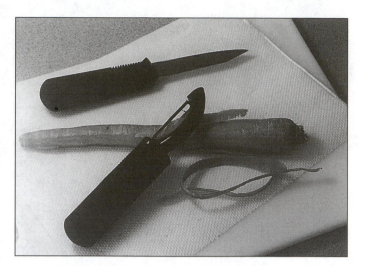

Figure 28-20. The rubber-ribbed handle of a Good Grips® cushioned-grip peeler is easier to hold, and it is dishwasher safe. (Photo by J.K.)

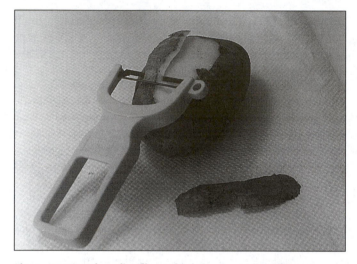

Figure 28-19. A loop-handle peeler lets you grasp with less force than is needed for a straight-handled tool. (Photo by J.K.)

turkey, or a combination of meats, you can use one of several methods for handling the meat: mix the meat and other ingredients with both hands, one hand, or with a fork; or use a standard electric mixer. Mix only until blended or the meat will toughen. (A hand mixer is not recommended, because it is not powerful enough to handle the heavy mixture.) Pack the mixture into a loaf pan, or shape it in a free-form loaf and put in a shallow baking/roasting pan. If you are living alone or with one other person, divide the mixture into two loaves, bake both, then freeze one for later use.

The lift-out tray insert of the low-fat meatloaf pan shown in Figure 28-23 makes it unique. The holes in the tray allow fat to drain while the meatloaf cooks. Handles on opposite ends of the microwave pan model help you lift meatloaf out of the pan. **Manufacturers/distributors:** 61, 142, 289. Cost is $10 and up for plastic or metal pans with or without a non-stick finish from housewares stores and mail-order firms. **Sources:** 65, 71, 173, 256, 270, 283, 378, 415.

Meatballs are easy to make with one or both hands. You may

brown and add them to prepared gravies or soups for a quick, economical meal. You can avoid handling a knife at the table by making them bite-size. Fix them ahead of time, on the stove or baked in the oven, cool, then store in freezer bags for instant use.

If you have strong grasp in one hand, try shaping meatballs with meatball scissors. This utensil resembles an ice cream scoop with "bowls" 1" to 2" in diameter, but operates like scissors. Dip the bowl into the meat mixture; press the looped handles together to form ball; then open them to release the meatball. **Manufacturers/distributors:** 142, 289. Cost is about $2 a pair and up from housewares stores and mail-order firms. **Sources:** 71, 256, 270.

BASTING

A baster safely "spoons" off excess fat when you are cooking meats and poultry. It increases safety by reducing the need to lift and handle hot containers. Try one to dispense sauces or marinades when barbecuing, basting baked fruits and meats, spooning off drippings, watering plants, and even filling a steam iron. **Manufacturers** include 112, 142, 289 (plastic); 289, 434 (metal). Cost of plastic or metal basters is $2 and up from housewares stores and mail-order firms. **Sources:** 231, 270, 283.

BAKING

CAKES

Inverting a cake pan to release the cake requires dexterity and the use of both hands. A layer-cake pan with a removable bottom simplifies cake removal. Let the cake cool, then loosen it around the edges. With one hand, flip the entire cake onto a plate or rack with one hand, and press gently on the bottom to release the outer ring. Once the ring is removed, slip a flat metal spatula between the pan and the cake to release the bottom. **Manufacturers:** 112, 273.

A spring-form pan with a removable bottom is easier to handle,

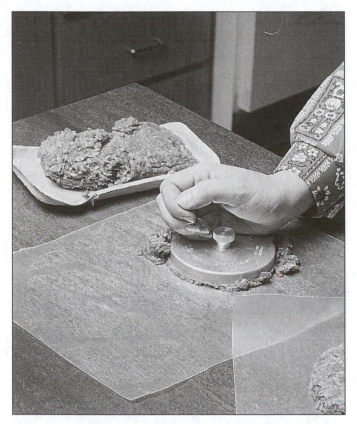

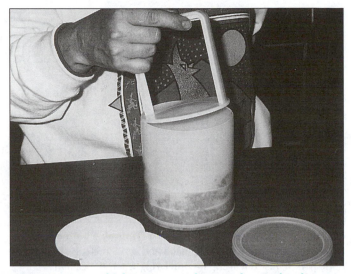

Figure 28-22. A multiple patty press forms and stores hamburgers or ground turkey for freezing. (Patty press by Tupperware®, Orlando, FL. Photo by J.K.)

Figure 28-21. A patty press shapes meat into patties of a uniform thickness and diameter. (Photo courtesy of the O.T. Dept., Howard A. Rusk Institute of Rehabilitation Medicine.)

because you may bake and serve the cake in the same pan by just releasing the outer ring when the cake has cooled (Figure 28-24). **Manufacturers:** 142, 273, 289. Cost of a spring-form pan with non-stick interior and/or tube and flat inserts is about $8 and up from housewares stores and kitchen specialty firms. **Sources:** 65, 71, 231, 256, 283, 427.

COOKIES

When you select cookie sheets, choose ones with low or angled sides that are easier to grasp. Insulated cookie sheets reduce burning on the bottom of baked goods because there is air space between two layers of metal that form the sheet. **Manufacturer:** 273. Cost is $9 each and up from housewares stores and kitchen specialty firms. **Sources:** 71, 231, 256, 270, 427. Insulated cake pans are also available from the same sources.

A cookie scoop makes quick work of measuring the right amounts of dough for drop cookies, whether working with one or two hands (Figure 28-25). Insert bowl of scoop into dough, then squeeze the handle to release the dough onto cookie sheet. This scoop may also be used to shape meat, melon, or sherbet balls. **Manufacturers:** 142, 289, 321. Cost is $4 and up in metal or plastic from housewares stores and mail-order firms. **Sources:** 231, 256, 270, 283, 364, 415.

PIES

Frozen pastry pie shells, graham cracker, or cookie-crumb ready-prepared crusts, refrigerated pie crust sheets as well as indi-

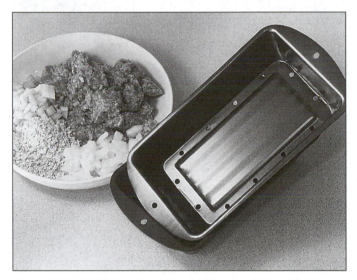

Figure 28-23. The lift-out tray insert of this low-fat meatloaf pan makes it unique. (Photo by J.K.)

vidual crumb or pastry shells are available at your supermarket.

A zippered pie crust maker makes the perfect sized 8" or 9" crust without the sticking or tearing of pastry on pastry cloths. Simply place the dough in the polyethylene bag and roll it out. It is helpful when you are working with one hand, have poor vision, or incoordination. A loop slipped through the zipper tab makes it easier to open or close if your pinch is weak. Cost is about $3 and up for 11" and 14" diameter polyethylene bags from housewares stores and mail-order firms. **Sources:** 59, 270, 415.

If you work with one hand, you can guide a rolling pin by resting your hand on the center. A rolling pin for use with one hand, also called a pizza rolling pin, is carried by gourmet and self-help and mail-order firms. **Manufacturers:** 142, 289. Cost is about $5 and up from housewares and self-help firms. **Sources:** 6, 120, 231, 252, 264, 283, 408.

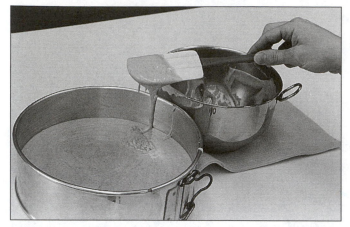

Figure 28-24. A spring-form pan with a removable bottom is easier to handle, because you may bake and serve the cake in the same pan by just releasing the outer ring when the cake has cooled.

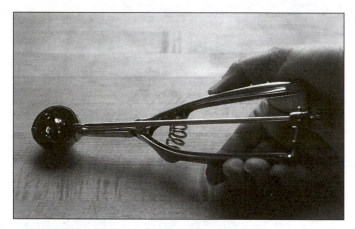

Figure 28-25. A cookie scoop makes quick work of measuring the right amounts of dough for drop cookies, whether working with one or two hands. (Photo by J.K.)

EGGS

TIPS FOR BREAKING EGGS

With weak hands, hold the clean, fresh uncracked egg about 12" above an empty bowl. Then, drop the egg so it falls on its side into the center of the bowl. The shell will crack into two parts. Remove the eggshell by catching it on your thumb.

With one hand, hit the egg sharply against the edge of the bowl. Then use your thumb and index finger to push the top half of the shell up, while your ring and little finger hold the lower half down.

Another way is to place the egg in a ½ cup measure, hit it with the heel of your hand, then lift out the shell with a fork.

A one-handed beater quickly whips up eggs and liquids (Figure 28-26). Press down on the handle. The spring action reverses blades as you release pressure. The base fits in a cup or small bowl and washes easily by hand. Top-rack dishwasher safe. **Manufacturer:** 278, 289. Cost is $6 and up from housewares stores and self-help firms. **Sources:** 71, 120, 408.

To separate eggs for a recipe or because you wish to reduce your cholesterol intake, use a funnel or an egg separator. The white

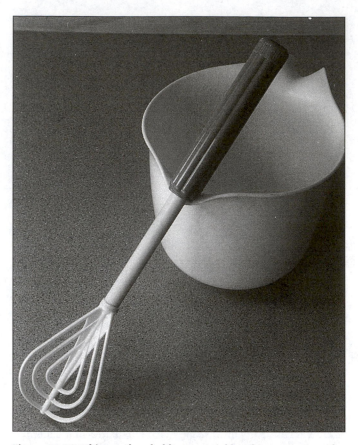

Figure 28-26. This one-handed beater quickly whips up eggs and liquids. (Photo by J.K.)

slips out through a slot while the yolk remains in the separator. **Manufacturers:** 112, 142, 273. Cost is about $1 and up for an egg separator from housewares stores and mail-order firms. A more elaborate egg separator for doing up to 10 eggs at a time is available by mail-order for about $16. You crack open the shell and drop the entire contents down the shoot. Whites go into outer bowl while yolks remain in inner chamber. **Source:** 71.

If you wish to reduce cholesterol intake, consider using egg substitutes. Made with the egg whites but not the yolks, they have less fat than whole eggs and no cholesterol. Egg substitutes may be used for omelets and scrambled eggs, or in baked goods, sauces, casseroles, and puddings. Because they are pasteurized, substitutes are safe in mayonnaise and eggnog. They are not recommended as a substitute for whole eggs in popovers or choux paste dough (cream puffs), as their leavening power is not good. Check package directions before using an egg substitute. Egg substitutes are available in the frozen and refrigerated foods section of your supermarket. Look for both plain and flavored versions.

You may also reduce the fat and cholesterol in your recipes by using two egg whites for each large egg required. If you miss the color, use two egg whites plus one whole egg in place of two whole eggs in recipes.

BOILING AND POACHING

Removing eggs from boiling water is easier and safer if you use tongs. Look for a pair with a curved surface that grasps egg securely. Let the water cool before emptying pan.

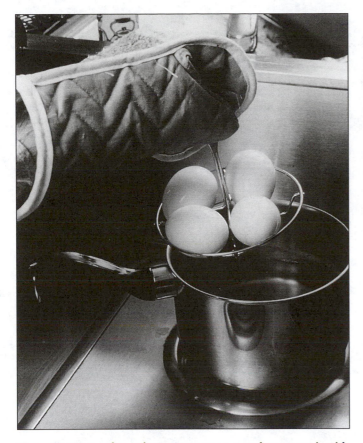

Figure 28-27. Another safe way to remove eggs from a pan is with an egg holder. (Photo courtesy of the O.T. Dept., Howard A. Rusk Institute of Rehabilitation Medicine.)

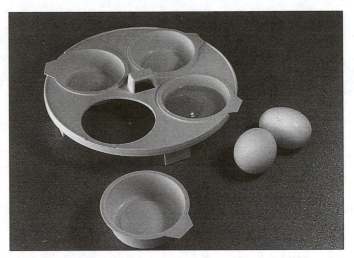

Figure 28-28. Egg poachers are available for range top and microwave cooking. (Photo by J.K.)

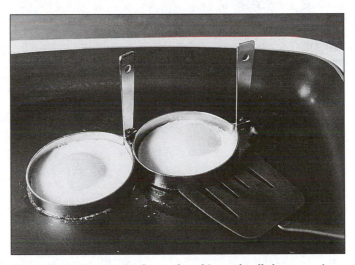

Figure 28-29. An egg ring keeps the white and yolk from running and is especially helpful if you have poor coordination or loss of vision. (Photo by J.K.)

Another safe way to remove eggs from a pan is with an egg holder (Figure 28-27). Cost is about $3 and up from housewares stores.

When removing cooked eggs from the shell is difficult because of incoordination or limited use of your hands, try coddling or poaching them. An egg coddler cooks the broken egg in a covered small cup immersed in hot water. **Manufacturer:** 142. Cost is about $4 and up from housewares stores.

Egg poachers are available for range top and microwave cooking (Figure 28-28). A microwave poacher cooks eggs in 45 seconds to 2 minutes. The non-stick surface lets eggs slide out easily. Dishwasher safe. **Manufacturers:** 112 (stove-top poacher), 121 (microwave poacher), 142 (stove-top), 273, 278 (non-stick range-top poacher). Cost is about $4 and up from housewares stores and mail-order firms. **Sources:** microwave poachers—173, 387, 415; range-top poachers—71, 290, 364, 378, 415.

An egg ring keeps the white and yolk from running and is especially helpful if you have poor coordination or loss of vision (Figure 28-29). Slip the spatula under the egg and ring before you flip or remove the egg from the pan. **Manufacturer:** 142, 321. Cost is about $1 each and up from mail-order firms and housewares stores.

SEASONINGS

Enhance the flavors of foods with fresh herbs. Many varieties are available by the bunch or in airtight bags in the produce section of large supermarkets. Local garden nurseries and some supermarkets sell potted herb plants to keep on your kitchen windowsill or back deck for quick harvesting. Herbs are also available through mail-order firms. **Source:** 367.

If you are on a low-salt or weight-control diet, herbs add spice to eating. The varieties carried by local grocers and nurseries usually include thyme, dill, basil, rosemary, parsley, and chives. An herb and spice chart will help you increase use of flavorings.

Several devices make it easier to handle fresh garlic. A garlic peeler, the "e-z-rol," releases peel when you place cloves in a flexible rubber tube and roll it back and forth under your hand (Figure 28-30A). Unit is dishwasher safe. **Manufacturer:** 293B. Cost is about $6 from housewares stores and gourmet kitchen firms. **Sources:** 65, 231.

The Garlic Machine lets you press fresh garlic, even if your hands are weak (Figure 28-30B). Place peeled garlic cloves into the clear cylinder, and twist the T-handle until the desired amount of minced garlic is released through the perforated base. An air-

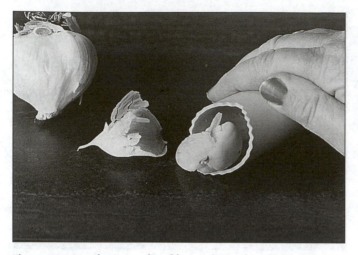

Figure 28-30A. The "e-z-rol" rubber garlic peeler quickly releases the covering of fresh garlic cloves when it is rolled on a hard surface with downward pressure. (Peeler by The Omessi Group Ltd., Northridge, CA. Photo by J.K.)

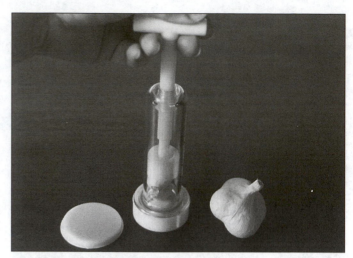

Figure 28-30B. The Garlic Machine lets you press fresh garlic, even if your hands are weak. (Garlic machine from Chef 'n Corp., Seattle, WA. Photo by J.K.)

tight cover stores peeled garlic in the refrigerator. It disassembles for cleaning. **Manufacturer:** 64. Cost is about $13 and up from kitchen and gourmet firms.

If you find it difficult to operate a standard pepper mill, try a manual squeeze or electric pepper mill. Cost is about $16 from gourmet stores and mail-order firms. **Sources:** 65, 290.

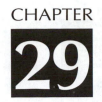

Cooking Techniques

RANGE-TOP COOKING

When selecting a pan for range-top cooking, consider these factors:

- Handles should be heat proof and firmly attached. Look for handles that extend far enough from the pan that you can securely grasp them with or without a pot holder.
- Weight should be comfortable for you to manage with safety and ease.
- Depth should be appropriate for the kind of cooking you are doing. Deep pans reduce spilling but are often heavier and make it harder to turn or handle food.
- Non-stick finishes clean easily. To prevent scratching the coatings, use plastic or wooden utensils, and follow instructions for washing.

A splatter shield is a three-piece, hinged, aluminum shield that you place on the range top to surround a pan (Figure 29-1). It deflects splatters and keeps walls clean while food cooks. Parts (each 10¼" x 9") separate for easy cleaning and storage. Dishwasher safe. Cost is $5 and up from housewares stores and mail-order firms. **Sources:** 71, 173, 270, 415.

A splatter screen fits over 9" to 11" saucepans and skillets to catch grease, yet allows air to circulate (Figure 29-2). The mesh shields you from fat coming in direct contact with your face, arms, and body, especially if you sit or work close to the range. If you have marked loss of vision, poor coordination, or move slowly, a splatter screen is an essential safety aid. Placed over a pan, it can also be used as a bread or roll warmer. Dishwasher safe. **Manufacturers:** 142, 278, 287. Cost is about $3 each and up from housewares stores and mail-order firms. **Sources:** 270, 378, 415.

The sloped sides of a sauté skillet let you easily stir ingredients or slide a spatula under the food (Figure 29-3). Skillets come with and without non-stick finishes. **Manufacturers:** 18, 84, 131, 273, 287, 329, 351, 391. Cost is about $10 and up from housewares stores and kitchen specialty firms. **Sources:** 65, 71, 231, 283, 427.

If you have incoordination, weakness, or arthritis in your arms and hands, a two-handled pan or a pan with an assist handle gives you more control when lifting (Figure 29-4). These pans are designed with heat-proof handles on both sides for easier lifting and durable, non-stick finishes.

A stir-fry pan makes quick work of cooking main dishes or vegetables. Deep, sloped sides allow you to stir food without spilling. Select one with a wood or heat-proof handle that stays cool and a non-stick surface that cleans easily. If you have weakness in your arms, look for a stir-fry pan with an assist handle. **Manufacturers:** 18, 142, 213, 273, 287, 351. Cost is about $10 and up from housewares stores and kitchen specialty firms. **Sources:** 71, 231, 283, 359, 364, 427.

If weakness is a major problem, you may distribute the effort of lifting with a unit like the panhandler or grip stick (Figure 29-5). It lets you pick up a pan with one hand if you have full strength in that arm or distribute the weight of the filled pan between both arms. The clamping device closes automatically onto the side of a saucepan, but it can also be used for baking tins, casseroles, pie pans, or mixing bowls. Do not use the grip stick if you have marked incoordination, because changes in pressure on the handle might allow the pan to slip. Cost is about $7 and up. **Sources:** 71, 173.

To stabilize a pan while stirring with one hand or with poor coordination, keep a filled teakettle on the back burner (Figure 29-6). Turn the handle of the pan until it rests against the tea kettle. Stir, rotating toward the kettle.

If working with one hand or if you have loss of coordination or vision, a pan holder is designed to keep the pot stationary on the range top (Figure 29-7). Three suction cups attach the steel frame to the range-top surface. Two vertical rods keep pans from turning. This aid comes in folding and non-folding models. Cost is about $13 from self-help firms. **Sources:** 5, 13, 120, 290, 370, 408.

Skillets and spatulas with rubber-coated handles provide a more secure grip. **Manufacturers:** 273, 301.

A square flat griddle lets you slip a spatula under the food more easily if you have limited motion or marked weakness. Non-

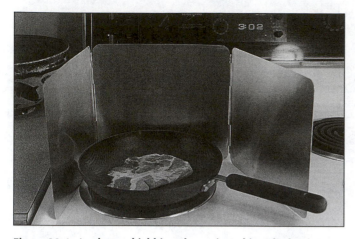

Figure 29-1. A splatter shield is a three-piece, hinged, aluminum shield that you place on the range top to surround a pan. (Photo by J.K.)

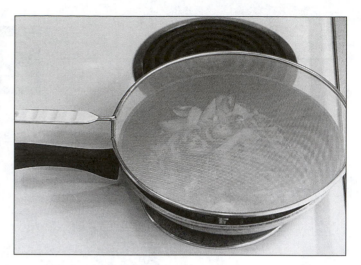

Figure 29-2. A splatter screen fits over 9″ to 11″ saucepans and skillets to catch grease, yet allows air to circulate. (Photo by J.K.)

stick surfaces clean without scrubbing. **Manufacturers/distributors:** 273, 287, 400. Cost is about $15 and up from housewares stores and mail-order firms. **Sources:** 65, 231, 283. If you have marked incoordination but no loss of strength and want a heavy flat pan for stability, look for a cast-iron, flat skillet. **Manufacturer:** 63.

A safety spoon clips to the side of the pan so it does not slide down but is ready for you to grab. The handle is heat-resistant. Cost is about $1.50 from mail-order firms specializing in products for people with loss of vision. **Sources:** 240, 261.

If lifting a pan or casserole is difficult, you might try a kitchen roll-about—an elevated wooden platform with wheels and a handle. Slide the pan or casserole dish onto the platform to move it across the counter or table. Platform surface has a heat-resistant cork pad. Cost is about $20 from self-help firms. **Sources:** 5, 120, 264, 370, 408.

OVEN COOKING

A cradle or adjustable rack placed in a roasting pan holds meat roasts above the pan's surface (Figure 29-8). During roasting, the fat drips down into the pan so there is less fat on the meat when served. When the meat is done, lift the roast off the rack with two large meat forks, or use two pot-holdered hands to transfer the whole rack to a platter. **Manufacturers** of rack or pan with rack: 112, 131, 142, 273, 287. You may purchase a rack alone for about $9 and up. **Sources:** 59, 65, 71, 270, 283, 364, 407.

A stand-up or vertical roaster rack is a metal rod with a base that you place in the roasting pan (Figure 29-9). It allows poultry to cook faster and evenly while juices and fat drip into a catch pan. Slide the unstuffed chicken or Cornish hen onto the rod, going through the body cavity. When the roast is done, you can carve it while it's still on rack or remove it to a platter. Some units are convertible to use for baking potatoes or shish kebabs. Dishwasher safe. The poultry rack is also available in plastic for microwave use. **Manufacturers:** 142, 154, 287, 289. Cost is about $6 and up from housewares stores and mail-order firms. **Sources:** 59, 71, 270, 378.

Hint: When foods are prepared in the oven, let someone else remove the pan when done, or turn off the oven and leave it until cool enough for you to safely handle. For cakes, turn off the oven and pull the cake out onto the oven door to cool for about 10 minutes. Then put it on the counter or slide it on top of a folded newspaper or magazine onto your lap.

A roast sling is placed under the roast in the roasting pan before cooking (Figure 29-10). The chain-link handles extend outward from either side. Wear oven-mitt pot holders to grasp the sling handles when transferring cooked meat from the pan to a carving board or platter. **Manufacturers/distributors:** 142, 289. Cost is about $5 and up from housewares stores. **Source:** 256.

Oven cooking bags permit you to roast meat or poultry in one container, with vegetables if desired, and without basting, Cleanup is minimal, because there is no pan to scrub. Read the directions on the package to adapt your favorite recipe. Remove as much fat and skin as possible. Mix sauce ingredients right in the bag. After cooking, allow the bag to cool at least 5 minutes; open it carefully on the side away from you to avoid the hot steam.

CASSEROLES

Main-dish casseroles help reduce meal preparation time and cleanup. They may be made in advance so that you are free to fix side dishes or to take a rest before mealtime.

If your arms and hands are weak, choose casserole dishes that you can safely and easily manage. Most microwave-safe casserole dishes are constructed of lightweight materials, and some may be used in a conventional oven. Look for casseroles with handles that extend out from the sides for a secure grasp. Paella and oven pancake pans come with extended handles and cost about $17 and up from housewares stores and mail-order firms. **Manufacturers:** 287, 343. **Sources:** 71, 231. You may also transfer a heated casserole into a basket holder with handles for easier carrying.

Individual casseroles are easier to lift than a heavy single pan when hands and arms are weak (Figure 29-11). The single-serving, glass-ceramic cookware shown is designed for mixing, cooking in a standard or microwave oven, serving, and storing in refrigerator or freezer. The small handle helps you grip the casserole with one

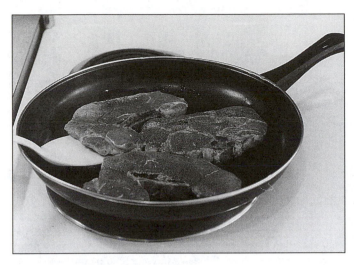

Figure 29-3. The sloped sides of a sauté skillet let you easily stir ingredients or slide a spatula under the food. (Photo by J.K.)

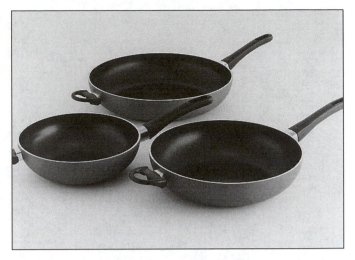

Figure 29-4. If you have incoordination, weakness, or arthritis in your arms and hands, a two-handled pan or a pan with an assist handle gives you more control when lifting. (Photo courtesy of Regal® Ware, Inc., Kewaskum, WI.)

hand and balance it with the other. **Manufacturers:** 28, 79. Cost is about $6 each from housewares stores.

Create variety by adding some of these simple garnishes and toppings to casseroles:

- Grated or sliced low-fat cheeses (parmesan, mozzarella, or cheddar).
- Flavored and unflavored bread crumbs, croutons, or dry prepared stuffing.
- Parsley flakes, dill weed, oregano, or chives.
- Crisp unsugared cereals.
- Refrigerated biscuits.

When a recipe calls for finely crushed crackers or stuffing and it is not an item you can buy ready-to-use, then use your food processor or blender or see Chapter 28 for doing it with a rolling pin.

Scooping up hot baked potatoes from a regular or microwave oven may be difficult, even dangerous, if you have poor vision, weak hands, or incoordination (Figure 29-12). A potato baking rack simplifies the job. Press the raw potatoes onto the rack, then bake them in the oven. Use a long-tined fork to retrieve the holder when the potatoes are done. Available in metal for conventional oven and plastic for microwave use. The handle folds for storage. **Manufacturers:** 112, 181. Cost is about $5 and up from mail-order firms. **Sources:** 231, 270, 378, 415. Making up your own variety of potato toppings creates easy fast-food meals at home. Adding milk or cheese to the toppings creates a balanced main meal without meat.

BROILING

Broiler pans that come with ovens are often heavy and hard to clean. In some ovens, the broiling unit is on the bottom, which requires that you bend and lift to broil. If you work from a wheelchair or use only one hand, you may want to consider alternatives to your oven broiler, such as top of the stove broiling, a portable broiler, or an outdoor grill. For information on countertop ovens

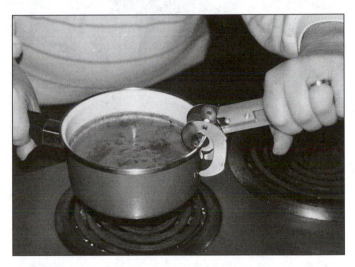

Figure 29-5. If weakness is a major problem, you may distribute the effort of lifting with a unit like the panhandler or grip stick. (Photo by J.K.)

and broilers, see Chapter 20.

If bending is difficult, use long-handled barbecue tools for the broiler. With a long fork, you can turn foods while seated or standing. If lifting is difficult, remove cooked food with tongs, then leave the pan in the broiler until it cools.

A lightweight, non-stick broiling pan may be used with or without the perforated tray insert. Two handles make it easier to manage. If you are working with one hand, look for a small rectangular broiling pan that is easy to grip. **Manufacturers:** 112, 273. Cost of small broiler pans is about $12 and up from housewares stores and mail-order firms. **Sources:** 71, 185, 270, 283, 287, 378, 427.

When using the broiler, here are some safety tips to consider:

- To avoid spills and burns, leave the hot broiler pan in the oven, and transfer the food directly from the pan to the serving platter.
- Aluminum-foil broiling pans are not recommended if you have

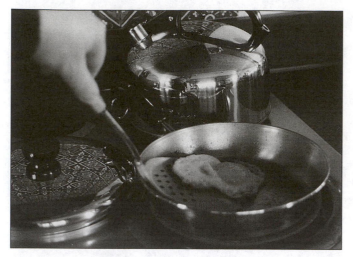

Figure 29-6. To stabilize a pan while stirring with one hand or with poor coordination, keep a filled teakettle on the back burner.

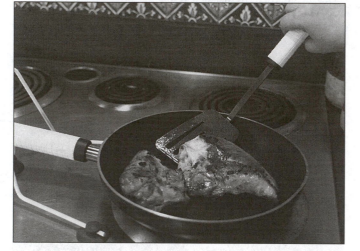

Figure 29-7. If working with one hand or if you have loss of coordination or vision, a pan holder is designed to keep the pot stationary on the range top.

weakness or incoordination, because foil pans tend to bend and require careful handling.

- Ask someone to help you remove a hot pan from the oven, or turn off the oven and wait until the pan cools enough for you to safely handle it.

Hint: To prevent steaks and chops from curling while broiling, trim the fat with a sharp knife or shears. Then slash meat edge every 2 to 3 inches.

An oven push-pull or rack jack allows you to pull the shelf out to a more comfortable angle for lifting (Figure 29-13). The curved notch in the device catches the front lip of the oven rack. If you have weak grasp, slip a dowel through the hole in the handle for a surer grip. **Manufacturers/distributors:** 142, 289. Cost is about $2 from housewares stores.

A hardwood oven paddle, called a pele, extends your reach by 15" (Figure 29-14). Slip the metal or wood tray under a pan or casserole only to slide it toward you, not to support the pan while taking it out of the oven. **Manufacturer:** 142. A similar pizza pad-

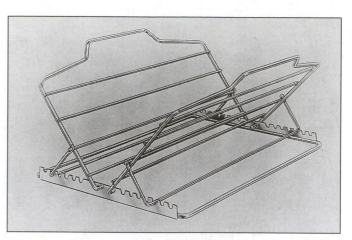

Figure 29-8. A cradle or adjustable rack placed in a roasting pan holds meat roasts above the pan's surface. (Photo courtesy of Mirro/Foley, Manitowoc, WI.)

dle has a wider base but shorter depth and may be used with toaster ovens. **Manufacturer:** 142. Cost of either unit is about $2 and up from housewares stores and mail-order firms.

FROZEN FOODS

To safely remove a frozen dinner from the oven, slide a cookie sheet under it. Be sure the sheet is completely under the dinner so it does not slide off. (Follow package directions. Do not put the cookie sheet under the tray while heating, unless directions state otherwise.)

GRILLING AND BARBECUING

The pleasure of barbecuing can easily be achieved indoors or out. Some range tops come with built-in grill units. If you have loss of vision or marked incoordination, it would be safer to have someone else do the grilling. If you or anyone else in the group has COPD and is using oxygen, stay out of the area where the grilling is being done.

Outdoor grills are available in many styles from hardware and department stores (Figure 29-15). A hibachi grill may be set on a table where you can sit and cook, or you may select a full-size gas or electric grill. **Manufacturers** of grills include 220, 397, 420. **Sources:** 245, 356, 359, 374, 381.

Here are a few tips for selecting a grill:

- Check out the working height and comfort before purchasing. If you are working from a chair or wheelchair, make sure that there is adequate clearance for your feet and foot pedals and that you can reach across the grill without touching the surface.
- Select a grill that you can operate safely without getting too close to the flame.
- Make sure that your legs will be protected from the heat.

Tabletop electric grills permit indoor cooking and come in a variety of styles and prices, from about $25 and up. **Manufacturers** include 131, 166, 260, 391. **Sources:** 71, 167.

Long-handled barbecue tools increase safety and simplify cooking at the grill. **Manufacturers/distributors:** 142, 289. Cost

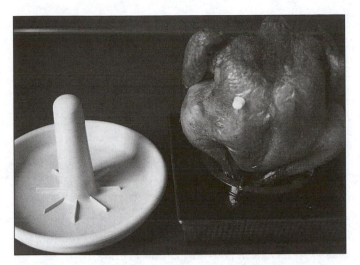

Figure 29-9. A stand-up or vertical roaster rack is a plastic or metal rod with a base that you place in the roasting pan. (Photo by J.K.)

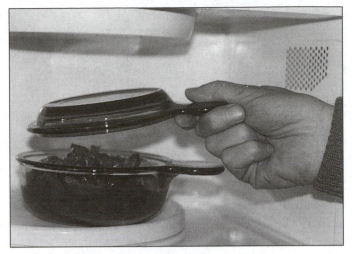

Figure 29-11. Individual casseroles are easier to lift than a heavy single pan when hands and arms are weak. (Visions® Heat 'n Eat dishes. Photo courtesy of Corning® Inc., Corning, NY.)

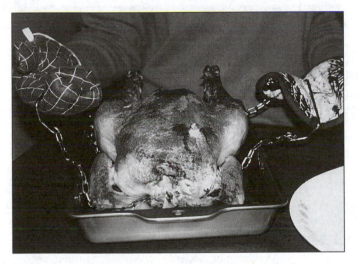

Figure 29-10. A roast sling is placed under the roast in the roasting pan before cooking. (Photo by J.K.)

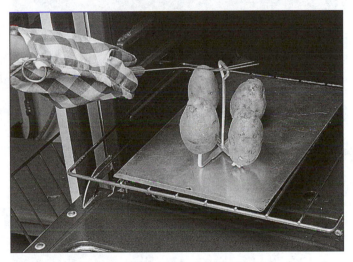

Figure 29-12. A potato baking rack simplifies the job of scooping up hot baked potatoes from a regular or microwave oven. (Photo by J.K.)

is about $5 each and up. **Sources:** 82, 242, 245, 359, 374, 390. You may want to add a storage unit for tools and foods. Cost is about $13 from mail-order firms, or one may come as an optional accessory with a grill unit.f **Manufacturer:** 397.

A grill grid or topper keeps foods like shrimp, vegetables, and kebabs from breaking or falling through the grill rack (Figure 29-16). **Manufacturers** include 142. Cost is about $8 and up for a 10½" x 10¾" size or $10 and up for a 12" x 16" size, from hardware stores and mail-order firms. **Sources:** 65, 82, 169, 242, 245, 270, 364, 427.

Kebabs may be easier to grill than individual pieces. A kebab basket eliminates the need to skewer pieces. Cost is about $8 and up from hardware stores and mail-order firms. **Sources:** 71, 369. Vegetables, fish, and meats may also be wrapped in foil and grilled.

HANDLING HOT LIQUIDS

A heat/flame diffuser, or simmer ring, reduces splatter and helps prevent the bottom of your pan from scorching (Figure 29-

17). It deflects heat coming in contact with your pan, even when melting heat-sensitive foods like chocolate, and is especially helpful if you move slowly or wish to avoid use of a double boiler or carrying of a separate pan of water from the sink to the stove. Place the ring directly over the gas or electric burner, then place the saucepan with contents on the ring to cook as directed. The diffuser, or formed ring, is made of two pieces of perforated sheet metal pressed together, leaving an air pocket between the metal pieces. Select a diffuser with a long wooden or heat-proof handle. **Manufacturers:** 181, 278. Cost is about $3 and up from housewares stores and mail-order firms. **Sources:** 71, 240, 247, 261.

If your upper extremities are weak or poorly coordinated, it is safer to ladle, rather than lift and pour, hot liquids. A double-lipped ladle lets you pour from either side, so it also may be helpful if arm motion is limited. **Manufacturer:** 112. Cost is about $2 and up from housewares stores.

Placed in the bottom of a saucepan before heating, a disk called a pot watcher prevents boil-overs. When the mixture comes to a

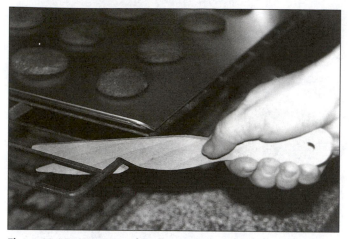

Figure 29-13. An oven push-pull or rack jack allows you to pull the shelf out to a more comfortable angle for lifting. (Photo by J.K.)

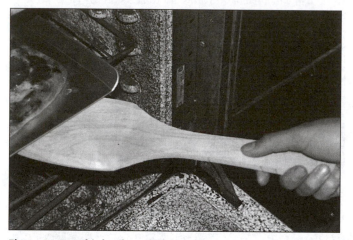

Figure 29-14. This hardwood oven paddle, called a pele, extends your reach by 15". (Photo by J.K.)

boil, you will hear the rattling of the disk in the saucepan. It does not, however, prevent the bottom from scorching. **Manufacturer:** 142. Cost is about $2 and up from housewares stores and mail-order firms. When adding liquids to a pan, it is safer to bring the liquid to the stove or oven than to move the pan to a counter or sink. It also prevents spilling, especially if you have any incoordination or difficulty walking and carrying.

DRAINING

Steaming or microwaving vegetables reduces the need to handle and drain pots of water. See Chapter 28 for more tips.

A slotted spoon is a safe tool for transferring hot foods from a pan to the serving dish. Cost is about $2 and up from housewares stores. **Manufacturers:** 112, 142, 270, 307, 321, 339.

You may remove fat or oil from a pan with a folded paper towel when working with a microwave oven or electric skillet. If using an electric skillet, turn off the control, then prop up one end of the appliance so that the fat runs to the lower end of the pan for absorbing with the paper towel. This method is not recommended when using a pan on the range top.

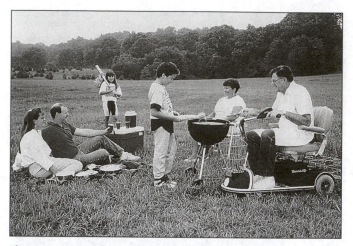

Figure 29-15. Outdoor grills are available in many styles from hardware and department stores. (Photo courtesy of Electric Mobility Corp.®, Sewell, NJ.)

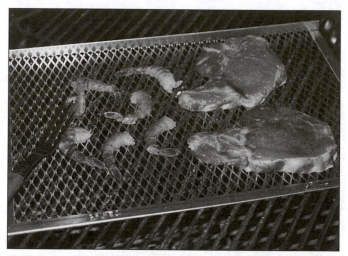

Figure 29-16. A grill grid or topper keeps foods like shrimp, vegetables, and kebabs from breaking or falling through the grill rack. (Photo by J.K.)

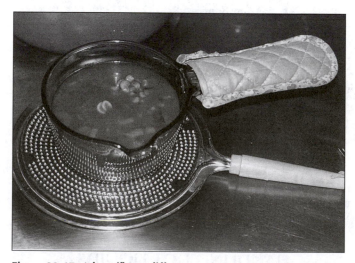

Figure 29-17. A heat/flame diffuser, or simmer ring, reduces splatter and helps prevent the bottom of your pan from scorching. (Photo by J.K.)

You may remove fat or oil from a pan with a folded paper towel when working with a microwave oven or electric skillet. If using an electric skillet, turn off the control, then prop up one end of the appliance so that the fat runs to the lower end of the pan for absorbing with the paper towel. This method is not recommended when using a pan on the range top.

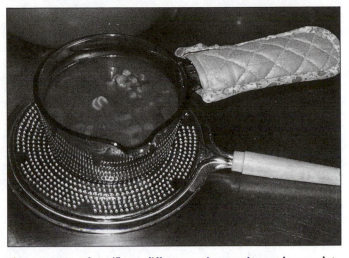

Figure 29-18. A heat/flame diffuser, or simmer ring, reduces splatter and helps prevent the bottom of your pan from scorching. (Photo by J.K.)

Serving
and Entertaining

If your arms and shoulders are weak or you have poor coordination or arthritis, resting both elbows on a surface when lifting or serving foods may help provide more leverage and stability.

HANDLING BEVERAGES

Whenever possible, select beverages in smaller containers to reduce the weight when pouring. Or when practicable, divide the contents into smaller containers. Look for lightweight plastic pitchers with handles through which you can slip your whole hand. **Manufacturers** include 343, 404. Cost is about $2 and up from housewares stores and mail-order firms.

When pouring from one container to another, a funnel may increase your chances of a spill-free transfer of liquids. Look for a funnel with an easy-to-grasp handle.

Adding a handle to milk or juice cartons and two-liter soda bottles makes pouring easier and reduces spills if your hands are weak or affected by arthritis, or if you are working with one hand (Figure 30-1). **Manufacturer:** 126. Cost is about $3 from housewares stores and mail-order firms. **Sources:** 173, 231, 270. The Soda Fresh handle replaces the cap on a 1- or 2-liter bottle, giving you not only a hand-hold for pouring but a method of locking in the fizz without having to tightly recap a bottle. A hole in the handle is also a bottle cap remover. **Manufacturer:** 216. Cost is about $4 from housewares stores and mail-order firms. **Sources:** 231, 378.

An ice cube bottle eliminates the frustration of filling and carrying ice cube trays to the refrigerator, wiping up the spills, then later trying to release frozen cubes (Figure 30-2). You simply fill this container half-way, lay it on its side to freeze, then hit the bottle against a hard surface to free the cubes. **Manufacturer:** 107. Cost is about $3 each from housewares stores and mail-order firms. **Sources:** 71, 240.

SERVING FOODS

A raised trivet is easier to slip pot-holdered hands underneath than a hot mat when setting down a pan or casserole (Figure 30-3). Look for wood and metal trivets in gourmet and kitchen specialty stores.

Roast forks have a wide surface and sharp prongs to help you lift a roast from the pan to a serving platter (Figure 30-4). **Manufacturers:** 142, 289. Set of two forks is about $5 and up from housewares stores and mail-order firms. Also see the roast-lifter sling in Chapter 29.

A meat lifter or broad spatula helps remove fish in one piece from a poaching liquid or baking pan (Figure 30-5). **Manufacturers:** 112, 273, 289. Cost of lifter is about $3 and up from housewares stores.

A spreading spatula, a utensil that fans out to three times its width as you press a lever, lets you get under and more securely transfer food from a skillet to a platter or plate. **Manufacturer:** 142. Cost is about $4 from housewares stores and mail-order firms.

Serving tongs grasp more securely than spoons, spatulas, or forks for handling salad, pastry, and other foods with one hand, loss of vision, or incoordination. Tongs of silver-plate, wood, or acrylic are available from housewares stores and gourmet or mail-order firms. **Manufacturers:** 142, 289. Cost is about $2 and up. **Sources:** 231, 364.

Some cake and pie servers may be used with one hand and are also helpful if you have incoordination or loss of vision (Figures 30-6A and 30-6B). A "first slice" pie insert eases the serving of pies and quiches. Cost of metal insert is about $3 from gourmet kitchen firms. **Sources** include 410.

Also look for a first-slice server. The wedge-shaped, metal insert fits into a pie plate before the crust is added. When ready to serve, you cut on either side of it, then lift the first piece out. Cost is about $3 from housewares stores and mail-order firms. **Sources:** 256, 261.

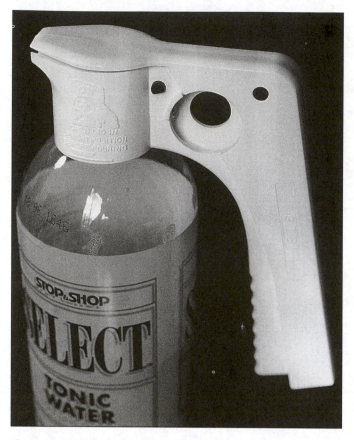

Figure 30-1. Adding a handle to milk or juice cartons and two-liter soda bottles makes pouring easier and reduces spills. (Soda Fresh handle by Kayser Housewares, Pine Brook, NJ. Photo by J.K.)

When serving ice cream or frozen yogurt, ask for help, or try a battery-powered ice cream scoop. Pushing a button on the handle heats the scoop to the optimum temperature, then turns off, so the cast-aluminum scooping surface can easily cut through frozen desserts. Cost is about $13 from department stores and mail-order firms. **Sources: 194, 270, 364.**

Additional serving aids are shown in Chapter 28 and Chapter 29.

ENTERTAINING

"Get me to the table on time" was the silent cry of many dishes in the not too distant past. Today with convenience foods, convection or microwave speed, and a variety of portable appliances, you can entertain guests at your own pace. The following tips will help make entertaining easier:

- Start with careful planning. Begin at least 2 or 3 days before the event.
- Conserve your energy. Shop ahead. Then, when it is time to cook, you are ready and able.
- Select the casual approach. Focus on the fun, not the trappings. Let the warmth of your hospitality be the most important seasoning on your menu.
- Choose recipes with which you are familiar and that can be prepared ahead of time. Simplicity is in!

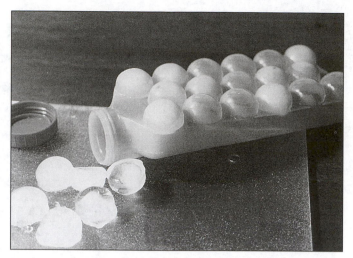

Figure 30-2. Simply fill this container half-way, lay it on its side to freeze, then hit the bottle against a hard surface to free the cubes. (Ice cube bottle by East Hampton Industries, E. Hampton, NY. Photo by J.K.)

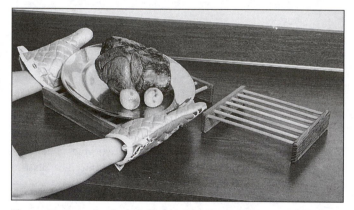

Figure 30-3. A raised trivet is easier to slip pot-holdered hands underneath than a hot mat when setting down a pan or casserole. (Photo by J.K.)

- Plan menus that your guests can help prepare. Portable appliances let company cook at the table.
- When someone offers to bring part of the meal, delegate that which is hardest for you. If cutting up vegetables for a salad is difficult, ask for help. If baking is tiring, enlist a volunteer.
- Reduce cleanup with easy-care tableware, including disposables.
- When the day comes, use all the techniques you have learned to reduce your work load. A wheeled cart or lapboard helps reduce steps. Setting up the meal as a buffet means that you don't have to set the table or carry everything to the dining room. If the weather is good, eat outside, letting everyone carry something out.

Food warmers and coolers allow you to serve foods more slowly, because they hold food at correct serving temperatures. Insulated containers of stainless steel, plastic, and foam, or with "microcore hot or cold packs," keep foods hot or chilled for hours. **Manufacturers: 17, 79.** Cost is about $15 and up. **Sources: 71, 270, 359, 374.** Electric heating units keep foods hot and range in size from 10" squares to wheeled carts. Some cordless models are

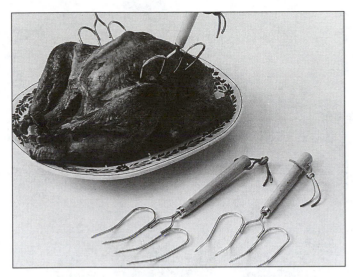

Figure 30-4. These roast forks have a wide surface and sharp prongs to help you lift a roast from the pan to a serving platter. (Photo courtesy of the O.T. Dept., Howard A. Rusk Institute of Rehabilitation Medicine.)

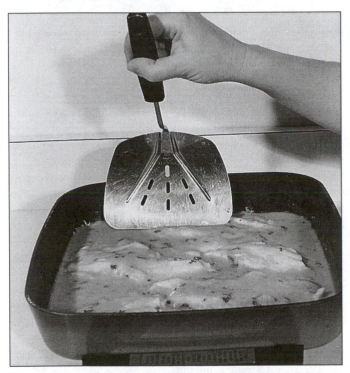

Figure 30-5. A meat lifter or broad spatula helps remove fish in one piece from a poaching liquid or baking pan. (Photo courtesy of the O.T. Dept., Howard A. Rusk Institute of Rehabilitation Medicine.)

heated in the microwave and retain heat for up to 45 minutes. If necessary, ask someone to transfer it to the table. Cost is about $20 for a small unit and up. **Manufacturers:** 131, 346. Cost is about $25 and up. **Sources:** 71, 167, cordless unit—364, 410.

Hot or cold drinks may be prepared ahead of time. An insulated pump-top pitcher holds hot soup for a first course, gravy, or sauce up to 30 minutes or a refreshing cool beverage for later. If you have weakness or incoordination in your arms, look for a unit

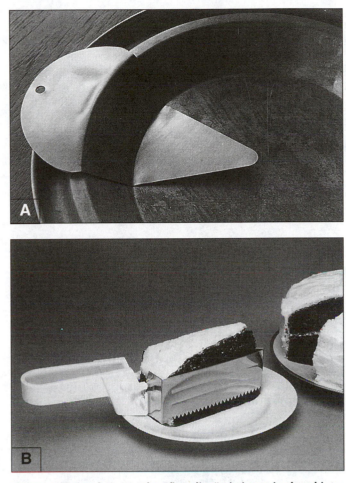

Figures 30-6A and 30-6B. The "first slice" pie insert is placed into the pan before shell and other ingredients. When pie is ready to serve, cuts are made along each side; insert is lifted out, and the remainder of the pie is easily cut and served. (Photo by J.K.)

with a non-breakable liner. **Manufacturers** include 70, 397. Cost is about $8 and up from housewares stores and mail-order firms.

An electric fondue pot lets you entertain with at-the-table cooking by your guests (Figure 30-7). An easy-to-turn control adjusts temperature; there is no need to refill with fuel. Ahead of time, you can cut up the bread, meats, and vegetables for a main dish or fruit and cake for a dessert fondue. Provide plates and long forks; then dip in. **Manufacturers:** 299, 346, 422. Cost is about $30 from housewares stores and mail-order firms. **Source:** 359.

Hint: Before cubing or slicing meat for a fondue, put it in the freezer for one hour or, if frozen, let it partially thaw. The firmer texture allows you to cut it more easily. Try the Swedish rehab knife (see Chapter 28) or a serrated blade for most efficient cutting.

An electric wok opens new vistas of dining at your table (Figure 30-8). The aluminum pan comes in a 6½- to 7-quart size and has a removable automatic heat control. The non-stick surface makes for easy cleaning. Wok shape is designed for stir-frying, poaching, steaming, or simmering foods. **Manufacturers:** 131, 346, 422. Cost is about $30 and up from housewares stores. **Source:** 364.

Rather than set a big table, a buffet lets your guests bring their meals to individual eating places.

A 20" high tubular steel and glass sofa table pulls in close to a

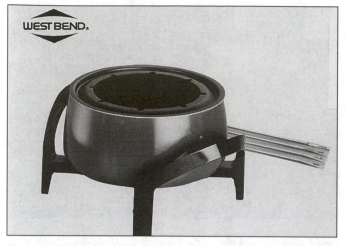

Figure 30-7. An electric fondue pot lets you entertain with at-the-table cooking by your guests. (Wok by the West Bend® Company, West Bend, IL. Photo by J.K.)

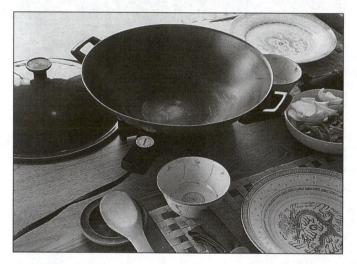

Figure 30-8. An electric wok opens new vistas of dining at your table. (Wok by the West Bend® Company, West Bend, IL. Photo by J.K.)

chair or slides under a couch. Cost is about $10 each and up for single-height or slightly higher for adjustable-height models (from 20" to 28"), from housewares stores and mail-order firms. Another solution is nested or folding tables that come out for company and keep the floor area free when not in use. For eating out on a deck, look for folding tables that attach to the deck railings and allow

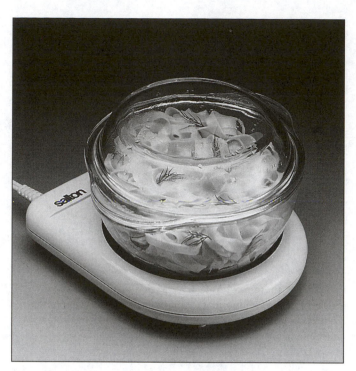

Figure 30-9. This electric Hot Spot® keeps a casserole warm while you prepare the remainder of the food or wait for guests to assemble. (Photo courtesy of Salton-Maxim®, Mt. Prospect, IL.)

access with a chair or wheelchair. **Source:** 387.

Inexpensive bamboo or plastic paper plate holders let you use disposable tableware indoors or out without the problem of spilling or soggy drips on tabletops. Cost is about $1 to $6 per set from housewares stores and mail-order firms. **Sources:** 59, 242.

The electric Hot Spot® keeps a casserole warm while you prepare the remainder of the food or wait for guests to assemble (Figure 30-9). Cost is about $20 from housewares stores. **Manufacturer:** 346.

Grilling and barbecuing can be done indoors or out. See Chapter 29. Ranges come with built-in grills. **Manufacturers:** 150, 205. Join outdoor chefs for easy entertaining. Hibachi stoves may be put on a table for easy reach, or a larger unit may be located on a deck or in your backyard. Take along a comfortable folding stool or chair for sitting by a campfire cook-out. Then grill the main course with long-handled barbecue tools. See Chapter 28. Let other guests bring along a "share-a-picnic" dish or two. Relax, eat, and enjoy. Cleanup is minimal.

A

Sources for Equipment and Tools

When purchasing items illustrated or discussed in *Mealtime Manual for People with Disabilities and the Aging*, let your "fingers do the walking." Check your telephone book first; then try local department, housewares, hardware, stationery, and specialty stores. You can also request a catalog from a listed mail-order firm. If a company does not have the item you request, it can often be ordered from their distributor. If necessary, call or write the manufacturer, whom in most cases will take a personal order or recommend a local or mail-order source. Telephone numbers are given for armchair shopping. For toll-free calls when the company is located in your state, check with your 800 directory information service.

"Kitchen/gourmet firm" is a company that specializes in aids for the cook and homemaker. "General mail-order firm" is an enterprise that carries a line of usually inexpensive items, including kitchen and household aids. A "self-help or rehabilitation firm" specializes in articles designed to aid in increased independence.

For suggestions on protecting yourself when ordering by mail, see Chapter 25. Warranties and Guarantees are discussed in Chapter 20.

Note: the addresses given here were current at time of publication. If you have a problem locating a company or product, please write what is required on the suggestion card, and I will answer your question or try to give you an alternate source.

1. **Abilitations by Sportime**
One Sportime Way
Atlanta, GA 30340
800-850-8602 (orders)
800-850-8603 (service)
Fax: 770-449-5700
Email: orders@sportime.com
Rehabilitation equipment firm.

2. **Access Industries, Inc.**
2509 Summer Ave.
Memphis, TN 38112
800-925-3100
901-323-5438
Fax: 901-323-5559

3. **Accent Books and Products**
P.O. Box 700
Bloomington, IL 61702

4. **Access to Independence**
1310 Mendoza St.
Madison, WI 53714
608-242-8484 x132
TTY: 608-242-8485

5. **Access to Recreation, Inc.**
P.O. Box 5072-430
Thousand Oaks, CA 91362-5072
800-634-4351
805-498-7535
Fax: 805-498-8186
Self-help firm.

6. **Access With Ease™**
1755 South Johnson, Box 1150
Chino Valley, AZ 86323
602-636-9469
Self-help firm.

7. **Accessible Work Systems, Inc.**
2295 CR 292
Bellevue, OH 44811
800-344-9301
Fax: 419-483-4872

8. **Achievement Products Inc.**
P.O. Box 9033
Canton, OH 44711
800-373-4699
330-453-2122
Fax: 330-453-0222
Rehabilitation firm.

9. **Acme International Inc.**
1006 Chancellor Ave.
Maplewood, NJ 07040
201-416-0400

10. **Acrylic Designs, Inc.**
100 River St.
Springfield, VT 05156
802-885-8579

11. **Action Products, Inc.**
22 North Mulberry St.
Hagerstown, MD 21740
800-228-7763
301-797-1414
Fax: 301-733-2073

12. **ActiveAid®, Inc.**
One ActiveAid Rd.
P.O. Box 359
Redwood Falls, MN 56283-0359
800-533-5330
507-644-2951
Fax: 507-644-2468

13. **AdaptAbility®**
Mill St.
P.O. Box 515
Colchester, CT 06415-0515
800-243-9232
203-537-3451
Fax: 800-566-6678
TDD: 800-688-4889
Self-help firm.

13B. **Addison-Wesley Longman, Inc.**
Route 128
Reading, MA 01867
800-447-2226
Fax: 617-944-9338

14. **Advantage Bag Company™**
22633 Ellinwood Dr.
Torrance, CA 90505
800-556-6307
310-540-8197
Fax: 310-316-2561

15. **Aids for Arthritis, Inc.**
3 Little Knoll Ct.
Medford, NJ 08055
609-654-6918
Self-help firm.

16. **AliMed®, Inc.**
297 High St.
Dedham, MA 02026-9135
800-225-8392
617-329-2900
Fax: 617-329-8392
Rehabilitation firm. Direct-to-You
consumer catalog.

17. **Aladdin Industries, Inc.**
Aladdin Mail Order
P.O. Box 100960
Nashville, TN 37224
800-251-4535
Fax: 615-748-3105

18. **All-Clad Metalcrafters, Inc.**
R.D. #2, Box 151
Canonsburg, PA 15317
412-745-8300

19. **AlumiRamp, Inc.**
90 Taylor St.
Quincy, MI 49082
800-800-3864
517-639-8777
Fax: 800-753-7267
http://www.inmax.com/alumniramp

19A. **Amadeus Press**
133 SW Second Ave., Ste. 450
Portland, OR 97204-3527
800-327-5680

20. **Amana Refrigeration, Inc.**
Hwy. 220
Amana, IA 52204
800-847-3783

21. **AARP Pharmacy Service Center**
7609 Energy Parkway, Ste. 1003
Baltimore, MD 21226-1755

22. **American Foundation for the Blind**
11 Penn Plaza, Ste. 300
New York, NY 10001
212-502-7600
TDD: 212-502-7662

23. **American Printing House for the Blind**
1839 Frankfort Ave.
P.O. Box 6085
Louisville, KY 40206-0085
800-223-1839
502-895-2405
Fax: 502-895-1509

24. **American Standard, Inc.**
1 Centennial Plaza
P.O. Box 6820
Piscataway, NJ 08855-6820
800-442-1902
908-980-3485

25. American Walker
900 Market St.
Oregon, WI 53575
800-828-6808
608-835-9255
Fax: 608-835-5234

26. Amigo® Mobility International, Inc.
6693 Dixie Highway
Bridgeport, MI 48722
800-821-9130
517-777-0910
Fax: 517-777-8184

27. A M K Designs, Inc.®
P.O. Box 16232
Duluth, MN 55816-0232
218-525-6723

28. Anchor Hocking Plastics
P.O. Box 2830
St. Paul, MN 55102-0830
612-227-7371

29. Ansell Perry, Inc.
1875 Harsh Ave. SE
P.O. Box 550
Massillon, OH 44648-0550
800-321-9752
330-833-2811
Fax: 330-833-5991

30. Apex Medical Corporation
P.O. Box 1235
800 S. Van Eps Ave.
Sioux Falls, SD 57101-1235
800-328-2935
605-332-6689
Fax: 605-332-6818

31. Apothecary Products
11531 Rupp Dr.
Burnsville, MN 55337
800-328-2742
EZ-Dos products, available
through local pharmacies.

32. Arcmate
637 Vinewood St.
Escondido, CA 92029-1926
888-637-1926
760-489-1140
Fax: 760-746-1926

33. Arrow Plastics Manufacturing Company
701 East Devon Ave.
Elk Grove Village, IL 60007
708-595-9000
Fax: 708-595-9122

34. Asko, Inc.
903 North Bowser, Ste. 200
Richardson, TX 75081-1805
800-367-2444

34B. Avery Publishing Group, Inc.
120 Old Broadway
Garden City Park, NY 11040
800-548-5757
516-741-2155
Fax: 516-742-1892

34C. Avon Books
1350 Ave. of the Americas
New York, NY 10019
800-238-0658
212-261-6800

35. The Bacova Guild, Ltd.
295 Fifth Ave.
New York, NY 10016-7130
212-481-8920
and
Hot Springs, VA 24445
540-839-2103

36. The Bag Lady
Box 531
West Stockbridge, MA 01266
413-637-3534

37. Bausch & Lomb®, Inc.
1400 North Goodman St.
Rochester, NY 14692
800-553-5340

38. Becton-Dickinson® Consumer Products
Becton-Dickinson and Company
1 Becton Dr.
Franklin Lakes, NJ 07417-1883
800-365-3321
201-847-7100

39. Best-Priced Products
P.O. Box 1174
White Plains, NY 10602
800-824-2939
914-472-2715
Fax: 800-356-8587
Rehabilitation firm.

39B. Berkeley Putnam Publishing Group
200 Madison Ave.
New York, NY 10016

40. Bissell® Healthcare Corp., Inc.
744 West Michigan Ave.
Jackson, MI 49201
800-788-2267
517-789-3241
and
Bissell® Healthcare Corp.- Canada
1224 Dundas St. East, Unit 5
Mississauga, ON L4Y 4A2

41. Black & Decker® (U.S.) Co.
Home Appliances
6 Armstrong Rd.
Shelton, CT 06484
800-231-9786
203-926-3218

42. Blair
220 Hickory St.
Warren, PA 16366

43. Brandt Industries, Inc.
4461 Bronx Blvd.
Bronx, NY 10470-1496
800-221-8031
718-994-0800
Fax: 718-325-7995

44. The Braun Corporation®
1014 South Monticello
P.O. Box 310
Winamac, IN 46996
800-843-5438
Fax: 219-946-4670
Email: braun@pwptc.com
http://www.braunlift.com

45. Braun®, Inc.
66 Broadway, Rte. 1
Lynnfield, MA 01940
800-BRAUN-11
617-592-3300
and
Braun® (Canada) Ltd.
Mississauga, ON L5T 1V5

46. Brita (USA) Inc.
The Clorox Company
1221 Broadway
Oakland, CA 94612
510-271-7000

47. BRK Electronics
Now: First Alert, Inc.
3901 Liberty Street Rd.
Aurora, IL 60504
708-851-7330

48. Brookes Publishing Company
c/o The Naples Press Distribution
Center
1083 Industrial Park M100
York, PA 17405
301-337-9580

49. Brookstone Company
1555 Bassford Dr.
Mexico, MS 65265-1382
800-351-7222

50. Bruce Medical Supply
411 Waverly Oaks Rd.
P.O. Box 9166
Waltham, MA 02254-9166
800-225-8446
617-894-6262
Fax: 617-894-9519
Self-help firm.

50B. Bruno® Independent Living Aids
1780 Executive Dr.
P.O. Box 84
Oconomowoc, WI 53066
800-882-8183
414-567-4990
Fax: 414-567-4341
http://www.bruno.com

51. Bull Publishing
110 Gilbert Ave.
Menlo Park, CA 94025
800-676-2855
415-322-2855

51B. Burke, Inc.
1800 Merriam Ln.
Kansas City, KS 66106
800-255-4147
Fax: 913-722-2614

52. Business and Institutional Furniture Co., Inc.
611 North Broadway
Milwaukee, WI 53202-5004
800-558-8662
Fax: 800-468-1526

53. Cabela's®, Inc.
812 13th Ave.
Sidney, NE 69160
800-237-4444
Fax: 800-496-6329
TDD: 800-695-5000

54. Cadie Products Corporation
41 Beech St.
Paterson, NJ 07509
201-278-8300

55. Caframo Ltd.
P.O. Box 70, Airport Rd.
Wiarton, ON N0H 2T0
519-534-1080
Fax: 519-534-1088

56. Camp® International, Inc.
A Bissell® Healthcare Company
2010 High St.
Jackson, MI 49204-0089
800-492-1088
517-787-1600
Rehabilitation firm.

57. Care Catalog Services
1877 Northeast 7th Ave.
Portland, OR 97212-3905
800-443-7091
503-288-8174
Fax: 503-287-3956
Rehabilitation firm.

58. Care Products
158 North Main St.
Florida, NY 10921
800-446-5206
914-651-3332

59. Carol Wright® Gifts
340 Applecreek Rd.
P.O. Box 82588
Lincoln, NE 68501-8918
402-474-4465
General mail-order firm.

60. Casual Collections
5301 South Southcenter Blvd.
Seattle, WA 98188
800-886-6878

61. Chadwick-Miller, Inc.
Pequot Industrial Park
300 Turnpike St.
P.O. Box 515
Canton, MA 02021
617-828-8300

62. Channing L. Bete Company
200 State Rd.
South Deerfield, MA 01373-0200
800-628-7733
Fax: 800-499-6464

63. Chantry®
1164 NE Cleveland St.
Clearwater, FL 34615
941-446-1960

64. Chef'n Corporation
2001 Western Ave., Ste. 555
Seattle, WA 98121
206-448-1210

65. The Chef's Catalog
3215 Commercial Ave.
Northbrook, IL 60062-1900
800-338-3232
Fax: 800-967-2433
Kitchen/gourmet firm.

66. Chicago Cutlery® Housewares
General Housewares Corp.
Consumer Services Dept.
1536 Beech St.
Terre Haute, IN 47804-4066
800-457-2665, ext. 273

67. Chicago Metallic
Div. of CM Products, Inc.
800 Ela Rd.
Lake Zurich, IL 60047-2340
847-438-3400

68. Chicago Wirecraft
1534 South Ashland Ave.
Chicago, IL 60608
312-243-5940
Fax: 312-243-5945

69. Clairson International
Closet Maid®
P.O. Box 4400
Ocala, FL 32674
904-351-6100

70. Coleman® Company, Inc.
P.O. Box 1042
Maple Plain, MN 55348
800-685-5235

71. Colonial Garden Kitchens
P.O. Box 66
Hanover, PA 17333-0066
800-245-3399
Kitchen/gourmet firm.

72. Calphalon Corporation
Now: Commercial Aluminum
Cookware Company
P.O. Box 583
Toledo, OH 43696-0583
800-809-7267 (24 hr. service number)
419-666-8700
Fax: 419-666-2859
http://www.calphalon.com

73. Community Kitchens
2 North Maple Ave.
Ridgely, MD 21660
800-535-9901

74. Concept Design
dba Creative Work Systems
13 Lund Rd.
Saco, ME 04072-1806
207-282-4173
Fax: 207-282-8380

75. Consumer Care Products, Inc.
P.O. Box 684
Sheboygan, WI 53092-0684
920-459-8353
Fax: 920-459-9070

75B. Consumers Reports Books®
Division of Consumers Union of
U.S., Inc.
101 Truman Ave.
Yonkers, NY 10903
914-378-2000

76. The Container Store
200 Valwood Parkway
Dallas, TX 75234
800-733-3532
Fax: 800-786-5858

76B. Contemporary Books, Inc.
2 Prudential Plaza, Ste. 1200
Chicago, IL 60601
800-621-1918 (orders)
312-540-4500
Fax: 312-782-3987

77. Cook's Club™ Inc.
Lechters
1 Cape May St.
Harrison, NJ 07029-2404
201-481-1100

77B. Cool Hands Communications
1098 NW Boca Raton Blvd.
Boca Raton, FL 33432
800-428-0578

78. Copco Division
Wilton Enterprises
2240 West 75th St.
Woodbridge, IL 60517
800-772-7100
708-963-7100

79. Corning/Revere Consumer
Information Center
P.O. Box 1994
Waynesboro, VA 22980
800-340-5471
Fax: 540-949-9118

80. Cosco®, Inc.
2525 State St.
Columbus, OH 47201
812-372-0141

81. Country Technology, Inc.
P.O. Box 87
Gays Mills, WI 54631
608-735-4718
Fax: 608-735-4859

82. Crate & Barrel
P.O. Box 9059
Wheeling, IL 60090-9059
800-323-5491

83. Crump Products, Inc.
952 South 3rd St.
Louisville, KY 40203
502-583-6046
Fax: 502-583-0748

84. Cuisinarts, Inc.
150 Milford Rd.
East Windsor, NJ 08520
800-726-0190

85. Cuisine de France
Subsidiary of the Forschner Group,
Inc.
Shelton, CT 06484
203-929-6391

86. Damaco Freedom on Wheels
5105 Maureen Lane
Moorpark, CA 93021
800-432-2434
805-532-1832
Fax: 805-532-1836

87. Damark International Inc.
7101 Winnetka Ave. North
P.O. Box 9437
Minneapolis, MN 55440-9437
800-729-9000

88. Danamar Productions
106 Monte Vista Place
Sante Fe, NM 87501
505-986-9072
Video on stroke rehabilitation.

89. Dazey Corporation
One Dazey Circle
Industrial Airport, KS 66031
800-255-6120
913-782-7500
Fax: 913-829-1485

90. Dazor® Manufacturing
Corporation
4483 Duncan Ave.
St. Louis, MO 63110
800-345-9103

91. Deflecto® Corporation
P.O. Box 50057
Indianapolis, IN 46250

92. DeLonghi America, Inc.
625 Washington Ave.
Carlstadt, NJ 07072
800-322-3848

93. Delta® Faucet Company
Div. of Masco Corp. of Indiana
55 East 111th St.
P.O. Box 40980
Indianapolis, IN 46280
800-345-3358
317-848-1812

94. Deni® Better Living by Design
Keystone Manufacturing Co., Inc.
P.O. Box 863
20 Norris St.
Buffalo, NY 14207
716-875-6680
Fax: 716-875-6969

95. Design Ideas
P.O. Box 2967
Springfield, IL 62708
800-426-6394
Fax: 217-753-3080

96. The Disability Bookshop
P.O. Box 129
Vancouver, WA 98666-0129
800-637-2256
206-637-2256
Fax: 206-696-3210

97. Dixie USA, Inc.
P.O. Box 55549
Houston, TX 77255-9937
800-347-3494
800-688-2507 (orders)
713-688-4993
Fax: 713-688-5932 (orders)

98. Domestications
825 Baltimore St.
Hanover, PA 17331-4100
800-746-2555
717-633-3060
Fax: 800-338-1635

99. The Door Store
Call for store nearest you.
800-433-4071

100. Dr. Leonard's® Health Care Products
42 Mayfield Ave.
P.O. Box 7821
Edison, NJ 08818-7821
800-785-0880
Self-help firm.

101. Dow Brands
P.O. Box 68511
Indianapolis, IN 46268-0511

102. E.I. Dupont de Nemours & Company
Product Information Center
1007 Market St.
Wilmington, DE 19898
800-441-7515

103. Duro-Med® Industries, Inc.
1788 West Cherry St.
P.O. Box 547
Jesup, GA 31598-0546
800-526-4753
912-427-7358
Fax: 800-479-7968

104. Dycem®
P.O. Box 6920
83 Gilbane St.
Warwick, RI 02887
800-458-0060
401-738-4420
Fax: 401-739-9634
E-mail: DYCEM_USA@IDS.NET

105. Dynamic Rehab Videos and Rentals
307 Spruce Ave. South
Thief River Falls, MN 56701
218-681-4240
218-681-1624 (after 5pm)
Upper extremity amputee video.

106. Early Winters/Norm Thompson
P.O. Box 3999
Portland, OR 97206-3999
800-458-4438

107. East Hampton Industries, Inc.
81 Newtown Lane
East Hampton, NY 11937
800-645-1188
516-324-2224 (in NY)
Fax: 516-324-2248

108. Easy Street
8 Equality Park West
Newport, RI 02840-2603
800-959-EASY

109. Econol® Elevator Lift Corporation
Box 584
Cedar Falls, IA 50613
319-277-4777
Fax: 319-277-4778

110. Eddie Bauer®, Seattle
1330 Fifth and Union
P.O. Box 3700
Seattle, WA 98130-0006
800-426-8020
Fax: 206-869-4629
800-641-2564 (for retail store locations)

111. EdgeCraft Corporation
825 Southwood Rd.
Avondale, PA 19311
800-342-3255
610-268-0500
Fax: 610-268-3545

112. Ekco® Housewares, Inc.
9234 West Belmont Ave.
Franklin Park. IL 60131
312-678-8600

113. Electric Mobility® Corporation
#1 Mobility Plaza
Sewell, NJ 08080
800-662-4548
609-468-0270
Fax: 609-468-3426
http://www.emobility.com
and
Electric Mobility® of Florida
7910 Ulmerton Rd. East
Largo, FL 33771
800-MOBILITY
and
Electric Mobility® of California
5666 Corporate Ave.
Cypress, CA 90630
800-225-6919

114. Electrolux® Corporation
2300 Windy Ridge Parkway
Atlanta, GA 30339
800-243-9078
905-542-0250 x211
and
Electrolux® Canada
2470 Milltower Ct.
Mississauga, ON L5N 6H3
800-668-0763

115. Elkay® Manufacturing Company
2222 Camden Ct.
Oak Brook, IL 60521
800-635-7500

116. Embracing Concepts, Inc.
40 Humbolt St., Ste. 220
Rochester, NY 14609
800-962-5542
716-654-9090
Fax: 716-458-0593

117. Empak
Consumer Products Division
4571 Valley Industrial Blvd. South
Shakopee, MN 55379
612-445-4110

118. Emson
Division of E. Mishan & Sons
230 Fifth Ave.
New York, NY 10001
212-689-9094

119. Enabler Wheelchairs, Inc.
5105 Maureen St.
Moorpark, CA 93021
800-432-2434
Fax: 805-532-1836

120. Enrichments® for Better Living
A Bissell® Healthcare Co.
P.O. Box 5050
Bolingbrook, IL 60444-9973
800-323-5547
Fax: 800-547-4333
Self-help firm.

121. Ensar Corporation
135 East Hintz Rd.
Wheeling, IL 60090-6036
312-520-1000

122. Etac USA, Inc.
2325 Parklawn Dr., Ste. J
Waukesha, WI 53186
800-678-3822
414-796-4600
Fax: 414-796-4605

123. The Eureka® Company
1201 East Bell St.
Bloomington, IL 61701
800-282-2886

124. European Kitchen Bazaar, Inc.
P.O. Box 4099
Waterbury, CT 06704
800-243-8546

125. Everest & Jennings®, Inc.
3601 Rider Trail South
Earth City, MO 63045
800-235-4661
314-512-7000
Fax: 800-542-7648

126. Evlo Plastics, Inc.
310 Industrial Lane
P.O. Box 2295
Sandusky, OH 44870-2295
419-626-2430
Fax: 419-626-8183

127. Evo™ Pen
200 East 33rd St.
New York, NY 10016
212-213-1065
Fax: 212-213-1065

128. Excel Cutlery, Inc.
99 Quentin Roosevelt Blvd.
Garden City, NY 11530
515-794-3355
Fax: 516-794-5250

129. EZ-Por
Div. of Packaging Corp. of America
1500 Soth Wall Rd.
Wheeling, IL 60090
847-459-1900

130. Fairway King
4300 North Sewall
Oklahoma City, OK 73118
800-222-1145
405-528-8571
Fax: 405-235-7483

131. Farberware®, Inc.
Div. of Kidde, Inc.
1500 Bassett Ave.
Bronx, NY 10461-3295
212-863-8000

132. Fashion-Ease
Div. of M&M Health Care Apparel Co.
1541 60th St.
Brooklyn, NY 11219
800-221-8929
718-871-8188

133. Fat Finder®
41-905 Boardwalk, Ste. B
Palm Desert, CA 92260
800-323-8042

134. Fernanda Manufacturing
120 Marcus Blvd.
Deer Park, NY 11729
516-254-2070

135. Fingerhut® Corporation
11 McLeland Rd.
St. Cloud, MN 56372-0001

136. Fisher-Price® Company
7811 Girard Ave.
East Aurora, NY 14052-1879
716-687-3000

137. Fiskars®, Inc.
7811 West Stewart Ave.
Wausau, WI 54401
715-842-2091
Fax: 715-848-5528
and
#1-201 Whitehall Dr.
Markham, ON L3R 9Y3
Canada

138. Flaghouse, Inc.
150 North MacQuestern Parkway
Mt. Vernon, NY 10550
800-739-7900
800-265-6900 (Canada)
914-739-7922 (outside U.S.)
Fax: 800-739-7922
Rehabilitation firm.

139. Flexi-Mat Corporation
2244 South Western Ave.
Chicago, IL 60608
800-338-7392
312-376-5500
Fax: 312-376-0825

140. The Flinchbaugh™ Company, Inc.
390 Edberts Lane
York, PA 17403
800-326-2418
717-854-7720
Fax: 717-843-7355

141. Flotool International
15542 Mosher Ave.
Tustin, CA 92680
800-334-3062
714-850-9212
Fax: 714-850-9748

142. Fox Run Craftsmen
P.O. Box 2727
1907 Stout Dr.
Ivyland, PA 18974
215-675-7700
Fax: 215-675-4508
and
20A Voyager Ct. South
Etobioke, ON M9W 5M7
Canada
416-213-9880
Fax: 416-213-9886

143. Franco® Manufacturing Company
309 Fifth Ave.
New York, NY 10016
212-481-5400

144. Frank Eastern Company
599 Broadway
New York, NY 10012-3258
800-221-4914
212-219-0007 (NY)
Fax: 212-219-0722

145. **Franke, Inc.**
Kitchen Systems Div.
212 Church Rd.
North Wales, PA 19454
800-626-5771

146. **Freedom Designs**
2241 Madera Rd.
Simi Valley, CA 93065
800-331-8551

147. **Frigidaire®, Inc.**
Consumer Assistance Center
P.O. Box 7181
Dublin, OH 43017-0781
800-245-0600

148. **Fuller Brush® Company**
Check local Business Phone Book.

149. **Gabriel Manufacturing
Company**
P.O. Box 2381
Oshkosh, WI 54903
414-231-0155

150. **Gaggenau USA Corporation**
425 University Ave.
Norwood, MA 02062-2536
617-938-1655

151. **Garvey Company**
816 Transfer Rd.
P.O. Box 4306
St. Paul, MN 55104
800-328-6566
612-642-1272
Fax: 888-329-7868
Rehabilitation and self-help firm.

152. **Gavilan's®**
Gavilan Hills, CA 92599
909-943-2022
Fax: 909-943-5574

153. **Gaylord Brothers**
Box 4901
Syracuse, NY 13221-4901
315-457-5070

154. **Gemco® Ware, Inc.**
One Gemco Plaza
P.O. Box 813
Freeport, NY 11520-0813
516-623-9300
Fax: 516-378-6699

155. **G.E. Miller, Inc.**
45 Saw Mill River Rd.
Yonkers, NY 10701
800-431-2924
Rehabilitation firm.

156. **General Electric® Appliances**
Appliance Park
Louisville, KY 40225
G.E. Answer Center: 800-626-2000

157. **Gerber Products Company®**
445 State St.
Fremont, MI 49413-0001
800-4-GERBER

158. **Global Business Furniture**
National Order Processing Center
22 Harbor Park Dr., Dept. F
Port Washington, NY 11050
800-472-0101
Fax: 800-336-3818

159. **Goldstar Electronics
International Inc.**
1000 Sylvan Ave.
Englewood Cliffs, NJ 07632
800-292-3013

160. **Goodhope Bags Industries, Inc.**
623 Vineland
La Puente, CA 91746
818-369-0146

161. **Grayline Products, Inc.**
455 Kehoe Blvd.
Carolstream, IL 60188
800-222-7388

162. **Great Lakes Designs**
544 South Green Rd.
Cleveland, OH 44121
216-382-6961
Fax: 216-382-7756

163. **Guardian® Products**
Div. of Sunrise Medical Co.
4175 Guardian St.
Simi Valley, CA 93063
800-333-4000
Fax: 800-579-2828
and
Sunrise Medical Canada Inc.
265 Hood Rd., Unit 3
Markham, ON L3R 4N3

164. **Guilford Press, Inc.**
72 Spring St.
New York, NY 10012-9941
800-365-7006 (orders)
212-431-9800
Fax: 212-966-6708

165. **Haband for Her**
265 North 9th St.
Paterson, NJ 07530-0002

166. **Hamilton Beach-Proctor Silex,
Inc.**
4421 Waterfront Dr.
Glen Allen, VA 23060
800-486-0343
804-273-9777

167. **Hammacher Schlemmer**
Operations Center
9180 Le Saint Dr.
Fairfield, OH 45014-5475
800-543-3366

168. **Handi-Ramp®, Inc.**
1414 Armour Blvd.
Mundelein, IL 60060-4404
800-876-RAMP
847-816-7525
Fax: 847-816-7689
Email: handiramp.aol.com
http://www.marketzone.com/handi-ramp

169. **Handsome Rewards®**
19465 Brennan Ave.
Perris, CA 92599
909-943-2023
Fax: 909-943-5574

169B. **Hanley & Belfus, Inc.**
210 South 13th St.
Philadelphia, PA 19107
800-962-1892
Fax: 215-790-9330

170. **Hanna Andersson®**
1010 NW Flanders
Portland, OR 97209
800-222-0544
TDD: 800-435-9194 (9-5, PT, 7
days)
Fax: 503-321-5289 (24 hours, 7
days)

171. Hanover House®
340 Poplar Street
Hanover, PA 17331
717-633-3377
717-633-3366 (credit card orders
over $15)
General mail-order firm.

172. HarperCollins, Inc.
Order Entry Dept.
Keystone Industrial Park
Scranton, PA 18512
800-242-7737
Fax: 800-822-4090

173. Harriet Carter®
Dept. 16
North Wales, PA 19455
215-361-5151
General mail-order firm.

174. Health Enterprises
90 George Levin Dr.
North Attleboro, MA 02760
800-633-4243
Fax: 508-695-3061

175. HealthHouse USA
Box 9036
Jericho, NY 11753
516-334-9754 (orders, 24 hr/day)
516-334-2099 (service)

176. Heartland America
6978 Shady Oak Rd.
Eden Prairie, MN 55344-3453
800-229-2901
Fax: 800-943-4096

177. Hello Direct®, Inc.
5893 Rue Ferrari
San Jose, CA 95138-1858
800-HI-HELLO (800-444-3556)
Fax: 408-972-8155
E-mail: xpressit@hihello.com
http://www.hello-direct.com (ordering)

178. Herrschners
2800 Hoover Rd.
Stevens Point, WI 54492-0001
800-441-0838

178B. Henry Holt & Co.
115 West 18th St.
New York, NY 10011
800-488-5233
212-886-9200

**179. Hertz Furniture Systems
Corporation**
E55 Midland Ave.
Paramus, NJ 07652-9875
800-526-4677
Fax: 800-842-9290

180. Heuck Kitchen Tools
P.O. Box 23036
Cincinnati, OH 45223
513-681-1774

181. Hoan® Products Ltd.
Lifetime Hoan Corp.
P.O. Box 921
8-2 Corn Rd.
Dayton, NJ 08810
908-274-3434

182. Hoffritz®
Retail Mail Div.
515 West 24th St.
New York, NY 10011-1182
212-924-7300

**183. Hoky® International Marketing
Co., Inc.**
P.O. Box 810
Lakeville, MN 55044-0810

184. Holst®, Inc.
P.O. Box 1431
Midland, MI 48641-1431
517-832-1800
General mail-order firm.

185. Home Trends
1450 Lyell Ave.
Rochester, NY 14606-2184
716-254-6520
Fax: 716-458-9245
Housewares mail-order firm.

186. Home Care Products, Inc.
15824 SE 296th St.
Kent, WA 98042
800-451-1903
206-631-4633
Fax: 206-630-8196

187. Home-Sew
Bethlehem, PA 18010-0109
215-867-9717
Fax: 215-867-9717

188. Honeywell, Inc.
1985 Douglas Dr. North
Minneapolis, MN 55422
800-451-1903
Fax: 206-630-8196

189. The Hoover Company
101 East Maple
North Canton, OH 44720
216-499-9200

190. Hoyle Products, Inc.
P.O. Box 606
Fillmore, CA 93015
800-345-1950

191. Hutzler Gerda
Div. of Hutzler Manufacturing
Company
Canaan, CT 06018
860-824-5117

192. IKEA
410-931-8940 (East coast)
818-912-1119 (West coast)

193. Imperial Schrade Corporation
7 Schrade Ct.
P.O. Box 7000
Ellenville, NY 12428-0981
914-647-7600

194. Improvements
Quick and Clever Problem Solvers
Hanover, PA 17333-0084
800-642-2112
Fax: 800-757-9997

195. Inclinator® Company of America
P.O. Box 1557
Harrisburg, PA 17105
717-234-8065
Fax: 717-234-0941

196. Independent Living Aids, Inc.
27 East Mall
Plainview, NY 11803
800-537-2118
516-752-8080
Fax: 516-752-3135

197. In-Sink-Erator
4700 21st St.
Racine, WI 53406
800-558-5712

198. Interactive Technologies, Inc.
2266 Second St. North
N. St. Paul, MN 55109
800-777-5484
612-777-2690
Fax: 612-779-4890

199. Intermatic®, Inc.
Intermatic Plaza
Spring Grove, IL 60081
318-282-7300

200. Invacare® Corporation
899 Cleveland St.
P.O. Box 4028
Elyria, OH 44036-2125
800-333-6900
216-329-6000
Fax: 216-366-0729
800-668-5324 (Canada)
800-668-5354 (Ontario)
Email: selder@invacare.com
http://www.invacare.com

201. J.A. Henckels Zwilling, Inc.
Now: Zwilling, J.A. Henckels, Inc.
171 Saw Mill Rd.
Hawthorne, NY 10532-2191
914-592-7370
Fax: 914-592-7384

202. Jaeco Orthopedic Specialties
P.O. Box 75
Hot Springs, AR 71902-0075
501-623-5944

203. Jay® Medical Ltd.
Now: J Medical Kid Kan
P.O. Box 18656
4745 Walnut St.
Boulder, CO 80301
800-648-8282
303-442-5529
Fax: 800-442-3855

204. J.C. Penney® Company, Inc.
Call 800 number for referral to catalog division nearest you.
800-222-6161

205. Jenn-Air® Company
Division of Maytag Corp.
3035 Shadeland Ave.
Indianapolis, IN 46226-0901
800-536-6247

206. Jeremy P. Tarcher Inc.
11835 Olympic Blvd.
East Tower, Ste. 500
Los Angeles, CA 90064
213-935-9986
Fax: 213-935-9986

207. J.K. Adams
P.O. Box 248
Dorset, VT 05215
802-362-2303
Fax: 802-362-5472

208. Joan Cook®
119 Foster St.
P.O. Box 6038
Peabody, MA 01961-6038
800-935-0971 (orders)
508-532-6523 (service, 9-5 E.S.T.)
Fax: 800-933-3732

209. Jobar International
220 North Inglewood Ave.
Inglewood, CA 90300
310-671-1126
Fax: 310-671-8200

209B. Johns Hopkins University Press
2715 North Charles St.
Baltimore, MD 21218-4319
800-537-5487
410-516-6900

210. Johnny Appleseed's®, Inc.
30 Toser Rd.
Beverly, MA 01915-5593
800-225-5051

211. Johnson Smith Company
4514 19th St. Court East
Box 25500
Bradenton, FL 34206-5500
941-747-2356 (orders, 24 hrs.)
941-747-5566, ext. 5 (service)
Fax: 941-746-7896

212. Jokari/U.S. Inc.
1205 Venture Ct.
Carrollton, TX 75006

213. Joyce Chen Products
6 Fortune Dr.
Billerica, MA 01821
508-671-9500

214. Juno Lighting, Inc.
P.O. Box 5065
Des Plaines, IL 60017-5065
800-323-5068

215. M. Kamenstein, Inc.
565 Taxter Rd.
Elmsford, NY 10523
914-785-8036
Fax: 914-785-8095

216. Kayser Housewares
ISI North America, Inc.
Pine Brook, NJ 07058
201-227-2426

217. Ken McRight Supplies, Inc.
7456 South Oswego
Tulsa, OK 74136
918-492-9657
Fax: 918-492-9694

218. Kendall Futuro®
5405 Dupont Circle, #A
Milford, OH 45150
513-271-3782
Fax: 513-576-8274

219. Kenton Technology, Inc.
1448 North Rapids Rd.
Manitowoc, WI 54220

220. Kingsford
The Clorox Company
Oakland, CA 94612
800-677-2624

221. Kingstar International America, Inc.
P.O. Box 10157
Chicago, IL 60610-0157
800-336-6550
312-951-1115

222. KitchenAid® Home Appliance
KitchenAid Customer Satisfaction Center
2611 North M63 #139
Benton Harbor, MI 49022-2543
800-243-1180

223. Kohler® Company
444 Highland Dr.
Kohler, WI 53044
800-456-4537

224. Krups® North America
7 Reuten Dr.
Closter, NJ 07401
201-767-5600

225. Kwikset Corporation
516 East Santa Anna
Anaheim, CA 92803
714-535-8111

226. Lamson & Goodnow
Conway Rd.
Shelburne Falls, MA 01370
800-872-6564
413-625-6331

227. Land's End
Land's End Lane
Dodgeville, WI 53595-0001
800-356-4444

228. Larand International
506 Kenny Rd.
St. Paul, MN 55101
612-771-5537

229. Laurel Designs
Now: Innisfree Press

230. Le Cook's™ Ware Company
601 Gateway Blvd., Ste. 1150
San Francisco, CA 94008
415-244-0224
Fax: 415-435-1451

231. Lechters
1 Cape May St.
Harrison, NJ 07029-2404
201-481-1100
Check phone book for nearest
store.
Housewares store.

232. Lee Rowan Company
900 South Highway
Fenton, MO 63026
314-343-0700
Fax: 314-349-9650

233. Lefty's Corner
P.O. Box 615
Clark's Summit, PA 18411
717-586-5338
Catalog, $2 credit toward purchase.

234. Leichtung
The Workbench People
4944 Commerce Parkway
Cleveland, OH 44128
800-321-6840

235. Leifheit®
Items manufactured in Europe.
Available through local housewares
stores and mail-order firms.

236. Leisure Lift
1800 Merriam Lane
Kansas City, MO 66106
800-255-0285

237. Lifecare International Inc.
1401 West 122nd Ave.
Westminster, CO 80234-3421
800-669-9234
303-457-9234
Fax: 303-255-9000

238. Life Enhancements
1318 Southdale Center
Minneapolis, MN 55435
800-299-0578
612-920-0525
Fax: 612-721-8050
Self-help firm.

239. LIFESPEC Cabinet Systems Inc.
County Rd. 262
Oxford, MS 38655
601-234-0330

240. Lighthouse Consumer Products
100 Enterprise Place
P.O. Box 7044
Dover, DE 19903-7044
800-829-0500

241. Lightolier, Inc.
100 Lighting Way
Secaucus, NJ 07094-0508
201-864-3000

242. Lillian Vernon® Corporation
354 Main St.
New Rochelle, NY 10801-6306
Virginia Beach, VA 23479-0002
800-285-5555 (orders)
914-576-6400
TDD/TTY: 800-285-5536
Fax: 804-430-1010

242B. Lippincott-Raven Publishers
227 East Washington Sq.
Philadelphia, PA 19106-3708
800-777-2295
215-238-4200

243. Living Media, Inc.
219 Kitchawan Rd.
South Salem, NY 10590
914-533-2772

244. LK Manufacturing
P.O. Box 167
Huntington Station, NY 11746
516-420-8777

245. L.L. Bean® Inc.
1 Casco St.
Freeport, ME 04033-0001
800-221-4221
Fax: 207-552-3080
TTY: 800-545-0090

246. Lossing Orthopedic
P.O. Box 6224
Minneapolis, MN 55406
800-328-5216
612-724-2669

247. LS&S Group, Inc.
P.O. Box 673
Northbrook, IL 60065
800-468-4789 (orders)
847-498-9777 (information)
TTY: 800-317-8533
Fax: 847-498-1482
http://www.lssgroup.com

248. Lucent Technologies
600 Mountain Ave.
Murray Hill, NJ 07974-0636
1-888-4-LUCENT

249. Lumex®, Inc.
100 Spence St.
Bay Shore, NY 11706-2290
800-645-5272
516-273-2200
Fax: 800-273-5681

250. Lux® Products Corporation
6000-I Commerce Parkway
Mt. Laurel, NJ 08054
800-468-1317
609-234-7905

251. Luxo Lamp Corporation
63 Midland Ave.
P.O. Box 951
Port Chester, NY 10573
914-937-4433

251B. Macmillan Publishing, Inc.
Div. of Simon and Schuster
866 Third Ave.
New York, NY 10022
800-428-5331

252. Maddak®, Inc.
6 Industrial Rd.
Pequannock, NJ 07869
800-443-4926
973-628-7600
Fax: 973-305-0841
Email: tallete@webspan.net
http://www.maddak.com

252B. The Magellan Group
2512 East 43rd St.
P.O. Box 182236
Chattanooga, TN 37422
800-644-8100

253. Magic Chef®
Maycor
240 Edwards St. SE
Cleveland, TN 37311
423-478-6793

254. Magic Sliders LP
50 Main St.
White Plains, NY 106
914-682-9400
Fax: 914-682-0033

255. Magla® Products
3636 Taylorsville Hwy.
Statesville, NC 28577
704-873-6384
Fax: 704-873-8684

256. Maid of Scandinavia
Div. of Sweet Celebrations, Inc.
P.O. Box 39426
Edina, MN 55439-0426
800-328-6722
612-943-1688 (local)
Fax: 612-943-1688

257. Mapa Professional
512 East Tiffin St.
Willard, OH 44890
800-537-2897

258. Mary Maxim®
2001 Holland Ave.
Port Huron, MI 48060
800-962-9504

259. Master Manufacturing Company
Master Caster Division
9200 Inman Ave.
Cleveland, OH 44105
216-641-0500

260. Maverick Industries, Inc.
265 Ravitan Center Pkwy.
Edison, NJ 08837
908-417-9666

261. Maxi-Aids
Products for Independent Living
42 Executive Blvd.
P.O. Box 3209
Farmingdale, NY 11735
800-522-6294
718-846-4799
V/TTY: 718-441-1984
E-mail: maxiaids@haven.ios.com
http://www.maxiaids.com

262. M.B. Walton, Inc.
2021 West St.
River Grove, IL 60171
800-543-8105
708-452-4100
Fax: 708-452-9967 or 9968

263. McCarty's Sacro-Ease®
3329 Industrial Ave.
Coeur d'Alene, ID 83814
800-635-3557
Fax: 208-664-6891

264. Meacham Surgical
107 Meacham Ave.
Elmont, NY 11003
516-354-2950

265. Medical Line Warehouse
6130 Clark Center Ave., #103
Sarasota, FL 34238
800-247-2256

266. Medicine in the Public Interest, Inc.
192 South St., Ste. 500
Boston, MA 02111
617-728-7977
Fax: 617-728-9135

267. Medi-Mart® Centers
525 Third St.
Beaver, PA 15009
412-728-3851
Call for branch nearest you.

267B. Meredith Corporation
Better Homes and Gardens®
1716 Locust St.
Des Moines, IA 50336
800-678-8091
Fax: 515-284-3371

268. Merrillat® Industries, Inc.
P.O. Box 1946
Adrian, MI 49221
800-624-1250

269. Metro Marketing
P.O. Box 47170
Gardena, CA 90247
310-898-1888

270. Miles Kimball Company
41 West 8th St.
Oshkosh, WI 54906-0100
414-231-3800
General mail-order firm.

271. Mind Body, Inc.
535 Lippa Parkway, Ste. 110
Kihei, HI 96753

272. Minnesota Mining And Manufacturing
3M Center
St. Paul, MN 55101
612-733-1110

273. Mirro®/Foley/WearEver/Rema
1512 Washington
P.O. Box 1330
Manitowoc, WI 54221-1330

274. Mobil Chemical Co.
Div. of Mobil Oil Corp.
Plastics Division-Consumer Products
Pittsford, NY 14534

275. Modern Maid Company
Hefner and Washington
Topton, PA 19562-1499
610-682-4211

276. Moen® Division
377 Woodland Ave.
Elyria, OH 44306

277. Montgomery Ward
Direct Order Processing
6700 Shady Oak Rd.
Eden Prairie, MN 55344-3433
800-852-2711

277B. Mosby-Year Books, Inc.
Subs. of Time Mirror Co.
11830 Westline Industrial Drive
St. Louis, MO 63146
800-426-4545
314-872-8370

278. Mouli Manufacturing Corp.
#1 Montgomery St.
Belleville, NJ 07109
800-789-8285
201-751-6900
Fax: 201-751-0345

279. Moulinex® Appliances, Inc.
20 Caldari Rd.
Concord, ON L4K 4N8
Canada
416-221-3519

280. Mountainville Housecalls™
P.O. Box 331148
Fort Worth, TX 76163-1148
800-460-7282

281. MultiMark
Multi Marketing and
Manufacturing Co., Inc.
P.O. Box 1070
Littleton, CO 80160-1070
Phone/Fax: 303-347-1321

282. MOMA
Museum of Modern Art
MOMA Mail Order Dept.
11 West 53rd St.
New York, NY 10019-5401
212-708-9888

283. Nasco® Fort Atkinson
901 Janesville Ave.
P.O. Box 901
Fort Atkinson, WI 53538-0901
414-563-2446
Fax: 414-563-8296
and
Nasco® Modesto
4825 Stoddard Rd.
Modesto, CA 95356-9318
209-545-1600
Fax: 209-545-1669

284. National Association for Visually Handicapped
22 West 21st St., 6th Floor
New York, NY 10010
212-889-2209
and
3201 Balboa St.
San Francisco, CA 94121
415-221-3201

285. National Presto® Industries, Inc.
3925 North Hastings Way
Eau Claire, WI 54703-3703
715-839-2209

286. National Wheel-O-Vator Co., Inc.
509 West Front St.
Roanoke, IL 61561-0348
800-551-9095
Fax: 309-923-5091

286B. New Harbinger Publications
5674 Shattuck Ave.
Oakland, CA 94609
800-748-6273
510-652-0215

287. NordicWare®
Northland Aluminum Products, Inc.
P.O. Box 16074
Hwy. 7 at 100
Minneapolis, MN 55416
800-328-4310
Fax: 612-924-8561

288. Norelco®
Div. of Philips Electronics North
America Corp.
1010 Washington Blvd.
P.O. Box 120015
Stamford, CT 06912-0015
800-572-4116
Fax: 203-975-1812

289. Norpro®, Inc.
2215 Merrill Creek Parkway
Everett, WA 98203-5899
206-261-1000
Fax: 206-261-1001

290. North Coast Medical, Inc.
Functional Solutions for
Independent Living
Consumer Products Division
187 Stauffer Blvd.
P.O. Box 6070
San Jose, CA 95125
800-821-9319
Fax: 408-277-6824
Email: mcmcs@aol.com
http://www.blvd.com/northcoa.htm

290B. Norton, W.W., and Co., Inc.
500 Fifth Ave.
New York, NY 10110
800-223-2584

291. Nutone®
Madison and Red Bank Rd.
Cincinnati, OH 45227-1599
800-543-8687
513-527-5100

292. Obus Forme® Ltd.
550 Hopewell Ave.
Toronto, ON M6E 2S6
Canada
416-785-1386
Fax: 416-785-5862

293. Office Furniture Center
411 Waverly Oaks Rd. Rte. 60
Waltham, MA 02154
800-343-4222
617-893-5180

293B. The Omessi Group Ltd.
Northridge, CA 91326

294. One Step Closer
923 Brown Ave.
Stillwater, OK 74075
405-624-5886

295. Open Sesame
1933 Davis St., Ste. 279
San Leandro, CA 94577
800-673-6911
510-638-0770

295B. Optiway Technology Inc.
500 Norfinch Dr.
Downsview, ON M3N 1Y4
Canada
800-514-7061
416-739-8333
Fax: 416-739-6622

296. Oreck Corp.
100 Plantation Rd.
New Orleans, LA 70123-9989
800-286-8900

297. Ortho-Kinetics, Inc.
P.O. Box 1647
Waukesha, WI 53187-1647
800-558-7786
414-542-6060
Fax: 414-542-4258

298. Orvis® Company, Inc.
1711 Blue Hills Dr.
P.O. Box 12000
Roanoke, VA 24022-8001
800-541-3541

299. Oster®
Sunbeam Oster Household
Products, Inc.
Hwy. 15
North Laurel, MS 39440
601-649-6170

300. Oxmoor House
Division of Southern Progress
Corp.
2100 Lakeshore Drive.
Birmingham, AL 35209
800-633-4712
205-877-6000

301. Oxo International
230 Fifth Ave.
New York, NY 10001
800-545-4411

302. Palmer Industries, Inc.
P.O. Box 5707
Endicott, NY 13760
800-847-1304
607-754-1954 (NY)

303. Panasonic® Company
Kitchen Appliance Division
6550 Katella Ave.
Cypress, CA 90630
714-373-7757

304. The Paragon
P.O. Box 995
89 Tom Harvey Rd.
Westerly, RI 02891-0995
800-343-3095
Fax: 401-596-6104

305. Paragon® Industries
A Windmere Company
Malvern, PA 19355

306. ParaMedical Distributors
2020 Grand Ave.
Kansas City, MO 64141
816-421-6203

307. Pedrini USA Inc.
125 Cartwright Loop
Bayport, NY 11705
516-472-4501

308. Pelouze Scale Company
P.O. Box 1058
7560 West 100 Pl.
Bridgeview, IL 60455
800-654-8330
847-430-833-
Fax: 800-654-8330

308B. Penguin Books®
375 Hudson St.
New York, NY 10014
800-526-0275 (orders)
212-366-2607

309. Perfection Products, Inc.
22627 Lambert St., Ste. 620
Lake Forest, CA 92630
800-229-3489
714-770-3489
Fax: 714-770-4090

310. Pin Dot Products
2840 Maria Ave.
Northbrook, IL 60062
800-451-3553
708-509-2800
Fax: 708-509-2801

311. Playskool®
1027 Newport Ave.
Pawtucket, RI 02861
401-727-5000

312. The Plow and Hearth
Rte. 230 West
P.O. Box 5000
Madison, VA 22727
703-948-2272
Fax: 703-948-5369

313. Porta-Ramps
5592 East La Palma Ave.
Anaheim, CA 92807
800-654-RAMP
714-970-0683 (in CA)

314. J.T. Posey Company
5635 Peck Rd.
Arcadia, CA 91006-0020
800-447-6739
818-443-3143
Fax: 818-443-5014
Fax: 800-767-3933 (orders)

315. Power Access
106 Powder Mill Rd.
P.O. Box 235
Collinsville, CT 06022-0235
800-344-0088
860-693-0751
Fax: 860-693-0641
Email: powaccess@aol.com

316. Prairie View Industries, Inc.
714 5th St.
P.O. Box 575
Fairbury, NE 68352-0575
800-544-RAMP
402-729-4055
Fax: 402-729-4058

316B. Prentice-Hall Press
Div. of Simon and Schuster
160 Gould St.
Needham Heights, MA 02194-2310
617-455-1300

316C. Price Stern Sloan, Inc.
A member of Penguin Putnam, Inc.
200 Madison Ave.
New York, NY 10016

317. Pride Health Care, Inc.
182 Susquehanna Ave.
Exeter, PA 18643
800-800-1636
717-655-5574
Email: mmiller1@pridehealth.com
http://www.pridehealth.com

318. Proctor-Silex®, Inc.
Catalog Savings
263 Yadkin Rd.
Southern Pines, NC 28387-3428
800-486-0343

319. Prince Lionheart
24215 Westgate Rd.
Santa Maria, CA 93455

320. Progressive International Corp.
P.O. Box 97046
Kent, WA 98064
800-426-7101
206-850-6111
Fax: 206-852-2611

321. Progressus
40 St. Mary's Place
Freeport, NY 11520-4684
800-421-0351
716-691-0133
Fax: 716-691-0137

322. Promotheus Books
59 John Glenn Drive
Amherst, NY 14228-2197

323. Quickee Manufacturing Corporation
P.O. Box 156
Cinnaminson, NJ 08077
609-829-7900

324. R & G Manufacturing
Box 864
Moorhead, MN 56560
218-236-9686

325. Radio Shack®

326. Random House, Inc.
201 East 50th St.
New York, NY 10022
800-726-0600
(Imprints: Hearst, Knopf, Pantheon, Times Books.)

326B. Random House of Canada
1265 Aerowood Dr.
Mississauga, ON L4N 1B9
800-668-4247
905-624-0672
Fax: 905-624-6217

327. Raymo® Products, Inc.
212 South Blake
P.O. Box 248
Olathe, KS 66051-0248
913-782-1515

328. Redman Wheelchairs
945 East Ohio, Ste. 4
Tucson, AZ 84714
800-727-6684
520-294-2621
Fax: 520-294-8836
Email: radman@dakota.com.net
http://www.redmanpowerchairs.com

329. Regal® Ware, Inc.
1675 Reigle Dr.
Kewaskum, WI 53040-9400
414-626-2121

330. Regent Gallery
Now: Regent Sheffield Ltd.

331. Regent-Sheffield Ltd.
70 Schmidt Blvd.
Farmingdale, NY 11735
800-872-3343
516-293-8200
Fax: 516-293-7379

332. Regina® Company
266 Fernwood Ave.
Edison, NJ 08837-3839

333. Research Products Corporation
Box 1467
Madison, WI 53701-1467
608-257-8801

334. The Rival® Company
P.O. Box 19556
800 East 101 Terrace
Kansas City, MO 64131
800-343-0065
816-943-4100

335. Robinson Design Group
243 West Main St.
Springville, NY 14141
716-592-2891

335B. Rodale Press, Inc.
33 East Minor St.
Emmaus, PA 18098
800-527-8200
215-967-5171

336. Roho®, Inc.
100 Florida Ave.
Belleville, IL 62221-5430
800-850-7646
618-277-9150
Fax: 618-277-6518
Email: rohoinc@rohoinc.com
http://www.rohoinc.com

337. Roloke Company
5670 Hannum Ave.
Culver City, CA 90230
800-533-8212
213-649-1807

338. The Rosen Group
29 East 21st St.
New York, NY 10010
800-237-9932
212-777-3017
Fax: 212-777-0277

339. Rowoco®
Wilton Industries
2240 West 75th St.
Woodridge, IL 60517
800-772-7111
708-963-7149

340. Royal Appliance Manufacturing Company
650 Alpha Drive
Cleveland, OH 44143-2172
800-321-1134
800-661-6200 (Canada)

341. Rubbermaid® Commercial Products, Inc.
3124 Valley Ave.
Winchester, VA 22601
540-667-8700
and
Rubbermaid® Canada Inc.
2531 Stanfield Rd.
Mississauga, ON L4Y 1R6
416-279-6464

342. Rubbermaid® Health Products, Inc.
See Rubbermaid® Commerical Products, Inc.

343. Rubbermaid®, Inc.
1147 Akron Rd.
Wooster, OH 44691
800-998-8852
216-264-6464

344. Safety First, Inc.
210 Boylston St.
Chestnut Hill, MA 02167

345. The Safety Zone
Hanover, PA 17333-0019
800-999-3030
Fax: 800-338-1635

346. Salton/Maxim® Housewares Group
550 Business Center Dr.
Mt. Prospect, IL 60056
800-233-9054

347. Samsonite®
11200 East 45th Ave.
Denver, CO 80239-3018
303-373-2000
Fax: 303-373-6300

348. **Samsung® Electronics America Inc.**
Samsung Pl. and U.S. Hwy. No. 46
Ledgewood, NJ 07852
201-347-8004

349. **Sanyo® Fisher USA Corp.**
218 State Rd. 17, 4th Floor
Rochelle Park, NJ 07662-3333
800-524-0047
201-641-3000
Fax: 201-641-4798

350. **Sassy, Inc.**
1534 College SE
Grand Rapids, MI 49507
616-243-0767

351. **ScanPan USA, Inc.**
49 Walnut St., Ste. 3A
Norwood, NJ 07648-1329
201-767-6252

352. **Schlage® Lock Company**
2401 Bayshore Blvd.
San Francisco, CA 94134
415-467-1100

353. **Schulte—Distinctive Storage**
12115 Ellington Ct.
Cincinnati, OH 45249
513-489-9300

354. **Science Products**
Box 888
Southeastern, PA 19399
800-888-7400

355. **Scripto-Tokai**
11591 Etiwanda Ave.
Fontana, CA 92337-8202
909-360-2100

356. **Sears Roebuck® Health Care Catalog**
9804 Chartwell
Dallas, TX 75243
800-326-1750

357. **Seiko® Time**
1111 MacGauther Blvd.
Mahwah, NJ 07430
800-289-7345

357A. **Self-Counsel Press, Inc.**
1704 North State St.
Bellingham, WA 98225
800-663-3007
360-676-4530
Fax: 360-676-4549
E-mail: selfcoun@pinc.com
and
1481 Charlotte Rd.
North Vancouver, BC V7J 1H1
Canada

358. **SENSORFLO®**
The Speakman® Company
P.O. Box 191
Wilmington, DE 19899-0191
302-765-0200

359. **Service Merchandise Co. Inc.**
Customer Relations
P.O. Box 24600
Nashville, TN 37202-4600
For store nearest you or for catalog to order by mail, call 800-251-1212

360. **Seymour Housewares**
885 North Chestnut St.
Seymour, IN 47274
800-457-9881

361. **Sharp® Electronics Corp.**
Sharp Plaza
Mahwah, NJ 07430-2135
800-237-4277

362. **The Sharper Image**
P.O. Box 7031
San Francisco, CA 94120-7031
800-344-4444
415-445-6000

363. **Shepherd Products**
204 Kerth Ave.
St. Joseph, MI 49085
906-983-7351

364. **Signatures®**
19465 Brennan Ave.
Perris, CA 92599
909-943-2021
Fax: 909-943-5574

364B. **Simon & Schuster®, Inc.**
1230 Ave. of the Americas
New York, NY 10020
(Imprints: Free Press, Pocket, Scribners, Touchstone.)

365. **Simple Solutions, Inc.**
See Lechters

366. **Singer Company**
Ryobi Motor Products Corp.
1424 Pearman Dairy Rd.
Anderson, SC 29625

367. **Smith & Hawkens**
117 East Strawberry Dr.
Mill Valley, CA 94941
415-383-4050

368. **Smith & Nephew Rehabilitation**
One Quality Dr.
P.O. Box 1005
Germantown, WI 53022-8205
800-558-8633
414-251-7840
Fax: 800-545-7758
E-mail: www.easy-living.com
http://www.easy-living.com

369. **Solutions: Products That Make Life Easier®**
P.O. Box 6878
Portland, OR 97228-6878
800-342-9988, ext. 110

370. **Southside Apothecary**
1815 South Clinton Ave., Ste. 400
Rochester, NY 14618-5799
800-333-0979
716-271-7141
Fax: 716-271-0829

371. **Spanners Company**
17621 Sampson Ln.
Huntington Beach, CA 92647
714-841-6292
Fax: 714-841-1623

372. **Spenco® Medical Corporation**
P.O. Box 8113
Waco, TX 76714-8113
800-433-3334
817-772-6000
Fax: 817-772-3093
Email: spenco@spenco.com

373. **Spiegel, Inc.**
For catalog, write:
P.O. Box 182563
Columbus, OH 43218
and
P.O. Box 1496
Windsor, ON N9A 6RS
Canada
Or order by credit card:
800-345-4500

374. Sporty's Preferred Living Catalog
Clermont County Airport
Batavia, OH 45103-9747
800-543-8633
Fax: 513-732-6560

375. Stand Aid of Iowa, Inc.
P.O. Box 386
Sheldon, IA 51201
800-831-8580
712-324-2153 (in IA)
Fax: 712-324-5210
E-mail: standaid@rconnect.com

376. Stanley® Hardware
Division of the Stanley Works
480 Myrtle St.
New Britain, CT 06050
800-622-4393

377. Staples®, Inc.
100 Pennsylvania Ave.
P.O. Box 9328
Framingham, MA 01701-9328
800-333-3330
Call for catalog or store in area.

378. Starcrest of California®
19465 Brennan Ave.
Perris, CA 92379
714-657-2793

379. Steady Write® Ltd., Inc.
28091 Morro Ct.
Laguna Niguel, CA 92677
714-831-8527

380. SubZero Freezer Co., Inc.
P.O. Box 4130
Madison, WI 53744-4130
800-222-7820

381. Sunbeam® Appliance Co.
Sunbeam Oster Household
Products
1910 Highway 15 North
Laurel, MS 39441
800-597-5978

382. Support Plus
Division of Surgical Products, Inc.
99 West St.
Box 500
Medfield, MA 02052-05000
800-229-2910

383. Susquehanna Rehab
R.D. 2, Box 41
9 Overlook Dr.
Wrightsville, PA 17368
800-248-2011
Fax: 717-252-1768

384. Swing-A-Way® Manufacturing Company
4100 Beck Ave.
St. Louis, MO 63116

385. Tappan®
Westinghouse Frigidaire Consumer Services
6000 Perimeter Dr.
Dublin, OH 43017
908-753-4411
800-245-0600 (local sources)

386. Taylor & Ng®
Concept Housewares, Inc.
1730 Amphlett Blvd., Ste. 222
San Mateo, CA 94402
800-255-3129
415-655-7270
Fax: 415-655-7271

387. Taylor Gifts®
600 Cedar Hollow Rd.
P.O. Box 1770
Paoli PA 19301-0807
800-829-1133
610-293-3613
General mail-order firm.

388. Teledyne
1730 East Prospect Rd.
Fort Collins, CO 80553-0001
800-525-2774

389. Temco Home Health Care Products, Inc.
400 Rabro Drive
Hauppauge, NY 11788
800-645-8176

389B. Ten Speed Press
Box 7123
Berkeley, CA 94707
800-841-2665
510-559-1610

390. Tesa Tape/Tuck, Inc.
5825 Carnegie Blvd.
Charlotte, NC 28209
800-367-8825
704-554-0707
Fax: 800-284-2525

391. T-Fal® Corp.
25 Riverside Dr.
Pine Brook, NJ 07058

392. Theradyne
21730 Hanover Ave.
Lakeville, MN 55044
800-328-4014
612-469-4404

393. TheraFin Corp.
P.O. Box 848
19747 Wolf Rd.
Mokena, IL 60448
800-843-7234
708-479-7300
Fax: 708-479-1515
http://www.inmax.com
Rehabilitation and self help firm.

394. Therapro
225 Arlington ST.
Framingham, MA 01702
800-257-5376
508-872-9494
Fax: 508-875-2062

395. Thermador
5551 McFadden Ave.
Huntington Beach, CA 92649

396. Thermometer Corporation of America
New: Taylor Environmental Instruments
1123 West 22nd St., Ste. 103
Oak Brook, IL 60521
630-954-1250
Fax: 630-954-1275

397. The Thermos® Company
1555 Route 75 East
P.O. Box 600
Freeport, IL 61032-0600
800-553-6126
and
Canadian Thermos Products, Inc.
2040 Eglinton Ave. East
Scarborough, ON M1L 2M8

397A. Time-Life Books
2000 Duke St.
Alexandria, VA 22314

398. Through the Looking Glass
2198 6th St., Ste. 100
Berkeley, CA 94710-2204
800-644-2666
Fax: 510-848-4445

399. Toastmaster® Inc.
1801 North Stadium Blvd.
Columbia, MO 65202
314-445-8666
Fax: 314-876-0618

400. Tools of the Trade
Brand made for Macy's.
Check phone book for nearest
store.

400B. Tough Traveler
1012 State St.
Schenectady, NY 12307
800-408-6844
518-377-8526
Fax: 518-377-5434

401. Toshiba® America Consumer Products Inc.
82 Totowa Rd.
Wayne, NJ 07470
201-628-8000

402. Triad Communications
P.O. Box 13355
Gainesville, FL 32604-1355
904-373-5800

403. Tucker Housewares
AMS Industries
Subsidiary of Kidde Inc.
25 Tucker Drive
Leominster, MA 01453
800-225-7734
and
P.O. Box 5467
721 111 St.
Arlington, TX 76011
800-433-5158
and
4625 Interstate Way
West Kingman, AZ 86401
602-757-3261

404. Tupperware®
P.O. Box 2353
Orlando, FL 32802
Check local phone book.

405. Twentieth Century Plastics
205 South Puente St.
Brea, CA 92621
800-767-0777

406. Ultra Flo®

407. United States Purchasing Exchange®
13571 Vaughn St.
San Fernando, CA 91340
818-895-5555

408. Vandenburg ADL
P.O. Box 995
6811 West 167th St.
Tinley Park, IL 60477
800-872-2347
708-532-9344
Fax: 708-532-2676
Rehabilitation and self-help firm.

409. Velcro® USA, Inc.
406 Brown Ave.
Manchester, NH 03103
800-225-6640

410. The Vermont Country Store
P.O. Box 3000
Manchester Center, VT 05255-3000
802-362-2400
Fax: 802-362-0285

411. Viva Medical Sciences Corporation
812 Proctor Ave.
Ogdensburg, NY 13996
800-731-8482
Fax: 613-731-7486

412. Vornado Air Circulation
415 East 13th St.
Andover, KS 67002

413. Vortex Industries, Inc.
2520 West Hayes Ave.
P.O. Box 1133
Fremont, OH 43420
419-332-8999

414. Walk Away Walker, LLC.
P.O. Box 1131
Garden Grove, CA 92842
714-220-0155
Fax: 714-220-0610

415. Walter Drake® & Sons
Drake Building
Colorado Springs, CO 80940
719-596-3853
General mail-order firm.

416. Waring® Products Division
Dynamics Corporation of America
283 Main St.
New Hartford, CT 06057
203-379-0731

417. Washington Products, Inc.
1147 Oberlin Ave. SW
P.O. Box 644
Massillon, OH 44648
330-837-5101

418. Waupaca Elevator
P.O. Box 246
138 South Osborn
Waupaca, WI 54981
800-238-8739
715-258-5581
Fax: 715- 258-5004

419. WD-40® Company
1061 Cudahy Place
San Diego, CA 92110

420. Weber-Stephens Products Co.
200 East Daniels Rd.
Palantine, IL 60067
800-99-WEBER

421. Welbilt® Appliances
175 Community Drive
Great Neck, NY 11021
414-365-5040

422. The West Bend® Company
400 Washington St.
West Bend, WI 53095
414-334-2311

423. Westclox/Seth Thomas
P.O. Box 4125
Norcross, GA 30091-4125
770-447-5300

424. Whirlpool® Corp.
Consumer Assistance Center
200 M-63
Benton Harbor, MI 49022-2692
800-253-1301
616-927-7200
TDD: 800-723-7059
Fax: 616-923-3785
http://www.whirlpoolappliances.com

425. White-Westinghouse
Consumer Assistance Center
P.O. Box 7181
Dublin, OH 43017-0718
800-245-0600

426. (John) Wiley, Inc.
605 Third Ave.
New York, NY 10158-0021
800-225-5945 (orders)
212-850-6000

427. Williams-Sonoma
P.O. Box 7456
San Francisco, CA 94120-7456
415-421-4242
Kitchen/gourmet mail-order firm.

428. Winco, Inc.
5516 SW First Lane
Ocala, FL 34474-9307
800-237-3377
352-854-2929
352-854-9544
E-mail: winco-Medquip@world-net.att.net

429. Winsome Trading Inc.
7023 NE 175th St.
Bothel, WA 98011-3504
Fax: 206-483-4141

430. Woodcraft®
210 Wood County Industrial Park
P.O. Box 1686
Parkersburg, WV 26102-1686
800-225-1153

431. The Wooden Spoon
Route 145, Heritage Park
P.O. Box 931
Clinton, CT 06413-0931
800-431-2207

431B. Workman Publishing
708 Broadway
New York, NY 10003
800-722-7202
212-254-8098

431C. Writers Digest Books
1507 Dana Ave.
Cincinnati, OH 45207
800-289-0963
513-531-2690

432. Wusthof Trident of America, Inc.
200 Brady Ave.
P.O. Box 448
Hawthorne, NY 10532-0448
800-289-9878

433. Yield House®
Rte. 16, Box 5000
North Conway, NH 03860
800-258-0376
603-356-3141
Fax: 603-356-8942

434. Zim Manufacturing Company
6100 West Grand Ave.
Chicago, IL 60639
312-622-2500

435. Zyliss Housewares Ltd.
CH-3250 Lyss
Switzerland
Items sold through kitchen/gourmet firms and housewares stores.

APPENDIX

B

Helpful Organizations and Agencies

The following organizations and agencies offer information and additional support. Before contacting a national office, check with your local resources. Many groups have chapters that offer programs and services to nearby residents. These may include education, transportation, referral to other agencies, and funding.

AARP WIDOWED PERSONS SERVICE
601 E St. NW
Washington, DC 20049
Peer support for widows and widowers.

ABLEDATA
8455 Colesville Rd.
Suite 935
Silver Springs, MD 20910
800-227-0216
TTY: 301-608-8912
Fax: 301-608-8958
http://www.abledata.com
Computerized bibliographical resource
for people with disabilities.

ACCENT ON INFORMATION
P.O. Box 700
Bloomington, IL 61702
309-378-2961
Computerized information service for people with disabilities.

ACCESS/ABILITIES
P.O. Box 458
Mill Valley, CA 94942
415-388-3250
Computerized information service for people with disabilities.

ACTION
1100 Vermont Ave. NW
Washington, DC 20525
202-634-9380

ADMINISTRATION ON AGING
330 Independence Ave. SW
Washington, DC 20201
202-619-0724
E-mail: AoA_ESEC@Ban-Gate.AoA.DHS.Gov
http://www/AoA.DHHS.Gov

ALEXANDER GRAHAM BELL
ASSOCIATION FOR THE DEAF
3417 Volta Pl. NW
Washington, DC 20007-2778
202-337-5220

ALZHEIMER'S ASSOCIATION
919 North Michigan Ave., Ste. 1000
Chicago, IL 60611-1676
800-272-3900
Fax: 312-335-1110

ALZHEIMER'S DISEASE EDUCATION AND REFERRAL
CENTER
P.O. Box 8250
Silver Spring, MD 20892
800-438-4380
301-495-3311
Fax: 301-495-3334
E-mail: adear@alzheimers.org
http://www.alzheimers.org/adear

AMERICAN ACADEMY OF ALLERGY AND
IMMUNOLOGY
611 East Wells St.
Milwaukee, WI 53202
800-822-ASMA
414-272-6071

AMERICAN ALLERGY ASSOCIATION
Box 7273
Menlo Park, CA 94026
415-322-1663

AMERICAN AMPUTEE FOUNDATION
P.O. Box 25048
Hillcrest Station
Little Rock, AR 72225
501-666-2523

AMERICAN ASSOCIATION OF RETIRED PERSONS (AARP)
444 North Capitol St. NW, Ste. 846
Washington, DC 20001-1512
800-424-3688
202-387-1968
Fax: 202-387-2193
Call to find local chapters.

AMERICAN ASSOCIATION ON MENTAL RETARDATION
1719 Kalorama Rd. NW
Washington, DC 20009
202-387-1968
800-424-3600

AMERICAN AUTOMOBILE ASSOCIATION (AAA)
8111 Gatehouse Rd.
Falls Church, VA 21047

AMERICAN CANCER SOCIETY
1599 Clifton Rd. NE
Atlanta, GA 30329
404-320-3333
800-ACS-2345
Fax: 404-329-5787

AMERICAN CHRONIC PAIN ASSOCIATION
P.O. Box 850
Rocklin, CA 95677
916-632-0922

AMERICAN COUNCIL OF THE BLIND
1010 Vermont Ave. NW, Ste. 1000
Washington, DC 20005
202-393-3666

AMERICAN DAIRY ASSOCIATION
O'Hare International Center
10255 West Higgins Rd., Ste. 900
Rosemont, IL 60018-5616
847-803-2000
Fax: 847-803-2077

AMERICAN DIABETES ASSOCIATION
1660 Duke St.
Alexandria, VA 22314
800-DIABETES (342-2383)
http://www.diabetes.org

AMERICAN DIETETIC ASSOCIATION
216 West Jackson Blvd., Ste. 800
Chicago, IL 60606-6995
312-899-0040

AMERICAN FOUNDATION FOR THE BLIND
11 Penn Plaza
New York, NY 10001
800-232-5463
212-502-7600 (NY)
Fax: 212-502-7773

AMERICAN HEART ASSOCIATION
National Center
7320 Greenville Ave.
Dallas, TX 75231-4596
800-AHA-USA1 (242-8721)
214-373-6300
Fax: 214-706-1341
E-mail: chuckh@amhrt.org
http://www.amhrt.org
8:30 A.M. to 5 P.M. central timeCheck phone book for local chapters.

AMERICAN HOME ECONOMICS ASSOCIATION
1555 King St.
Alexandria, VA 22314
703-706-4600

AMERICAN LUNG ASSOCIATION
1740 Broadway
New York, NY 10019-4374
800-LUNG-USA (586-4872)
212-315-8700
Fax: 212-265-5642

AMERICAN LUPUS SOCIETY
23751 Madison St.
Torrance, CA 90505
213-373-1335

AMERICAN MEDICAL ASSOCIATION
515 North State St.
Chicago, IL 60610
312-464-5000

AMERICAN OCCUPATIONAL THERAPY ASSOCIATION, INC.
4720 Montgomery Lane
Bethesda, MD 20814-3425
800-SAY-AOTA (members); 301-652-2682 (non-members)
TDD: 800-377-8555
Fax: 301-652-7711

APA INJURY HOTLINE
American Paralysis Association
Montebello Hospital
2201 Argonne Drive
Baltimore, MD 21218
800-526-3456 (National)
800-638-1733 (MD)
Computerized information service for people with disabilities.

AMERICAN PARAPLEGIC SOCIETY
7520 Astoria Blvd.
Jackson Heights, NY 11370-1178
718-803-3782

AMERICAN PARKINSON'S DISEASE ASSOCIATION
116 John St., Ste. 417
New York, NY 10038
800-223-2732

AMERICAN PHYSICAL THERAPY ASSOCIATION
1111 North Fairfax St.
Alexandria, VA 22314
800-999-3212
703-684-2782
Fax: 703-706-3396

AMERICAN PODIATRIC MEDICAL ASSOCIATION
9312 Old Georgetown Rd.
Bethesda, MD 20814301-571-9200

AMERICAN RED CROSS
17th and D Streets
Washington, DC 20006
202-737-6300
Call local chapter for listing of services.

AMERICAN SLEEP DISORDERS ASSOCIATION
1610 14th Street NW, Ste. 300
Rochester, MN 55901

AMERICAN SOCIETY ON AGING
833 Market St., Ste. 512
San Francisco, CA 94103
415-543-2617

AMERICAN SPEECH-LANGUAGE-
HEARING ASSOCIATION
10801 Rockville Pike
Rockville, MD 20852
800-638-TALK
V/TDD: 301-897-8682

AMPUTEE COALITION OF AMERICA
P.O. Box 2528
Knoxville, TN 37901-2528
Fax: 423-525-7917

AMYOTROPHIC LATERAL SCLEROSIS ASSOCIATION
21021 Ventura Blvd., Ste. 321
Woodland Hills, CA 91364
818-340-7500
E-mail: eajc27b@prodigy.com
http://www.alsa.org
Call or write for local chapter.

ARTHRITIS AND HEALTH RESOURCE CENTER
486 Washington St.
Wellesley, MA 02181
617-431-7080

THE ARTHRITIS FOUNDATION
1330 West Peachtree St.
Atlanta, GA 30309
800-283-7800
Fax: 770-442-9742 (Publications orders)

ASSISTIVE DEVICE DATABASE SYSTEM (ADDS)
American International Data Search, Inc.
2326 Fair Oaks Blvd., Ste. C
Sacramento, CA 94825
916-925-4554
Computerized information system for people with disabilities.

ASSOCIATION FOR PERSONS
WITH SEVERE HANDICAPS
29 West Susquehenna Ave., Ste. 210
Baltimore, MD 21204-5201

ASSOCIATION FOR RETARDED CITIZENS
P.O. Box 6109
2501 Ave. J
Arlington, TX 76011
817-640-0204

ASSOCIATION OF RADIO READING SERVICES
National Office
1133 20th St. NW
Washington, DC 20036
800-255-2777

ASTHMA AND ALLERGY FOUNDATION OF AMERICA
1125 15th St. NW, Ste. 502
Washington, DC 20005
800-727-8462
202-466-7643
Fax: 202-466-8940

BENEVOLENT PROTECTIVE ORDER OF ELKS
P.O. Box 159
Winston, NC 27986
919-358-7661

BETTER VISION INSTITUTE
P.O. Box 77097
Washington, DC 20013
800-424-VICA
703-243-1528

BEVERLY FOUNDATION
44 South Mentor Ave.
Pasadena, CA 91106
818-792-2292
Fax: 818-792-6117
Develops programs and opportunities for "creative aging."

B'NAI BRITH
Call local office for listing of services.

CANADIAN PARAPLEGIA ASSOCIATION
520 Sutherland Drive
Toronto, ON M4G 3V9
416-422-5640

CHILDREN OF AGING PARENTS
2761 Trenton Rd.
Levittown, PA 19056
215-945-6900
800-227-7294

CHRONIC FATIGUE AND IMMUNE DYSFUNCTION SYN-
DROME ASSOCIATION OF AMERICA
P.O. Box 220398
Charlotte, NC 28222-0398
800-442-3437
Fax: 704-365-9755
E-mail: cfids@vnet.net

CHRONIC FATIGUE IMMUNE DYSFUNCTION SYNDROME
SOCIETY
P.O. Box 320108
Portland, OR 97223
503-684-5261

CLEARING HOUSE FOR THE HANDICAPPED
Office of Special Education and Rehabilitative Services
U.S. Department of Education
330 C St. SW
Room 3132, Switzer Building
Washington, DC 20202
202-732-1244
Information and referral to federal and private services for people
with disabilities.

CONSUMER INFORMATION CENTER
P.O. Box 100
Pueblo, CO 81009

CONSUMER PRODUCT SAFETY COMMISSION
Office of Information and Public Affairs
5401 Westbard Ave.
Bethesda, MD 20207
Consumer Product Safety Hotline
800-638-2772
TDD: 800-638-8270 (outside MD)

COUNCIL FOR EXCEPTIONAL CHILDREN
P.O. Box 3000, Dept EP
Denville, NJ 07834
800-247-8080
Fax: 201-489-1240
(FEN) http://www.families.com

COUNCIL OF BETTER BUSINESS BUREAUS
4200 Wilson Blvd., 8th Floor
Arlington, VA 22209
703-276-0133

COUNCIL ON AGING
600 Maryland Ave. SW
Washington, DC 20024
202-479-1200
Contact your state Agency on Aging for list of area offices.

CROHN'S AND COLITIS FOUNDATION OF AMERICA
386 Park Ave. South
New York, NY 10016-7374
800-932-2423
212-685-3440
Fax: 212-779-4098

DEPARTMENT OF AGRICULTURE
Home Economics Extension
Check local yellow and blue phone book pages.

DISABLED OUTDOORS FOUNDATION
320 Lake St.
Oak Park, IL 60302
312-284-2206
and
708-524-0600

DISABILITY RIGHTS CENTER
2500 Hugh St. NW
Washington, DC 20007
202-337-4119

DIZZINESS AND BALANCE DISORDERS ASSOCIATION
Resource Center
1015 NW 22nd Ave., Room 300
Portland, OR 97210
503-229-7348

DOGS FOR THE DEAF, INC.
10175 Wheeler Rd.
Central Point, OR 97502
V/TDD: 503-826-9220
Fax: 503-826-6696

EASTERN PARALYZED VETERANS ASSOCIATION
75-20 Astoria Blvd.
Jackson Heights, NY 11370-1178
800-803-0414

EPILEPSY FOUNDATION OF AMERICA
4351 Garden City Drive
Landover, MD 20785-2267
800-332-1000
TTY: 800-332-2070
Fax: 301-577-4941
E-mail: postmaster@efa.org

EYE-OPENERS
For information on starting a group for the blind,
call 800-367-6274

FAMILY SERVICE ASSOCIATION OF AMERICA
44 East 23rd St.
New York, NY 10010
Check local listing in your telephone book, for supportive services and assistance in determining funds to which you may be
entitled.

FEDERAL COUNCIL ON AGING
330 Independence Ave. SW, Room 4280 HHS-N
Washington, DC 20201
202-245-2451

FEDERAL TRADE COMMISSION
Office of Public Affairs
Sixth St. and Pennsylvania Ave. NW, Room 421
Washington, DC 20580
202-326-2180

FOOD AND DRUG ADMINISTRATION
Office of Consumer Affairs
301-827-4420

FOOD AND NUTRITION INFORMATION CENTER
National Agricultural Library Building
Room 304
Beltsville, MD 20705
301-504-5719

FOSTER GRANDPARENT PROGRAM
400 Montauk Highway
West Islip, NY 11795
516-669-5355

FOUNDATION FOR HOSPICE AND HOME CARE
519 C St. NE
Washington, DC 20002
202-547-7424

FRATERNAL ORDER OF EAGLES
Call local chapter for listing of services.

FRIENDS FOR IMMEDIATE AND SYMPATHETIC HELP
(FISH)
Call local chapter for transportation, shopping and other services.

GRAY PANTHERS
P.O. Box 21477
Washington, DC 20009-9477
800-280-5362
202-466-3132
Fax: 202-466-3133
(An inter-generational movement.)

HOWARD A. RUSK INSTITUTE OF REHABILITATION
MEDICINE
New York University Medical Center
400 East 34th St.
New York, NY 10016

INDEPENDENT LIVING RESEARCH UTILIZATION PRO-
JECT
P.O. Box 20095
Houston, TX 77225
713-797-0200

INTERNATIONAL MEDICAL SOCIETY OF PARAPLEGIA
National Spinal Injuries Centre
Stoke Mandeville Hospital
Aylesbury
Buckinghamshire, England

INTERNATIONAL POLIO NETWORK
4207 Lindell Blvd., #110
St. Louis, MO 63108-2915
314-534-0475
Fax: 314-534-5070

JONI AND FRIENDS
P.O. Box 3333
Agoura Hills, CA 91301
818-707-5664
(Christian Fund for the Disabled-financial aid program for the
disabled.)

JUNIOR LEAGUE
Call local chapter for listing of services.

KIWANIS
Call local chapter for listing of services.

KNIGHTS OF COLUMBUS
Call local chapter for listing of services.

LEARNING DISABILITIES ASSOCIATION OF AMERICA
156 Library Rd.
Pittsburgh, PA 15234
412-341-1515

LIONS
Call local chapter for listing of services.

LOYAL ORDER OF MOOSE
Call local chapter for listing of services.

LUPUS FOUNDATION OF AMERICA, INC.
1717 Massachusetts Ave. NW, Ste. 203
Washington, DC 20036
800-558-0121

MAINSTREAM, INC.
1030 15th St. NW, Ste. 1010
Washington, DC 20005
202-898-0202
(Computerized information service for people with disabilities)

MAKE TODAY COUNT
1235 East Cherokee St.
Springfield, MO 65804-2203
800-432-2273
417-885-3324
417-885-2584
For persons with cancer and their families.

MARCH OF DIMES BIRTH DEFECTS FOUNDATION
1275 Mamaroneck Ave.
White Plains, NY 10605
914-428-7100

MENTAL HEALTH ASSOCIATION
1021 Prince St.
Alexandria, VA 22314
703-684-7722

MUSCULAR DYSTROPHY ASSOCIATION
3300 East Sunrise Dr.
Tucson, AZ 85718
800-572-9060
520-529-2000
Fax: 520-529-5300
Check phone book for local chapter.

NATIONAL ALLIANCE OF SENIOR CITIZENS
1700 18th St. NW, Ste. 401
Washington, DC 20009
202-986-0117
Fax: 202-986-2974

NATIONAL APHASIA ASSOCIATION
Murray Hill Station
P.O. Box 1887
New York, NY 10156-0611
800-787-6537
Fax: 303-771-1886

NATIONAL ARTHRITIS AND MUSCULOSKELETAL AND
SKIN DISEASES INFORMATION CLEARINGHOUSE
1 AMS
Bethesda, MD 20892-3675
301-495-4484
Fax: 301-587-4352

NATIONAL ASSOCIATION FOR THE DEAF
814 Thayer Ave.
Silver Springs, MD 20910
V/TDD: 301-587-1788
TTY: 301-587-1789
Fax: 301-587-1791

NATIONAL ASSOCIATION FOR
VISUALLY HANDICAPPED
22 West 21st St., 6th Floor
New York, NY 10010
212-889-3141
and
3201 Balboa St.
San Francisco, CA 94121
415-221-3201

NATIONAL ASSOCIATION OF PHYSICALLY
HANDICAPPED
76 Elm St.
London, OH 43140
614-852-1664

NATIONAL BRAILLE ASSOCIATION, INC.
3 Townline Circle
Rochester, NY 14623-2513
716-427-8260
Fax: 716-427-0263

NATIONAL CANCER INSTITUTE
Office of Cancer Communications
Building 31, Room 10A24
Bethesda, MD 20892
301-496-5583

NATIONAL CHOLESTEROL EDUCATION PROGRAM
4733 Bethesda Ave.
Bethesda, MD 20814
301-951-3260

NATIONAL CHRONIC PAIN OUTREACH ASSOCIATION
4922 Hampden Lane
Bethesda, MD 20814
301-652-4948

NATIONAL CHRONIC FATIGUE SYNDROME SOCIETY
919 Scott Ave.
Kansas City, KS 66105

NATIONAL CONSUMERS LEAGUE
1701 K St. NW, #1200
Washington, DC 20006
800-876-7060
202-835-3323
Fax: 202-835-0747

NATIONAL COUNCIL OF SENIOR CITIZENS
8403 Colesville Rd., Ste. 1200
Silver Springs, MD 20910-3314
301-578-8800

NATIONAL COUNCIL ON DISABILITY
800 Independence Ave. SW
Washington, DC 20591
202-267-3846

NATIONAL COUNCIL ON INDEPENDENT LIVING
2539 Telegraph Ave.
Berkeley, CA 94704
415-849-1243
TDD: 415-848-3101

NATIONAL COUNCIL ON THE AGING
600 Maryland Ave. SW, West Wing 100
Washington, DC 20024
202-479-1200

NATIONAL DIABETES INFORMATION CLEARINGHOUSE
1 Information Way
Bethesda, MD 20892-3560
E-mail: ndic@aerie.com
http://www.niddk.nih.gov

NATIONAL EASTER SEAL SOCIEETY
2302 West Monroe, Ste. 1800
Chicago, IL 60606-4802
800-221-6827
312-726-6200
TTD: 312-726-4258
Fax: 312-726-1494
E-mail: nessinfo@seals.com
http://www.seals.com
Call local chapter for listing of services.

NATIONAL EYE CARE PROJECT
P.O. Box 429098
San Francisco, CA 94142-9098
800-222-EYES

NATIONAL FEDERATION OF THE BLIND
1346 Connecticut Ave. NW
Washington, DC 20036

NATIONAL FIRE PROTECTION ASSOCIATION
Batterymarch Park
Quincy, MA 02269
800-344-3555

NATIONAL HEARING AID ASSOCIATION
20361 Middlebelt St.
Livonia, MI 48152
313-478-2610

NATIONAL INDEPENDENT DAIRY FOODS ASSOCIATION
321 D St. NE
Washington, DC 20002-5763
202-543-3838

NATIONAL INFORMATION CENTER FOR HANDICAPPED CHILDREN AND YOUTH
1555 Wilson Blvd., Ste. 508
Rosslyn, VA 22209
703-522-3332

NATIONAL INSTITUTE OF ALLERGY AND INFECTIOUS DISEASE
Building 31, Room 7A-50
Bethesda, MD 20892
301-496-5717

NATIONAL INSTITUTES OF ARTHRITIS, MUSCU-LOSKELETAL, AND SKIN DISEASES
National Institute of Health
Building 31, Room 9A04Bethesda, MD 20892
301-496-3583

NATIONAL INSTITUTES OF NEUROLOGICAL DISORDERS AND STROKE
Information Office
Building 31, Room 8A06
9000 Rockville Pike
Bethesda, MD 20892
301-496-5751
Fax: 301-402-2186

NATIONAL INSTITUTE ON AGING
Public Information Office
Federal Building, Room 6C12
9000 Rockville Pike
Bethesda, MD 20892
301-496-1752

NATIONAL INSTITUTE ON DEAFNESS AND OTHER COM-
MUNICATION DISORDERS
Information Office
9000 Rockville Pike
Bethesda, MD 20892
301-496-5751

NATIONAL JEWISH CENTER FOR IMMUNOLOGY AND
RESPIRATORY MEDICINE
1400 Jackson St.
Denver, CO 80206
800-222-5864

NATIONAL LIBRARY SERVICE FOR THE BLIND AND
PHYSICALLY HANDICAPPED
The Library of Congress
Washington, DC 20542202-287-5100
202-707-5100
TDD: 202-707-0744
Fax: 202-707-0712
E-mail: NLS@loc.gov
http://www.loc.gov/nis or http://www.lcweb.loc.gov/nis
Check services through local library.

NATIONAL MULTIPLE SCLEROSIS SOCIETY
205 East 42nd St.
New York, NY 10017
212-986-3240
Check phone book for local chapters.

NATIONAL ORGANIZATION ON DISABILITY
910 Sixteenth St. NW, Ste. 600
Washington, DC 20006
800-248-ABLE
202-293-5968
TTY: 202-293-5968
Fax: 202-293-7999

NATIONAL OSTEOPOROSIS FOUNDATION
1150 17th St. NW, Ste. 500
Washington, DC 20037
800-464-6700
202-223-2226

NATIONAL PARKINSON FOUNDATION
1501 NW 9th Ave. (Bob Hope Rd.)
Miami, FL 33136-9990
800-327-4545
305-547-6666

NATIONAL REHABILITATION ASSOCIATION
633 South Washington St.
Alexandria, VA 22314
703-836-0850
TDD: 703-836-0849

NATIONAL REHABILITATION INFORMATION CENTER
8455 Colesville Rd., Ste. 935
Silver Spring, MD 20910
800-346-2742
301-588-9284
TTD: 301-495-5626
Fax: 301-587-1967
http://www.naric.com/naric
AbleData computer-based search service, and publications.

NATIONAL SAFETY COUNCIL
1121 Spring Lake Dr.
Itasca, IL 60143-3201
800-227-0216
708-285-1121
Fax: 708-285-1315

NATIONAL SCLERODERMA FEDERATION, INC.
1377 K St. NW, Ste. 700
Washington, DC 20005
703-549-0666

NATIONAL SPINAL CORD INJURY ASSOCIATION
545 Concord Ave., #29
Cambridge, MA 02138-1122
800-962-9629
617-441-8500
Fax: 617-441-3449
Email: nscia@aol.com
http://www.spinalcord.org

NATIONAL SPINAL CORD INJURY HOTLINE
National Study Center for Emergency Medical Systems
22 South Greene St.
Baltimore, MD 21201
800-638-1733

NATIONAL STROKE ASSOCIATION
96 Inverness Dr. East, Ste. 1
Englewood, CO 80112-5112
V/TT: 800-STROKES
303-649-9299
Fax: 303-649-1329

NATIONAL WHEELCHAIR ATHLETIC ASSOCIATION
(NWAA)
1604 East Pike's Peak Ave.
Colorado Springs, CO 80909
719-635-9300

OFFICE OF CONSUMER AFFAIRS
For help in handling product and other problems. Check Yellow
Pages for local office and phone number.

OLDER WOMEN'S LEAGUE
666 11th St. NW, Ste. 700
Washington, DC 20001
202-783-6686
Fax: 202-638-2356

OPTIMIST
Call local chapter for listing of services.

OVEREATERS ANONYMOUS
6075 Zenith Ct. NE
Rio Rancho, NM 87124-6424
505-891-2664
Fax: 505-891-4320
For overweight individuals, peer support and programs to combat
compulsive overeating.

PARALYZED VETERANS OF AMERICA (PVA)
801 18th St. NW
Washington, DC 20006
202-USA-1300
Fax: 202-785-4452
TTY: 202-416-7622

PARKINSON'S DISEASE FOUNDATION
William Black Medical Research Building
Columbia University Medical Center
640-650 West 168th St.
New York, NY 10032
800-457-6676

PHYSICALLY IMPAIRED ASSOCIATION OF MICHIGAN
PAM Assistance Centre
Living and Learning Resource Centre
Media Centre
10235 U.S. 27
St. Johns, MI 48879
V/TDD: 517-224-0333

THE POLIO SOCIETY
4200 Wisconsin Ave. NW
Washington, DC 20016
(Send SASE with $1 postage)

POST-POLIO PROGRAM
National Rehabilitation Hospital
102 Irving St. NW
Washington, DC 20010

POST-POLIO STUDY
National Institutes of Health
Bldg. 10, Rm 4N248
Bethesda, MD 20892

PREVENT BLINDNESS AMERICA
500 East Remington Rd.
Schaumberg, IL 60173
800-221-3004
847-843-2020

PROMATURA
ProMatura Group
428 North Lamar Blvd.
Oxford, MS 38655
601-234-0158
Fax: 601-234-0288
E-mail: mwylde@promatura.com

REACH TO RECOVERY
777 Third Ave.
New York, NY 10017
For women who have had mastectomies; peer support, through
local cancer societies.

REHABILITATION SERVICES ADMINISTRATION
Department of Education
Switzer Building
330 C St. SW, Room 3024
Washington, DC 20202
202-732-1265

ROTARY CLUB
Call local chapter for listing of services.

SCLERODERMA FOUNDATION
Peabody Office Bldg.
1 Newbury St.
Peabody, MA 01960
Newsletter: "The Connector."

SHHH: SELF HELP FOR HARD OF HEARING PEOPLE
7910 Woodmont Ave., Ste. 1200
Bethesda, MD 20814
V/TDD: 301-657-2249
E-mail: national@shhh.org
http://www.shhh.org

SHRINERS BURNS INSTITUTES
Shrine International Headquarters
P.O. Box 31356
Tampa, FL 33631-3356

SPINA BIFIDA ASSOCIATION OF AMERICA (SBAA)
4590 MacArthur Blvd. NW, Ste. 250
Washington, DC 20007-4226
800-621-3141
202-944-3285
Fax: 202-944-3295

SPINAL INJURIES ASSOCIATION
Yeoman House
76 St. James Lane
London N10 3DF, England
London 444-2121

SPONDYLITIS ASSOCIATION OF AMERICA
P.O. Box 5872
Sherman Oaks, CA 91413

STATE SOCIETIES FOR THE BLIND
Check local yellow or blue phone book pages.

STROKE CONNECTION
800-553-6321

SUPERINTENDENT OF DOCUMENTS
United States Government Printing Office
Washington, DC 20402

THEOS FOUNDATION
The Penn Hills Mall Office Bldg.
Pittsburgh, PA 15235
For the widowed and their families.

UNITED CEREBRAL PALSY ASSOCIATION
7 Penn Plaza, Ste. 804
New York, NY 10001
212-268-6655

UNITED PARKINSON FOUNDATION
833 West Washington Blvd.
Chicago, IL 60607
312-733-1893
Fax: 312-733-1896

UNITED SENIORS HEALTH COOPERATIVE
1334 H St. NW, Ste. 500
Washington, DC 20005
202-393-6222
Fax: 202-783-0588
E-mail: 103134.2627@compuserve.com
http://www.usho-online.org

UNITED WAY
Call local office for listing of organizations and referral.

U.S. DEPARTMENT OF HOUSING
AND URBAN DEVELOPMENT
Office of the Secretary
Room 4276
451 Seventh St. NW
Washington, DC 20410-0001
800-795-7915
TDD: 800-927-9275

VISITING NURSE ASSOCIATION OF AMERICA
3801 East Florida Ave., Ste. 806
Denver, CO 80210
800-426-2547

THE WELL SPOUSE FOUNDATION
P.O. Box 801
New York, NY 10023
212-724-7209

YMCA/YWCA
Call local branch for listing of services and programs.

Disability, Health, and Family Services Periodicals

Subscription prices were current at time of publishing. Please contact publishers for any changes. Several publications have home pages on the World Wide Web. Check a copy of the magazine for ones not listed here.

ABILITY
1682 Langley Ave.
Irvine, CA 92714
714-854-8700
Fax: 714-251-7011
Bimonthly, about $30 per year.

ACCENT ON LIVING
P.O. Box 700
Bloomington, IL 61702-9956
309-378-2961
Quarterly, about $12 per year. For persons with varied disabilities.

AFB NEWS
American Foundation for the Blind
1 Penn Plaza
New York, NY
Free 12 page national newsletter published five times a year.

AMERICAN HEALTH
RD Publications, Inc.
P.O. Box 3016
Harlan, IA 51593-2107
Ten issues per year, about $15. Focus on health issues, including nutrition.

THE AMP NATIONAL AMPUTATION FOUNDATION
73 Church St.
Malvern, NY 11565
516-887-3600
Fax: 516-887-3667
Monthly.

ARTHRITIS TODAY
The Arthritis Foundation
1330 West Peachtree St.
Atlanta, GA
800-933-0032
Six issues per year, $20 (donation to The Arthritis Foundation) includes magazine and membership.

BE STROKE SMART
National Stroke Association Newsletter
300 East Hampden, Ste. 240
Englewood, CO 80110-2622
Quarterly, free with membership.

BETTER HOMES & GARDENS
Meredith Corp.
1716 Locust St.
Des Moines, IA 50336
515-284-3000
Monthly, about $16 per year.

BON APPETIT
5900 Wilshire Blvd.
Los Angeles, CA 90036-5013
Monthly, about $16 per year.

BREAKING NEW GROUND
Breaking New Ground Resource Center
Dept. of Agricultural Engineering
Purdue University
1146 Agricultural Engineering Bldg.
West Lafayette, IN 47907
317-494-5088
Free subscription. Of interest to the rural resident or farmer with a disability.

CALIPER
Canadian Paraplegia Association
      ince of Wales Dr., Ste. 320
      ON K2C 3W7
Can:
613-   3-1033
      3-723-1060
      ly, $10 individual, $13 institution.

CANADIAN LIVING
Telemedia Publishing
25 Sheppard Ave. West, Ste. 100
North York, ON M2N 687
Canada
and
400 Woodward Ave.
Buffalo, NY 14217
13 issues per year; $27.98 Canada, $37 U.S.

CANCER SMART
P.O. Box 808
Yorktown Heights, NY 10598-9322
Quarterly newsletter, $19 per year, published by the Memorial
Sloan-Kettering Cancer Center.

THE CAPSULE
Children of Aging Parents
Woodbourne Office Campus
Woodbourne Rd., Ste. 302A
Levittown, PA 19057
215-945-6900
Fax: 215-945-8720
Bimonthly newsletter, $20 includes information. Networking
resources plus information on Caregiver Support Groups nation-
wide.

CHATELAINE
McClean Hunter Ltd.
Customer Service Department
P.O. Box 1600
Postal Station A
Toronto, ON MSW 2B8
Canada
Monthly. $20 Canada, $42 U.S.

CHILD
P.O. Box 3173
Harlan, IA 51593-2364
Ten issues issues per year, about $10.

CHOICE MAGAZINE LISTING
P.O. Box 10
Port Washington, NY 11050
516-883-8280
Bimonthly, free magazine on cassette tape for visually impaired.

CFIDS CHRONICLE
Chronic Fatigue and Immune Dysfunction Syndrome
Association
P.O. 220398
Charlotte, NC 28222
800-442-3437

CONSUMER REPORTS
Consumers Union
101 Truman Ave.
Yonkers, NY 10703-1057
914-378-2000
11 issues per year plus Annual Buying Guide, about $24.

CONSUMERS DIGEST INC.
5705 North Lincoln Ave.
Chicago, IL 60659
312-275-3590
Fax: 312-275-7273
Six issues per year, about $16.

COOKING LIGHT: THE MAGAZINE OF FOOD AND FIT-
NESS
P.O. Box 830656
Birmingham, AL 3S282-9086
10 issues per year, about $16.

COOK'S ILLUSTRATED
Box 59048
Boulder, CO 80322-9048
303-447-9330
Six issues per year, about $25.

DIABETES FORECAST
American Diabetes Association
1600 Duke St.
Alexandria, VA 22314
703-549-1500
Fax: 703-836-7439
Monthly, $24.

DIABETES SELF MANAGEMENT
R.A. Rapaport Publishing, Inc.
150 West 22nd St.
New York, NY 10011-2421
212-989-0200
Monthly, about $18.

THE DISABILITY RAG AND RESOURCE
Avocado Press
Box 145
Louisville, KY 40201
502-459-5343
Bimonthly, about $17.50 per year U.S., $30 Canada.

EATING WELL: THE MAGAZrNE OF FOOD AND HEALTH
Ferry Road
P.O. Box 54263
Boulder, CO 80323~263
Twelve issues a year, about $28.

EXCEPTIONAL PARENT: PARENTING YOUR CHILD WITH
A DISABILITY
Pys-Ed Corp.
209 Harvard St., Ste. 303
Brooldine, MA 02146-5005
800-247-8080
Monthly, about $28.

FAMILY CIRCLE
P.O. Box 10773
Des Moines, IA 50340-0773
Seventeen issues per year, about $17.

FRIENDLY WHEELS
Order through: Amigo Mobility International, Inc.
Source: 26
Three times per year, free, designed for platform mobility users.

GOOD HOUSEKEEPING
The Hearst Corp.
959 Fifth Ave.
New York, NY 10019
Monthly, about $20 per year.

GRAY PANTHERS NETWORK
National quarterly newspaper, $15 individual, $30 organization.

GRAY PANTHERS HEALTHWATCH
Bimonthly newsletter on health care issues, $12 year.

GRAY PANTHERS WASHINGTONWATCH
Bimonthly newsletter, $12 year.
Both available through:
Gray Panthers Office
1424 Sixteenth St. NW
Washington, DC 20036

HEALTH
P.O. Box 52431
Boulder, CO 80321-2431
Monthly, about $18 per year.

IN MOTION
Order through: Amputee Coalition of America.
Monthly, $25 per year includes membership.

LADIES' HOME JOURNAL
Meredith Corp.
P.O. Box 53940
Boulder, CO 80322-3940
Monthly, about $12 per year.

LADY'S CIRCLE
Lopez Publications, Inc.
East 35th Street
New York, NY 10016-3877
212-689-3933
Fax: 212-725-2239
Bimonthly, $12.

LIFELINE
National Chronic Pain Outreach Association, Inc.
4922 Hampden Lane
Bethesda, MD 20814
Quarterly newsletter.

LINK
The Amyotrophic Laterial Sclerosis Assocation
21021 Ventura Blvd., Ste. 321
Woodland Hills, CA 91403
Bimonthly, apply.

MAINSTREAM
Mainstream, Inc.
3 Bethesda Metro Center
Bethesda, MD 20814
301-654-2400
Bimonthly, $60 per year.

MODERN MATURITY
AARP Bulletin
American Association of Retired Persons
3200 East Carson St.
Lakewood, CA 90712
Bimonthly, $8 membership includes both publications.

NEW CHOICES FOR RETIREMENT LIVING
Retirement Living Publishing Company, Inc.
28 West 23rd St.
New York, NY 10010
212-366-8800
Fax: 212-336-8899
Monthly, about $16.
Topics include health and nutrition.

NEW MOBILITY
Miramar Communications, Inc.
23815 Stuart Ranch Rd.
Malibu, CA 90265-8987
Monthly, $15 per year.

NUTRITION ACTION HEALTHLETTER
Center for Science in the Public Interest
P.O. Box 96611
Washington, DC 20077-7216
Monthly, $24.

ON THE LEVEL
Vestibular Disorders Association
1015 NW 22nd Ave.
Portland, OR 97210-3079
Quarterly, $15 per year includes annual membership.

PARAPLEGIA NEWS
2111 East Highland Ave.
Phoenix, AZ 85016-4702
Monthly, about $21 per year.

PARENT NEWS
Center for Persons with Disabilities
Utah State University
Logan, UT 84322-6845
801-797-1991
Fax: 801-797-2044
Quarterly, free to parents and professionals.

PARENTING
Times Publishing Ventures
301 Howard St., 17th Floor
San Francisco, CA 94105-2252
415-546-7575
Fax: 415-546-0578
Ten issues per year, about $18.

PARENTS
685 Third Ave.
New York, NY 10017
212-878-8700
Monthly, about $20.

PARKINSON'S DISEASE FOUNDATION NEWSLETTER
Parkinson's Disease Foundation
640-650 West 168th Street
New York, NY 10032
Bimonthly, apply.

REHABILITATION GAZETTE/G.I.N.I.
4207 Lindell Blvd., #110
St. Louis, MO 63108-2915
314-534-0475
Fax: 314-534-5070
Semi-annual, about $12 per issue to individuals.

REMEDY
The Remedy Arthritis Newsletter Subscription Dept.
P.O. Box 57630
Boulder, CO 80323-7630
Bimonthly, about $18 per year.

SAVEUR
P.O. Box 5429
Harlan, IA 51593-2929
6 issues per year, $24. Focuses on techniques in cooking.

SPINAL CORD INJURY LIFE
National Spinal Cord Injury Association
545 Concord Ave., Ste. 29
Cambridge, MA 02138
Quarterly, about $25 per year, includes membership.
Nonmember, $30.

SPINAL NETWORK EXI8A
Total Resource Magazine for the Wheelchair Community
Miramar Communications, Inc.
23815 Stuart Ranch Rd.
Malibu, CA 90265-8987
Ouarterly, $15 per year, add $6 outside U.S.

STROKE CONNECTION
Courage Stroke Network
3915 Golden Valley Rd.
Golden Valley, MN 55422
$8 per year for an individual; $17 for a professional, includes membership in the Courage Stroke Network.

THROUGH THE LOOKING GLASS: PARENTING WITH A DISABILITY
2198 Sixth St., Ste. 100
Berkeley, CA 94710-2204
800-644-2666

WOMAN'S DAY
Filipachhi Hachette Magazines, Inc.
P.O. Box 56061
Boulder, CO 80322-6061
15 issues per year, about $16.

ZIEGLER MAGAZINE FOR THE BLIND
20 West 17th St.
New York, NY 10011
212-242-0263
Free general interest magazine, 10 issues per year, available on Braille or recorded disk.

INDEX

Tear-Out Suggestion Card

From time to time new information that may be of interest or help to you will become available. In order to let you know about it and more fully meet your needs as a homemaker, this tear-out page has been included.

In this third edition of *Mealtime Manual* we've been able to share some of the suggestions that came from readers of the previous edition; we also will be glad to try and answer your questions. Your participation has been valuable and we look forward to hearing from you. Please send suggestions, questions, and comments to:

SLACK Incorporated
6900 Grove Road
Thorofare, New Jersey 08086

Name:
Miss
Mrs. _____
Mr.

Street _____

City _____ State _____ Zip_____

Age: ❑ Under 20   ❑ 20 to 35   ❑ 35 to 50   ❑ 51 to 65   65 to 70   ❑ Over 70

How many do you cook for?   ❑ Myself   ❑ Husband and myself   ❑ Family (give number)_____

Handicap (if any): _____

Suggestions I have found helpful:_____

_____

_____

Other areas and problems I would like to see covered: _____

_____

_____

_____

continue on reverse side

NOTE TO EDUCATORS AND GROUPS: Slides, in color and black and white, illustrating many of the techniques and equipment shown in *Mealtime Manual* are available. For information and current costs, send listing of those you desire to the address listed above.

Ideas I would like to share: _____

_____

_____

_____

_____

_____

_____

_____

_____

_____

_____

_____

_____

_____

_____

Meal Preparation and Training: The Health Care Professional's Guide

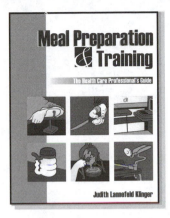

Meal Preparation and Training: The Health Care Professional's Guide
by **Judith L. Klinger**, OTR, MA, identifies and examines training techniques for the kitchen. *Meal Preparation and Training* is a great **companion guide** to *Mealtime Manual for People with Disabilities and the Aging* and is designed specifically for the therapist or health care professional. The techniques demonstrated may be utilized to teach those with physical limitations or the elderly how to understand and perform tasks successfully in the kitchen. Issues addressed in the book include kitchen planning, meal planning, nutrition, safety, stress, and more. The guide looks at how to deal with clients in their homes, working with children, hospice, individuals dealing with physical and cognitive disabilities, and the elderly from a health professional's perspective.

Meal Preparation and Training: The Health Care Professional's Guide
is divided into several sections. Section I assesses the situation—the types of patients as well as the caregivers and family then focuses on specific disabilities and problems, including a client with arthritis, chronic pain, etc. Section II involves the kitchen and the home, from safety and modifications to transporting items. Section III focuses on equipment, appliances, nutrition, shopping, and includes a guide to teaching recipes. Section IV provides help for the health care professional and caregivers with extensive support materials. These include funding, agencies and organizations, sources for equipment and materials, general references, and forms and plans for making equipment. The forms and plans may be photocopied, enlarged if desired, and are designed for use with clients.

Summary of Features

- **The guide gives recommendations for training and specific adaptations.**
- **Additional references on funding and resources are provided that will help the health care professional assist clients.**
- **Sources are included in the guide for developing homemaking activities geared toward varied physical and cognitive needs.**

☑ **Yes!** I would like to buy_____ copy(ies) of
Meal Preparation and Training: The Health Care Professional's Guide

Qty.	Title	Order#	Price	Total
_____	Meal Preparation and Training	33438	$28.00 ea.	_____

____Bill me (No billing will be done to post office boxes)
____Check Enclosed
____Charge My: ❏ AMEX   ❏ Visa   ❏ Mastercard
Exp. ____ Account No. _____
Signature._____

NJ Residents
Add 6% Sales Tax   _____
Handling Charge $4.50
TOTAL   _____

Please Print
Name: _____

Address: _____

City: _____ State: _____ Zip: _____

Phone: (____)_____ Fax: (____)_____

All Prices Are Subject To Change.   Shipping Charges May Apply.

SLACK Incorporated, Professional Book Division, 6900 Grove Road, Thorofare, NJ 08086-9447
Call 800-257-8290 or 609-848-1000, Fax 609-853-5991, E-Mail orders@slackinc.com or http://www.slackinc.com